Minimally Invasive Techniques of Oculofacial Rejuvenation

Thieme

Minimally Invasive Techniques of Oculofacial Rejuvenation

Stephen Bosniak, M.D.
Attending Oculofacial Surgeon
Manhattan Eye, Ear & Throat Hospital
New York, New York

Marian Cantisano-Zilkha, M.D., Ph.D.
Director of Ophthalmic Plastic Surgery
Center for Clinical Studies
Botafogo Ophthalmology Clinic
Rio de Janeiro
Brazil

Thieme
New York • Stuttgart

Thieme Medical Publishers, Inc.
333 Seventh Ave.
New York, NY 10001

Associate Editor: Owen Zurhellen
Consulting Editor: Esther Gumpert
Vice-President, Production and Electronic Publishing: Anne Vinnicombe
Production Editor: Becky Dille
Marketing Director: Phyllis Gold
Sales Director: Ross Lumpkin
Chief Financial Officer: Peter van Woerden
President: Brian D. Scanlan
Compositor: Thomson Press International
Printer: Four Colour Imports, Inc.
Library of Congress Cataloging-in-Publication Data

Bosniak, Stephen L.
Minimally invasive techniques of oculofacial rejuvenation / Stephen Bosniak, Marian Cantisano-Zilkha.
p. ; cm.
Includes bibliographical references and index.
ISBN 1-58890-231-5 (alk. paper) — ISBN 3-13-138321-6 (alk. paper) 1. Facelift. 2. Face—Surgery.
3. Ophthalmic plastic surgery. 4. Endoscopic surgery. 5. Surgery, Plastic.
[DNLM: 1. Face—surgery. 2. Orbit—surgery. 3. Reconstructive Surgical Procedures—methods.
4. Surgical Procedures, Minimally Invasive—methods. WE 705 B743m 2005] I. Cantisano-Zilkha, Marian.
II. Title.
RD119.5.F33B67 2005
617.5'20592—dc22

2004026298

Important note: Medical knowledge is ever-changing. As new research and clinical experience broaden our knowledge, changes in treatment and drug therapy may be required. The authors and editors of the material herein have consulted sources believed to be reliable in their efforts to provide information that is complete and in accord with the standards accepted at the time of publication. However, in the view of the possibility of human error by the authors, editors, or publisher of the work herein or changes in medical knowledge, neither the authors, editors, nor publisher, nor any other party who has been involved in the preparation of this work, warrants that the information contained herein is in every respect accurate or complete, and they are not responsible for any errors or omissions or for the results obtained from use of such information. Readers are encouraged to confirm the information contained herein with other sources. For example, readers are advised to check the product information sheet included in the package of each drug they plan to administer to be certain that the information contained in this publication is accurate and that changes have not been made in the recommended dose or in the contraindications for administration. This recommendation is of particular importance in connection with new or infrequently used drugs.

Printed in China

5 4 3 2 1

TMP ISBN 1-58890-231-5
GTV ISBN 3 13 138321 6

Dedication

To my mother Thelma who would have loved to see this book.

To my father Samuel who has always treasured the written word.

To Kevyn Aucoin who continues to inspire us.

SB

To Stephen Bosniak, my mentor and source of inspiration.

To my parents, Dr. Luiz and D. Duca for showing me the nuances between strength and tenderness.

To my brother Luiz Eduardo and his children Raiane and João Pedro Cantisano, my eternal sources of joy.

MCZ

Contents

Section II Less Invasive Surgical Options

Section III Perioral Rejuvenation

Section IV Complementary Treatment Modalities

Appendix

Foreword

Drs. Stephen Bosniak and Marian Cantisano-Zilkha bring a 10-year history of collaboration to this book. They have shared a most interesting professional journey in which they have investigated many of the emerging therapies and techniques of minimally invasive oculo-facial rejuvenation. Both of them have demonstrated the curiosity and insight to think and rethink their approaches to achieve optimal results through minimal intervention. During their investigations, they have met many innovators from different disciplines. These associations have allowed Drs. Bosniak and Zilkha to gather this distinguished group of fellow travelers who have also looked beyond what is conventionally accepted. Each of the authors brings a perspective that has been forged and tempered during each author's own journey of innovation. Together in this published text, they are defining the breadth of this area of emerging knowledge.

The organization of the text flows from noninvasive facial rejuvenation by photo, radiofrequency, and chemical modalities to the role of botulinum toxin in the first section. The second section is devoted to less invasive surgical procedures, with an excellent chapter on periobital surgery. The chapter on endoscopic techniques is a serviceable effort whereas the chapters on midface augmentation are well organized and cogently presented. Inclusion of the S-Lift technique by its modern developers makes this section especially strong. The third section includes perioral efforts, with a substantial emphasis on the rapidly expanding field of cosmetic dentistry. Finally, the fourth section moves to complementary treatments, including phototherapy of cancerous and precancerous facial lesions as well as a brief primer on traditional Chinese medicine. An appendix designed primarily for the lay reader is a valuable tool to help physicians frame treatment plans. Many of our patients have a surprisingly sophisticated understanding of their problems and want to participate in the choice of their therapy.

We all credit ourselves with having inquiring minds. Drs. Bosniak and Cantisano-Zilkha and their collaborators are colleagues who actually do think beyond the boundaries of conventional practice. For those who want an understanding of what are the most current techniques for minimally invasive oculo-facial rejuvenation and a glimpse of what might be, this text is a stimulating read.

Sterling S. Baker, M.D.

Foreword

I am greatly honored to have been asked by Dr. Stephen Bosniak and Dr. Marian Cantisano-Zilkha to write a foreword to their new book. I have admired their combined energy and medical expertise for many years. They are dedicated to their research and teaching and have been highly innovative in their assessments of new techniques and their adjunctive application for the maximum benefit of each individual patient.

The timing of presentation of their book could hardly be better. Not only are the aging "baby boomer" clientele well informed and seeking successful strategies for low downtime rejuvenation, but the aesthetic physicians providing these services have unprecedented access to new and successful technologies as a means to this end. This book supplies the information which both patient and physician will need.

What do today's cosmetically concerned adults actually want? Mainly they want to restore the natural appearance of their face from 10 to 15 years ago without looking "pulled", "done", or obvious. Today's aesthetic consumer is well informed but still requires more information about treatment efficacy and safety than previous generations of clients who may not have been so aware of what questions to ask. They are also interested in how adverse events, should they occur, would be managed.

This book is a wonderful, up-to-date reference for physicians and surgeons in this rapidly expanding field. The topics that have been selected for the chapters carefully reflect the aims of treatment that are desired by the aesthetically concerned public.

There is in-depth discussion of combination treatments to achieve the optimum results for the cosmetic patient—the all-important aim of cosmetic physicians and surgeons. This book is also written to be a valuable and important resource across all cosmetic specialties and disciplines.

Jean Carruthers, M.D., F.R.C.S.(C), F.R.C. OPHTH.
Fellow of the American Society of Ophthalmic Plastic and Reconstructive Surgery
Diplomat of the American Boards in Cosmetic Surgery
Cosmetic Surgeon
Clinical Professor
Department of Ophthalmology
University of British Columbia
Vancouver, Canada

Preface

Patient expectations have risen, while their tolerance for downtime has diminished. Enhanced understanding about rejuvenation and the desire to please the patients have led to technological advances, which allow physicians and surgeons to deliver to patients what they want and need. In exchange for avoiding lengthy healing processes, these techniques often require multiple treatment sessions in intervals that allow for the body to recover and respond appropriately while substantially contracting healing time. These noninvasive procedures have a cumulative effect, work in a complementary fashion, and are not, in many cases, stand-alone therapies. Clear instances of complementary therapy are Botox pretreatment for filling agents, ablative and nonablative laser therapies, intense pulsed light (IPL), microdermabrasion, and radiofrequency therapies. Skin therapies and home care products enhance the effects of Botox neuromodulation and filling agents. And low-emission diode (LED) treatments enhance the effects of IPL. Any physician treating the cosmetic patient must understand the need for multiple therapeutic options.

The effects of noninvasive therapies can be further enhanced by minimally invasive surgical techniques. Laser-assisted blepharoplasty can be performed in a virtually bloodless field. Surgical outcomes can be improved and healing time can be minimized. Endoscopic browplasty and small-incision facelift techniques can add to the dimension of final correction. Once the rejuvenation goal is achieved with the aforementioned therapies, the result can be maximized and features can be enhanced, with micropigmentation (semipermanent makeup) of eyebrows, eyeline, and eyelashes.

Stephen Bosniak, M.D.
Marian Cantisano-Zilkha, M.D., Ph.D.

Acknowledgments

Our patients, who have given us their trust.

Joan and Dan Sabatino, Danielle Braz for their tireless efforts.

Dr. Ioannis Glavas, our exceptional fellow.

Julie Finelli, Cee Cee Yarabinee, Patti Doyle, and the Esthetica Salon and Spa.

Denice Monaco Salon and Spa.

Audrey Kitagawa for her insight and guidance.

Terri Amig for her pencil portraits.

Eric Sakas (Kevyn Aucoin Beauty).

Caroline, Laura, David, Karen, and Gary Patou.

Jordana, Vicki, and Mark Bosniak.

Robert and Alexandra Heitz for their joy and pride in our project.

Contributors

Stephen Bosniak, M.D.
Attending Oculofacial Surgeon
Manhattan Eye, Ear & Throat Hospital
New York, New York

Marian Cantisano-Zilkha, M.D., Ph.D.
Director of Ophthalmic Plastic Surgery
Center for Clinical Studies
Botafogo Opthalmology Clinic
Rio de Janeiro
Brazil

Kyle Seung Choe, M.D.
Laser Skin & Vein Center of Virginia
Virginia Beach, Virginia

Mark Duffy, M.D., Ph.D.
Green Bay Eye Clinic
Green Bay, Wisconsin

Ioannis P. Glavas, M.D.
Attending Physician
Department of Opthalmology
Manhattan Eye, Ear & Throat Hospital
New York, New York

Karyn Grossman, M.D., F.A.C.S.
Grossman Dermatology
Santa Monica, California

Eckart Haneke, M.D., Ph.D.
Institute of Dermatology
Klinikk Bunæs
Sandvika, Norway

Steven B. Hopping, M.D., F.A.C.S.
Clinical Professor
Department of Surgery
George Washington University
Washington, D.C.

Jon B. Marashi, D.D.S.

Girish S. Munavalli, M.D., M.H.S.
Clinical Professor
Department of Dermatology
Johns Hopkins University
University of Maryland
Maryland Laser, Skin, and Vein Institute
Hunt Valley, Maryland

Gary Null, Ph.D.
Adjunct Professor
Fairleigh Dickinson University
Hackensack, New Jersey
Research Fellow in Public Health Science
Institute of Applied Biology
New York, New York

Roxanne Stambuk Panicacci, M.D., Ph.D.
San Clemente, California

Peter Rinaldi, D.M.D.
New York, New York

Thomas Romo III, M.D.
Chief of Facial Plastic and Reconstructive Surgery
Lenox Hill Hospital and
Manhattan Eye, Ear & Throat Hospital
New York, New York

Tracey J. Rosenberg, M.D., D.D.S.
Assistant Clinical Professor
Oral and Maxillofacial Surgery
Columbia University Medical Center
New York, New York

Neil Scott Sadick, M.D., F.A.C.P., F.A.A.C.S.
Clinical Professor
Attending Physician
Department of Dermatology
New York Weill Cornell Medical Center
New York, New York

Ziya Saylan, M.D.
Cosmetic Surgery Clinic
Duesseldorf, Germany

Steven Schram, Ph.D.
New York, New York

Kenneth D. Steinsapir, M.D.
Los Angeles, California

Margaret A. Weiss, M.D.
Maryland Laser, Skin, and Vein Institute
Hunt Valley, Maryland

Robert A. Weiss, M.D.
Maryland Laser, Skin, and Vein Institute
Hunt Valley, Maryland

Haresh Yalamanchili, M.D
Division of Facial Plastic and Reconstructive Surgery
Department of Otolaryngology and Head-Neck Surgery
The New York Eye & Ear Infirmary
New York, New York

Section I

Noninvasive Approaches

1

Introduction to Alternative Techniques of Oculofacial Rejuvenation

Stephen Bosniak

A variety of noninvasive techniques now exist for rejuvenating facial skin. We can separate them into three categories: (1) improving skin texture and pigmentation, (2) rhytid ablation, and (3) skin tightening.

◆ Improving Skin Texture and Pigmentation

Intense pulsed light (IPL) is the workhorse in this category (see Chapter 2) for diminishing dyspigmentation, telangiectasis, and background erythema. Although improvement in skin texture is not its primary function, these changes do occur.

Recently, light-emitting diodes (LEDs) have added further subjective improvement, enhancing the results of IPL and providing a molecular basis for clinical benefits. LED photomodulation uses coded pulses of low energy, nonlaser, nonthermal, light energy to stimulate mitochondrial activity, increase collagen and fibroblast production, and decrease collagenase (metalloproteinase). The currently recommended regimen is 50 seconds weekly for 8 weeks.[1–3]

Nonablative neodymium:yttrium-aluminum-garnet (Nd:YAG) lasers create a perivascular inflammatory response and secondary neocollagenogenesis while protecting the skin surface with a cryogen spray. Our experience with 1320 nm (Cool Touch II) (Cutera, Brisbane, California) has been generally positive with properly selected patients of all skin types, particularly for patients with mild rhytidosis and irregular facial suface contours resulting from acne scarring.[4,5] They have enjoyed substantial improvement after 4 to 6 monthly treatments. A dynamic tetrafluoroethane spray is synchronized to be applied to the skin for 30 msec with a delay of 40 msec before each laser pulse to the skin (precooling), while monitoring the skin surface temperature with a thermal sensor in the laser handpiece.[6] The desired endpoint is 41 to 45°C. In a similar fashion, the depth of the treatment can be varied, applying the cryogen spray immediately following each laser pulse (postcooling). We employ one precooling and two postcooling applications in our treatment sessions. Postprocedure erythema is typically gone within 30 minutes, or less if a Natragel mask (Gel Concept, Whippany, New Jersey) is applied. Improvement in skin texture is not usually evident for 4 to 6 months after the initiation of treatment. Although recovery time is minimal, we feel that the drawbacks are the discomfort during the procedure (even with topical anesthetic), and the subtlety of the improvement.

Although we have had no experience with the 1540 nm Er:Glass laser (Aramis, Quantel Medical, Clermont-Ferrand, France), it may also be another potential nonablative tool for improving surface irregularities following acne and actinic changes.[7,8]

◆ Rhytid Ablation

The selection of instrumentation, power, and density is determined by the severity and expanse of rhytidosis and the patient's skin type. The erbium:yttrium-aluminum-garnet (Er:YAG) laser emits laser energy in the midinfrared light spectrum with a 2940 nm wavelength. This wavelength has 10 to 15 times more affinity for water than the carbon dioxide (CO_2) laser. Because its wavelength is at the peak of water absorption, it is a true epidermal ablation laser, producing only 5 to 20 μm of thermal damage.[9–11] Mild Er:YAG ablation may begin with topical anesthetic cream using 2 J/cm^2, a pattern 3, size 4, and one pass. This technique can be used for very mild rhytidosis and has minimal downtime. Additional passes and local anesthesia infiltration can be added for more profound rhytidosis. Three Er:YAG passes will ablate about the same depth of epithelium as one pass of the CO_2 laser will vaporize. Because the Er:YAG laser applications are more superficial with less transmission of thermal energy and no vasoablative properties, there is less erythema and more rapid healing; but Er:YAG laser treatments may be limited by bleeding, which rarely occurs with CO_2 laser resurfacing. Although theoretically the Er:YAG laser can ablate even very marked rhytids, the CO_2 laser is more effective for ameliorating severe photodamage and rhytidosis. There may also be a role for the combined use of CO_2 and Er:YAG resurfacing techniques. Ablating the epithelial debris with the Er:YAG between passes of the CO_2 laser may also have some benefit.

The Er:YAG laser may be used cautiously, with low fluences, on patients with darker skin types (Fitzpatrick III and IV). More darkly pigmented patients will frequently have a transient interval of postinflammatory hyperpigmentation beginning 2 to 4 weeks after the procedure. Topical antiinflammatory agents can be added after the second postprocedure week. Because the neck skin has fewer dermal appendages and reepithelializes slowly, it can also be treated, but with great caution, using lower fluences.

Perioperative Erbium:YAG Laser Care

Cleansing and lubrication are the key. Although the recovery time following Er:YAG ablation is significantly less and the sequelae less pronounced than following CO_2 laser resurfacing, the same general principles are followed in the perioperative period. Showering and hair shampooing with baby shampoo twice daily and using a vinegar face wash (1 tablespoon of white vinegar in 4 cups of lukewarm water) twice daily will keep the face clean and minimize crusting. Natragel masks are applied frequently to supplement cutaneous hydration.

Intense sun protection is essential for all patients during the first 8 to 12 weeks postprocedure. Although cosmetically inelegant, zinc oxide is a total physical sun block and a soothing topical agent. We encourage our patients to use it for at least 2 weeks before they begin using makeup with a sun protection factor (SPF 15). After resurfacing, the patient's skin is exceptionally sensitive and allergic; inflammatory reactions may be severe and can delay recovery. Our patients are instructed not to use *any* topical products, herbs, or botanicals without consulting us. Patients lasered in the perioral area are treated prophylactically with acyclovir 400 mg orally beginning 1 day preoperatively and continuing for 2 weeks postoperatively. If more than three passes of the Er:YAG are used, ciprofloxacin 500 mg b.i.d. is begun 1 day preoperatively and continued until the patient is reepithelialized in about 1 week.

The CO_2 laser emits laser energy with a wavelength of 10,600 nm. Water is the absorbing chromophore. But

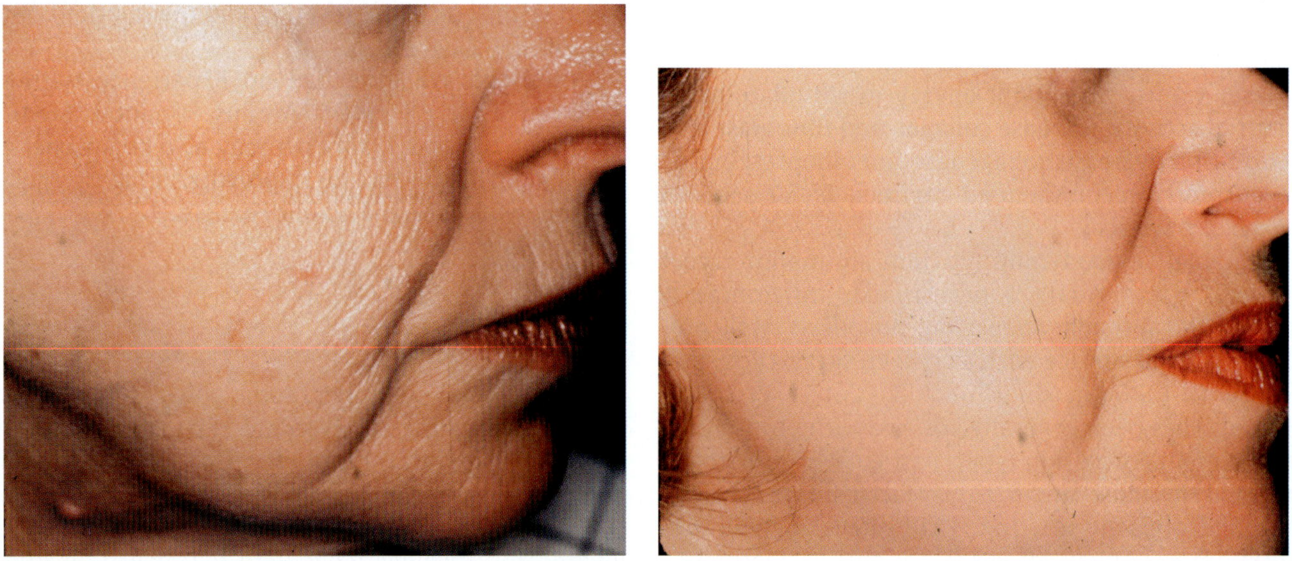

A B

Figure 1–1 **(A,B)** The facial skin is tighter and smoother, with improved contours following full-face CO_2 laser resurfacing (three passes of 300 mJ; pattern 3, size 8, density 6).

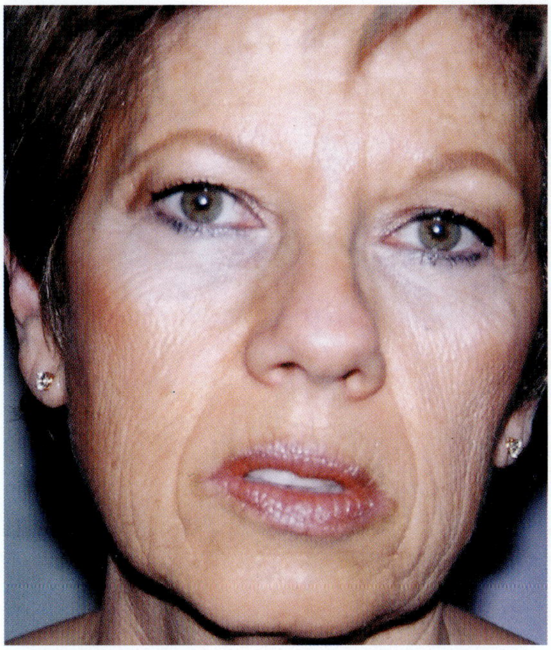

Figure 1–2 Marked rhytidosis with loss of skin elasticity and a blunting of facial contours was evident before carbon dioxide (CO_2) laser vaporization (full face: three passes of 300 mJ; pattern 3, size 8, density 6; eyelids: three passes 250 mJ and 200 mJ pattern 3, size 4, density 5). CO_2 laser-assisted upper lid blepharoplasty and internal brow suspension were performed at the same time. The patient has been pretreated with Botox neuromodulation of her lateral orbicularis, corrugator, procerus, depressor angulii oris, and platysma muscles.

unlike the Er:YAG, it causes tissue vaporization and dessication and 50 to 125 μm of thermal damage with each pass. These effects will generate much more new collagen production than the Er:YAG and create a tissue tightening not expected with the Er:YAG. CO_2 laser resurfacing can begin with one pass of 200 mJ (pattern 3, size 8, density 5 for the face). A maximum full-face treatment for a patient with marked solar damage would be three passes of 300 mJ. The higher the energy and the more passes, the greater the rhytid ablation, the more profound the tightening effect, and the longer the healing time. We do not treat the face segmentally (except for the eyelids and the upper lip) because this can leave demarcation lines. And the laser treatment is feathered inferior to the jawline by oblique applications or use of the Er:YAG. However, each segment of the face can be treated differently, with different pattern sizes, power, and densities.[9] Areas of more solar damage, rhytidosis, and actinic keratoses can be treated with higher fluences and more passes. The eyelids are treated with lower fluences and fewer passes (see Chapter 9). Applying a Natragel mask between CO_2 passes combined with Er:YAG ablation of debris appears to have beneficial effects on the postprocedure recovery (Figs. **1–1A,B; 1–2; 1–3; 1–4A,B; 1–5A,B**).

Perioperative Carbon Dioxide Laser Care

Following full-face CO_2 laser resurfacing the care is generally the same as following Er:YAG laser ablation, but more intense and the sequelae more dramatic.

During the first postoperative week, our standard protocol consists of applications of CU3 copper peptide cream four times daily with twice daily vinegar washes (1 tablespoon of white vinegar in 4 cups of lukewarm water). After the first postoperative week, Natragel mask applications are better tolerated and can be applied over CU3 cream (Fig. **1–3**). Protective makeup (with a physical sun block) is begun when epithelialization is complete and no crusting is apparent. Until that time the use of zinc oxide is encouraged. It is critically important that the patient has been emotionally prepared for several months of postprocedure erythema and instructed not to use *any* skin care products, herbs, or botanicals without having first discussed them with our staff.

All patients are treated prophylactically with acyclovir 400 mg q.i.d. and ciprofloxacin 500 mg b.i.d., beginning 1 day preoperatively and continued for 1 to 2 weeks postoperatively until they are completely reepithelialized. One dose of fluconazole 150 mg is given 1 day preoperatively.

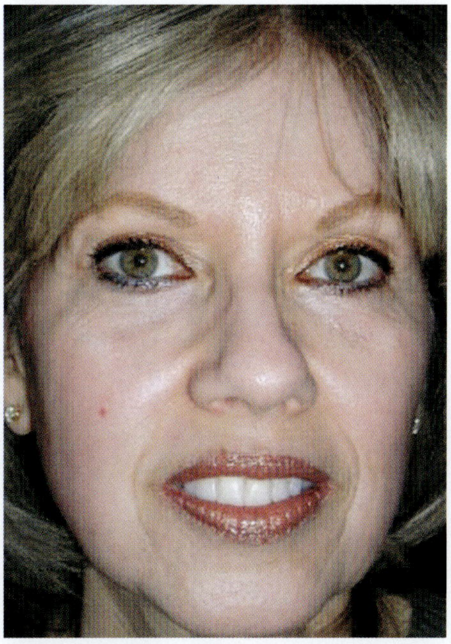

Figure 1–3 Two months after CO_2 laser resurfacing, moderate generalized erythema persisted. Six months later much of it has dissipated. Improved texture and contour are evident.

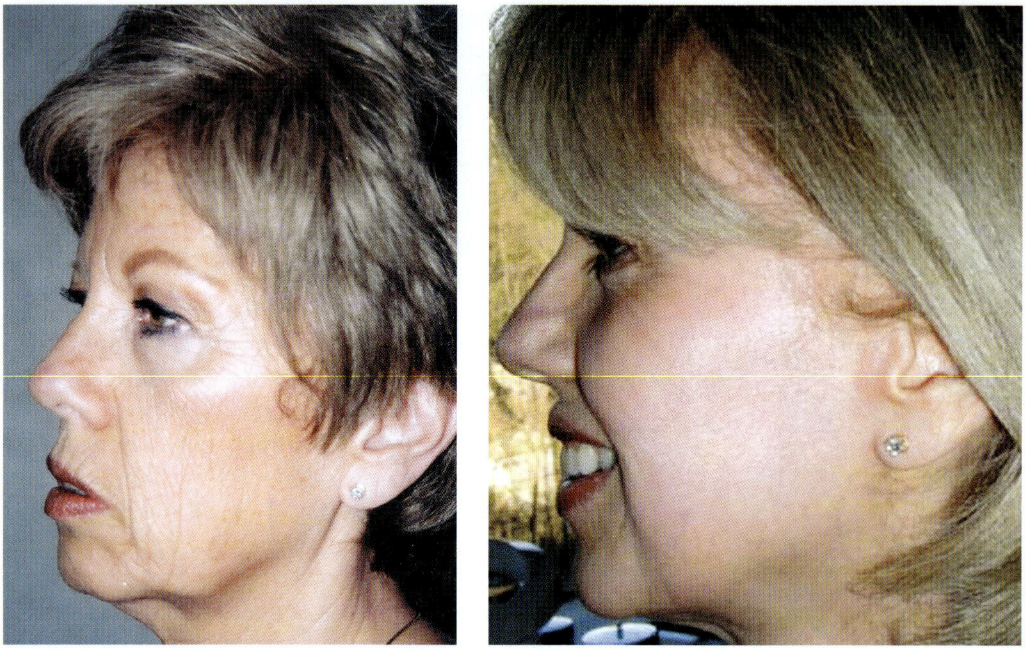

A B

Figure 1–4 (**A**) Lateral view of the same patient as shown in Figures 1–2 and 1–3. Marked facial rhytidosis and laxity are noted. (**B**) Six months following full-face CO_2 laser resurfacing, there is significant improvement of her rhytidosis and facial contours.

◆ Skin Tightening

The results of CO_2 laser resurfacing are the gold standard of nonincisional skin tightening (see earlier section) but a significant recovery period is required. A new generation of instrumentation utilizing radiofrequency energy has introduced the possibility of skin tightening without downtime (see Chapter 3, radiofrequency section). These techniques do not primarily ablate rhytids, but by tightening the cutaneous surface, we have seen improvement of skin folds and acne scarring (Figs. **1–6A,B; 1–7A,B**).

Since modifyings our treatment protocols by reducing the power of each application with the ThermaCool (Thermage Inc., Hayward, California) system outcomes have improved significantly.

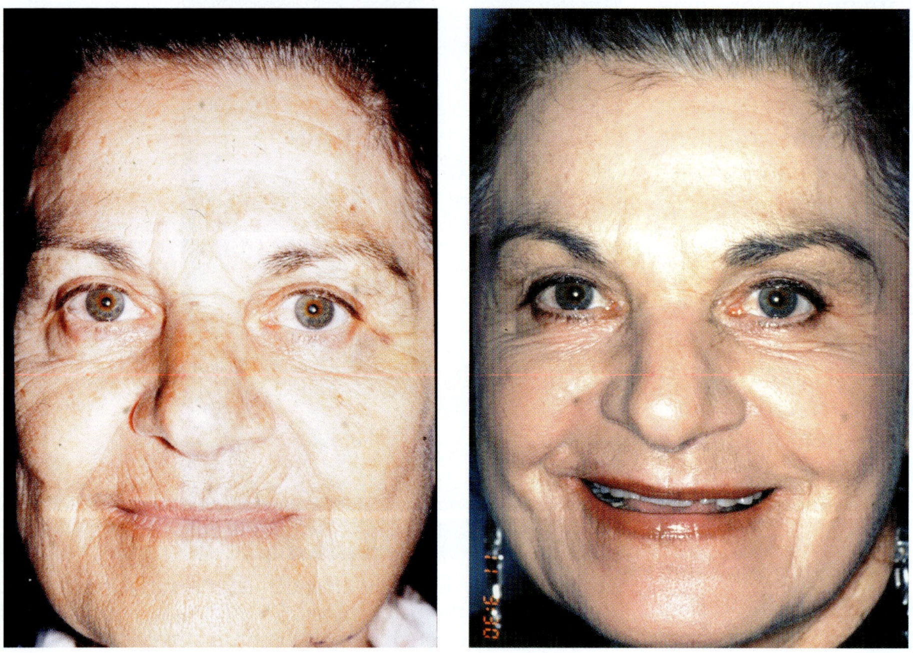

A B

Figure 1–5 (**A**) This 72-year-old woman exhibited marked actinic changes—dyschromia and rhytidosis—with blunting of her facial contours. (**B**) Full-face CO_2 laser resurfacing (300 mJ, 3 passes, pattern 3, size 8, density 6) resulted in dramatic improvement of her facial skin texture, pigmentation, elasticity, and contours. Her platysma and orbicularis muscles were pretreated with Botox to enhance the results. Micropigmentation of her eyebrows and eyelashes furthered the dramatic effect.

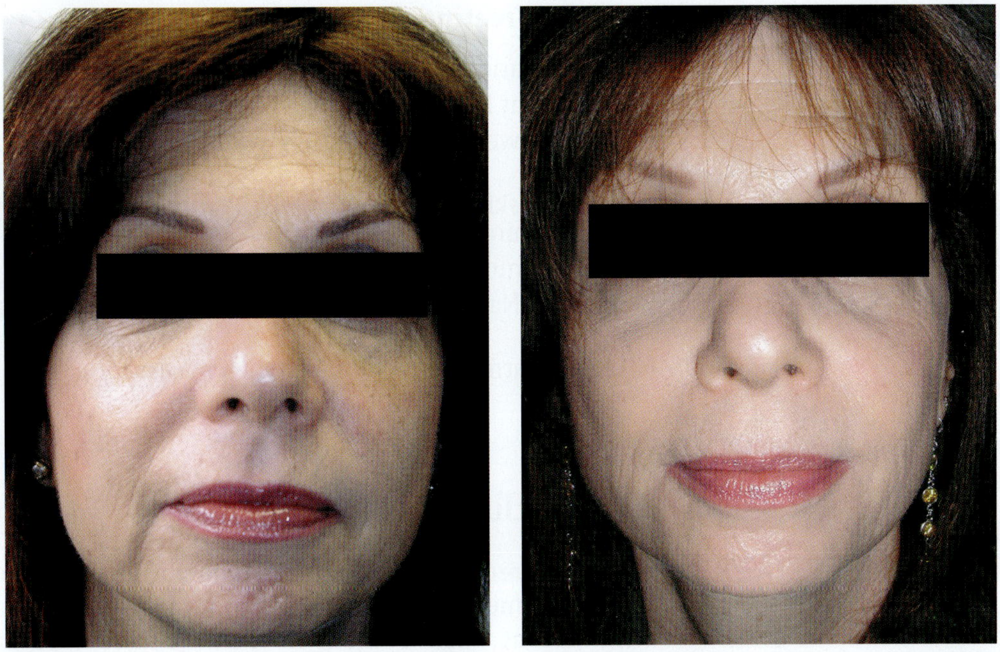

A B

Figure 1–6 (**A**) This 59-year-old woman manifested early descent of her malar fat pads, a deepening of her nasolabial folds and melojugal folds (marionette lines). (**B**) Four months following her Thermage procedure her nasolabial folds and melojugal folds are less apparent. Her depressor angulii oris and platysma muscles were pretreated with Botox.

Patient Preparation

We pretreat the patients with Botox 2 weeks before their "therma-lifting" procedure. If we are treating the forehead, we prepare the area with a neuromodulated brow lift. If we are treating the face and neck, we prepare these areas with neuromodulation of the platysma. In both cases relaxation of the muscles that depress the brow and the lower face in theory decrease resistance to collagen contraction and allow more efficient collagen remodeling.

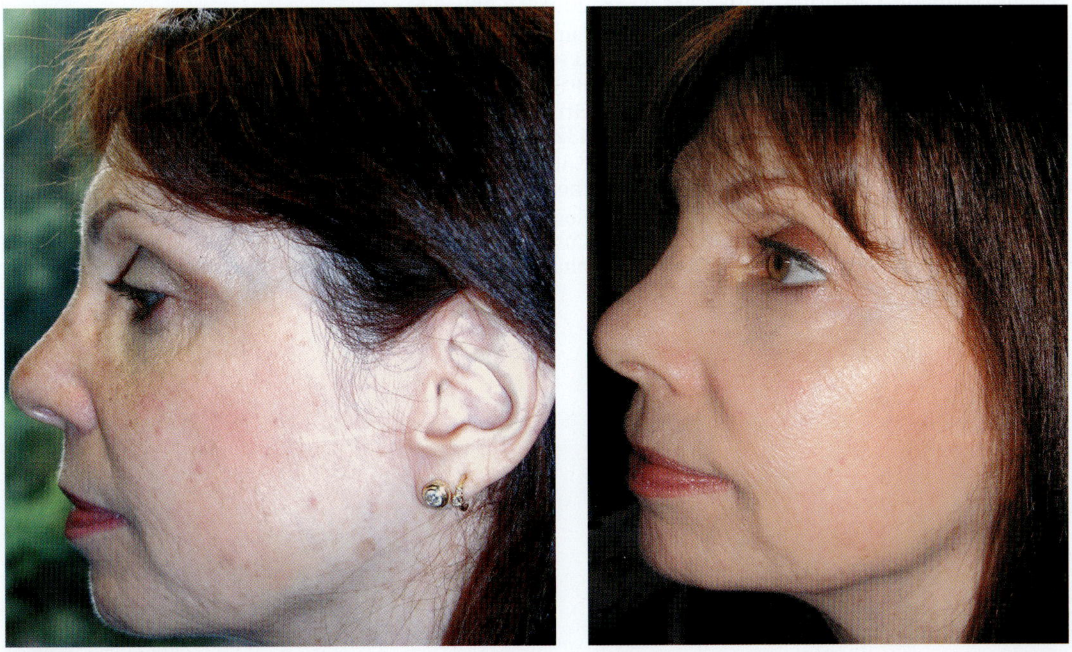

A B

Figure 1–7 (**A**) Side view of the same patient as in Figure 1–6 shows blunting of the jaw line and flattening of the malar eminence. (**B**) Following pretreatment of Botox to the platysma and depressor angulii oris muscles and Thermage to the face, an elevation of her malar contours is evident as well as a sharpening of her jaw line.

Face Treatment Protocol

First pass: setting 13.5; complete coverage
Second pass: setting 13.5; two rows of preauricular coverage

- Two rows above the jawline
- Two rows below the jawline
- One row from the corner of the mouth to the inferior tragus
- One row from the superior aspect of the nasolabial fold to the superior tragus

Third and fourth passes: setting 12.5; same passes as above

Forehead Treatment Protocol

First pass: setting 13.5; complete coverage
Second and third passes: setting 12.5; complete coverage

Neck Treatment Protocol

First, second, and third passes: setting 12.5; submental and lateral aspect of neck, avoiding midline

General Treatment Principles

1 Applications not overlapped
2. Allow at least 2 minutes before re-treating an area
3. Use lower power settings when applying multiple passes
4. Pinch skin between fingers in direction of desired tightening
5. Limit multiple passes to 5
6. Apply Natragel mask following completion of treatment
7. Re-treatment in 6 months when necessary

◆ Conclusion

It is apparent that a variety of nonablative techniques and treatments when used concomitantly can cause a significant improvement in facial skin texture and appearance. As other modalities become available, our menu of noninvasive therapies will expand.

References

1. McDaniel DH, Newman J, Geronemus R, Weiss RA, Weiss MA. Nonablative nonthermal LED photomodulation: a multicenter clinical photoaging trial [abstract 72]. American Society of Laser Medicine and Surgery annual meeting, Anaheim, California, April 2003
2. Geronemus R, Weiss RA, Weiss MA, Newman J. Nonablative LED photomodulation: light activated fibroblast stimulation clinical trial [abstract 73]. American Society of Laser Medicine and Surgery annual meeting, Anaheim, California, April 2003
3. Weiss RA, Weiss MA, McDaniel DH, Newman J, Geronemus R. Comparison of nonablative fibroblast photoactivation with and without application of topical cosmeceutical agents [abstract 74]. American Society of Laser Medicine and Surgery annual meeting, Anaheim, April 2003
4. Goldberg DJ. Subdermal resurfacing. Operative Techniques in Oculoplastic, Orbital and Reconstructive Surgery 1999; 2:188–193
5. Bosniak S, Cantisano-Zilkha M. A combined approach to noninvasive facial rejuvenation: home care, peels, neuromodulation, and laser-assisted subsurface collagen remodeling. Operative Techniques in Oculoplastic, Orbital and Reconstructive Surgery 2001;4:65–68
6. Goldberg DJ. Full-face nonablative dermal remodeling with a 1320 nm Nd:YAG laser. Dermatol Surg 2000;26:915–918
7. Fournier N, Dahan S, Barneon G, et al. Nonablative remodelling: clinical, hisologic, ultrasound imaging, and profilometric evaluation of a 1540 nm Er:glass laser. Dermatol Surg 2001;27:799–806
8. Lupton JR, Williams CM, Alster TS. Nonablative laser skin resurfacing using a 1540 nm erbium glass laser: a clinical and histologic analysis. Dermatol Surg 2002;28:833–835
9. Hruza GJ. Laser skin resurfacing. Arch Dermatol 1996; 132:451–455
10. Goldberg DJ. Er:YAG laser resurfacing: what is its role? Aesthetic Surg J 1998;18:255–260
11. Bosniak S. Laser resurfacing. In Bosniak S, Cantisano-Zilkha M. Cosmetic Blepharoplasty and Facial Rejuvenation. Philadelphia: Lippincott-Raven; 1999

2

Intense Pulsed Light for Full Facial Rejuvenation

Girish S. Munavalli, Margaret A. Weiss, and Robert A. Weiss

Nonablative broadband light and laser devices have grown in popularity in recent years. One such device, the intense pulsed light (IPL), was introduced in the mid-1990s and has become a well-recognized treatment modality to improve the appearance of the photoaged face. Photoaging consists of the characteristic clinical changes to facial and other sun-exposed skin caused by chronic exposure to ultraviolet (UV) light. These changes include the appearance of telangectasias, rough texture, fine and coarse wrinkles, yellow or sallow color, and mottled pigmentation.[1]

The overall appearance of aging skin is primarily related to the quantitative effects of sun exposure over time. UV radiation damages structural components of the dermis, chiefly collagen and elastic fibers. A common pathway whereby photoaging occurs is through UV-generated reactive oxygen species.[2] Facial appearance, however, is also affected by genetic factors, intrinsic factors, disease processes such as rosacea, and the overall loss of cutaneous elasticity associated with age. Signs of photoaging are becoming more evident in increasingly younger individuals, especially those regularly engaged in outdoor professions or recreational activities, as a consequence of exposure to increasingly high levels of UV radiation.[3] Treatment of these changes with nonablative devices has been termed photorejuvenation and can be approached in a rational, stepwise fashion (Table **2–1**).

Nonablative laser devices classically emit energy in coherent wavelengths within the near infrared to infrared spectrum (Table **2–2**). Intradermal water is the target chromophore and heat generated by this interaction causes thermal injury within the dermis, initiating a cascade of molecular repair events that promote collagen formation and deposition.[4] Clinically, this is manifested by subtle improvements in fine wrinkling and skin texture.

Alternatively, vascular-specific laser devices with wavelengths from 585 to 600 nm are also thought to cause thermal injury to dermal elements. These lasers are commonly used to treat the telangiectatic component. Energy is selectively absorbed by the target chromophore, hemoglobin. Light energy is converted to heat, which damages the vessel walls and radiates into the surrounding dermis, causing injury and repair with the formation of new collagen.[5]

By contrast, IPL is one proprietary noncoherent device in a class of several such devices, which emits a spectrum of wavelengths in the 515 to 1200 nm range. It allows for variation of pulse length/mode, delay between pulses, and fluence energy. Cutoff filters eliminate the lower range of wavelength of light emitted. Consequently, patients of darker skin types (Fitzpatrick III–IV) can be safely treated. Target lesions include blood vessels as well as lentigines. Selective thermal heating of chromophores including hemoglobin, water-containing tissue (collagen), and melanin is thought to induce neocollagenesis.[6] Intrinsic cooling provided by IPL devices allows for repair of photoaging structural changes in the skin without disruption of cutaneous integrity. The resulting patient treatment has a low-risk profile and minimal downtime.

◆ Technology

IPL devices consist of a flashlamp housed in an optical treatment head, in which reflecting mirrors are water cooled (Fig. **2–1**). Optically coated quartz filters are placed over the window of the optical treatment head

Table 2–1 Problem-Oriented Nonablative Treatment Algorithm for Facial Lesions

Lesion	Device
Facial telangiectasias	IPL, PDL
Mottled pigmentation	IPL, PDL, Microdermabrasion
Mild rhytids	IPL, CT2
Moderate rhytids	CT2

IPL, intense pulsed light; PDL, Pulsed dye laser (595 nm); CT2, CoolTouch II Laser (1320 nm)(Cool Touch Corp., Roseville, California).

to eliminate wavelengths lower than the filter. For faster recycling times, certain optical heads have water circulating around the flashlamp. The filter crystals must be optically coupled to the skin with a water-based gel.[3]

When filtered, the IPL device is capable of emitting a broad bandwidth of light from 515 to ~1200 nm. This bandwidth is modified by the application of filters, which exclude wavelengths lower than the filter to help protect against epidermal heating. Although the output is not uniform across this spectrum, it has been shown that during a 10 msec pulse relatively high doses of yellow light at 600 nm are emitted, with far less red and infrared, although output clearly is demonstrated beyond 1000 nm.[3]

Filters applied for vascular lesions are 515, 550, 570, and 590 nm. Longer filters 615, 645, 695, and 755 nm, which cut off much more of the yellow wavelengths, are used for various applications but most commonly for photoepilation. Importantly, IPL involves not only filtering and eliminating the lowest wavelengths emitted by the flashlamp but also the ability to easily manipulate pulse durations and to couple these pulse durations with precise resting or thermal relaxation times.

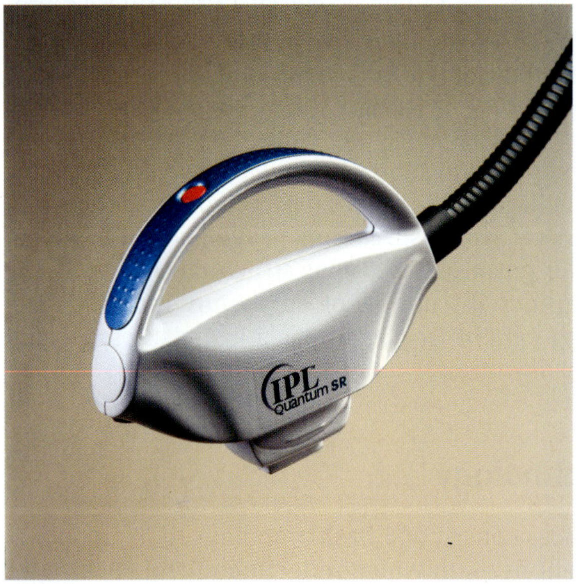

Figure 2–1 The head of the Lumenis Quantum intense pulsed light device (Lumenis Corp., Yokneam, Israel).

Table 2–2 Select Nonablative Devices, Including Coherent and Noncoherent Devices and Vascular Lasers

Wavelength	Coherent Devices
585–600 nm	Cynosure V-Star Candela V-Beam
1064 nm	Catera CoolGlide Lumenis One, Vasculight Laserscope Lyra, Gemini
1320 nm	CoolTouch II, III
1450 nm	Candela Smoothbeam
Wavelength	**Noncoherent Devices**
500–1200 nm	Lumenis PhotoDerm, Epilight, Vasculight, Quantum One Cutera Xeo Syneron Aurora Palomar Starlux

◆ Indications

Elements of IPL photorejuvenation treatment for the photoaged face include (1) identification of characteristic skin changes, both individual lesions and the photoaging complex; (2) identification of subpurpuric, subablative parameters; and (3) maintenance programs.[7,8]

One of the most frequently requested facial cosmetic procedures is elimination of facial telangiectasias. Removal of telangiectasias on the nose and cheeks results in a clinically smoother appearance to the skin texture.[9] To treat blood vessels by light energy, selective photothermolysis must be achieved. The filtered flashlamp noncoherent IPL source meets the requirements for selective photothermolysis by virtue of the absorption coefficient of blood in the vessel being higher than that of the bloodless dermis for a very broad range of wavelengths.[9]

Facial telangiectasias have been found to be generally more responsive to IPL treatment than leg telangiectasias. This is thought to be due to several factors: thinner overlying epidermis, thinner vessel walls rendering the endothelium more susceptible to thermal damage, higher relative amounts of oxyhemoglobin (better chromophore than deoxygenated hemoglobin), and lower hydrostatic pressures. As a result, the response of facial telangiectasias is more predictable with

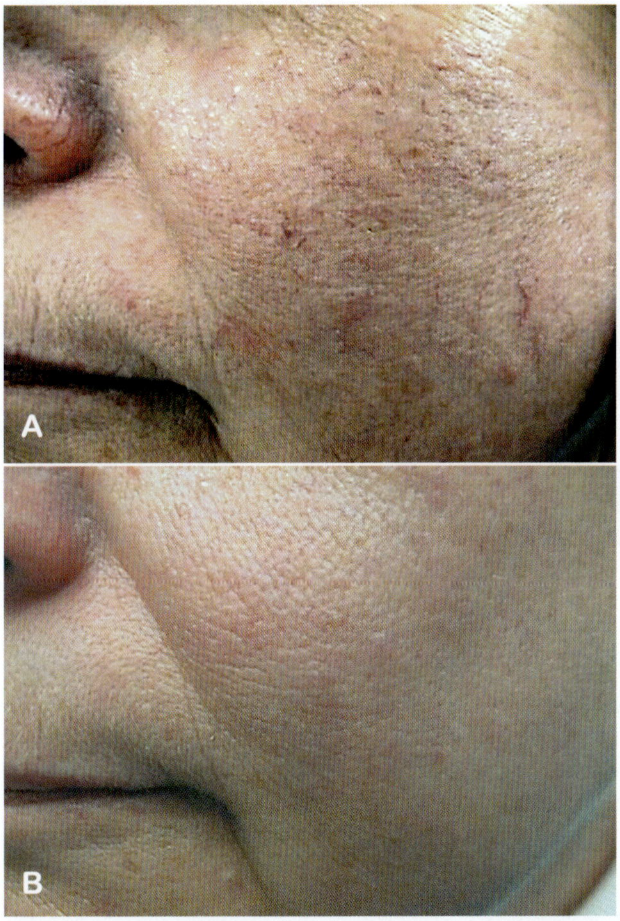

Figure 2–2 Successful treatment of cheek telangiectasias. (**A**) Prior to treatment. (**B**) After three treatments, spaced approximately 4 weeks apart.

an approximate 95% resolution rate after three treatments (Figs. **2–2A,B**).[8]

General parameters for the IPL treatment of facial telangiectasias includes a double pulse of 2.4 to 4.0 msec duration with a 560, 570, or 590 nm filter, depending on the degree of red coloration of the vessels. For example, a 590 nm filter would be used for less blue, brighter red (oxyhemoglobin-rich) vessels. Delay times between the pulses vary depending on the skin coloration. Darker skin types, such as Asian skin, require longer delays or 20 to 40 msec between pulses so that the heat generated within the vessel can be conducted safely to the surrounding tissues without potential damage to the epidermis. Delay times in the range of 10 to 20 msec are more common for lighter skin types.[9] Fluences typically between 20 and 30 J/cm^2 are used to start. If a pulse duration of >4 msec is used, then larger fluence of between 40 to 45 J/cm^2 can be used.[9]

The use of ice-cold coupling gel in conjunction with the chilled crystal tip of the IPL device is paramount to achieving optimal results with all IPL treatments, while helping to minimize the risk of epidermal damage, which results in blistering and burning. The ice-cold gel's purpose is twofold: (1) it serves as a focusing medium between the light emitted from the device to the air to the skin and (2) it serves as a heat sink to absorb heat that gets absorbed by or radiated to the epidermis from the target chromophores in the epidermis and dermis.

Clinical observation of subtle changes in vessel quality after treatment is paramount to achieving high-quality, reproducible results. Within seconds to minutes after a treatment, vessels should darken to a reddish-blue color (Fig. **2–3A,B**). This coloration can travel slightly beyond the treated area as the heat energy conducts along the vessel. Often, a mild "vessel blurring" or local urticaria-like reaction will be observed around the vessel. This reaction may take several minutes to manifest, and it is often necessary to wipe away coupling gel for better visualization. Using this approach, excellent results can be achieved (Fig. **2–4A,B**). Risk of adverse effects is greatly minimized by observation of several test pulses at different fluences prior to treating the entire affected area. The incidence of purpura is very low in this setting, and lower than that observed with classic pulsed-dye lasers. Patients should be told in advance to expect lesion clearance in one to three treatments. Perinasal telangiectasias often take multiple treatments, a presumed consequence of their relatively high-pressure, high-flow state secondary to their branching proximity to the angular artery.

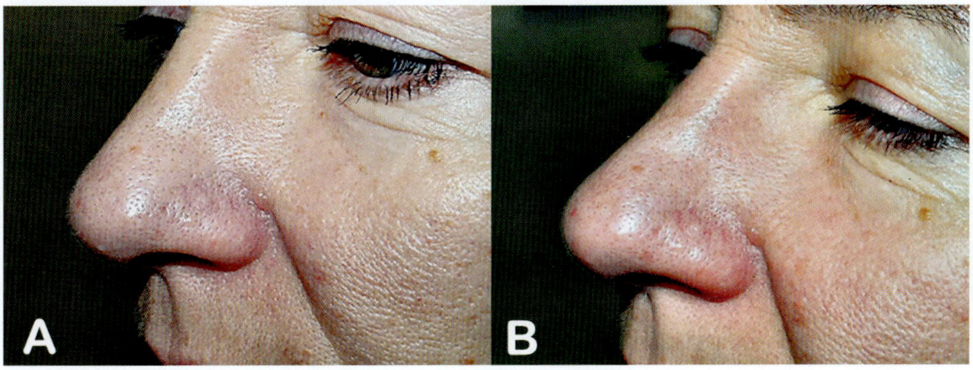

Figure 2–3 Note the subtle darkening of the left nasal alar vessels. (**A**) Before treatment. (**B**) Immediately following a pulse with an intense pulsed light device.

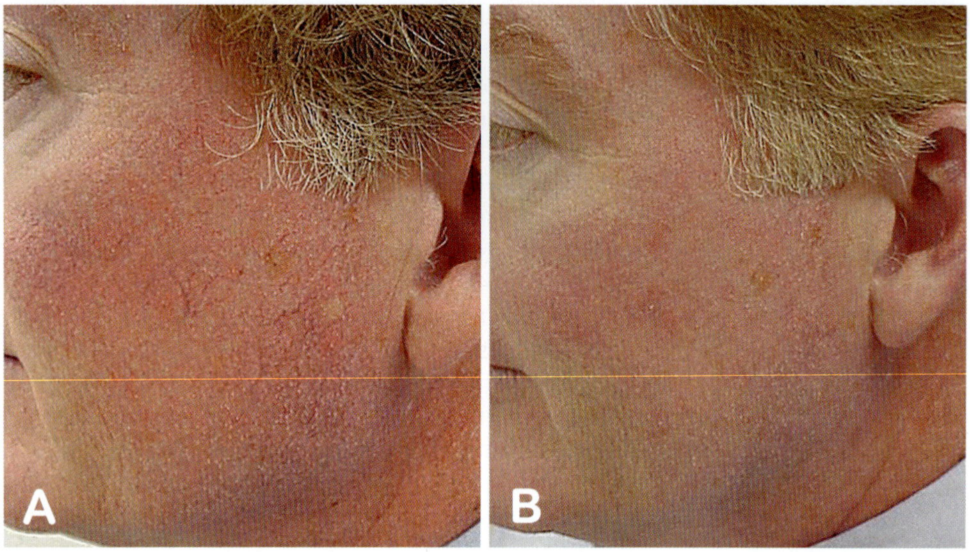

Figure 2–4 Successful treatment of left cheek telangiectasias. (**A**) Prior to treatment. (**B**) Six weeks after a single treatment.

Solar lentigines, known to patients as sun spots and liver spots, are another characteristic lesion observed on the photoaged face. These classically present as gradually appearing, well-defined light and dark brown round macules and patches on the malar cheeks and forehead. Often mistaken for moles by patients, these lesions are very effectively treated with IPL devices (Fig. **2–5A,B**). Suggested parameters for treatment are fluences of 24 to 33 J/cm^2, using a 560 or 590 nm cutoff filter with a 4 msec double pulse with 20 to 40 msec delays.[10] Treatment results in an immediate darkening of the lesion, a

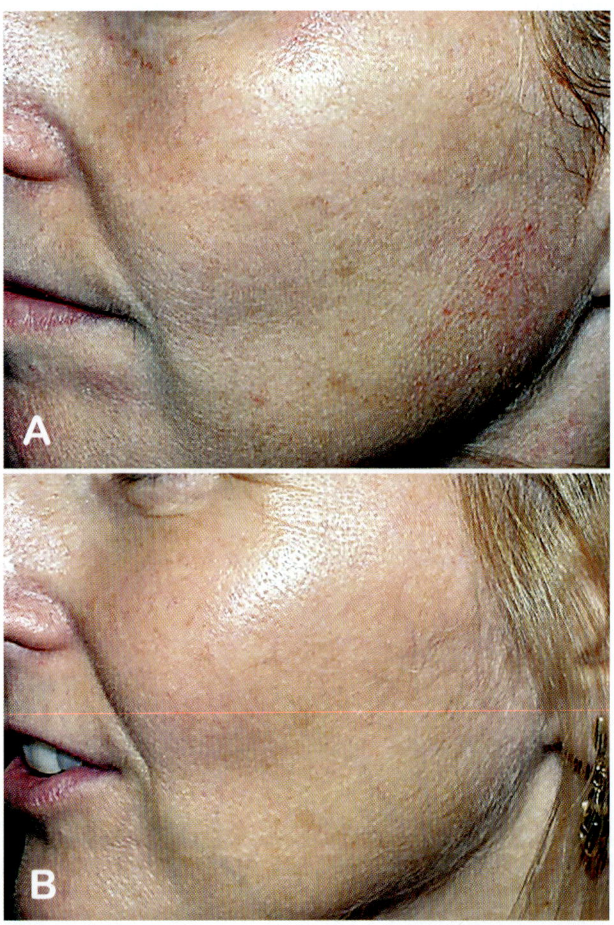

Figure 2–5 A marked reduction in lentigines. (**A**) Prior to treatment. (**B**) Four weeks after a single treatment.

Table 2–3 General Guidelines for Intense Pulsed Light Treatment

Initial Treatment
Elicit history of any recent tanning (natural or self-tanning products)
Start conservatively with lower fluences, 22–25 J/cm^2
Examine results of a test spot (laterally or inconspicuously placed) and adjust parameters according to immediate clinical response
Endpoint of therapy is mild edema and moderate erythema, vessel darkening/blurring, and lentigines darkening
Subsequent Treatments
From previous treatment, note history of purpura, swelling, or blister formation
Grade improvement in the following: skin texture, pigmentation, redness/flushing, pore prominence
Purpura, prolonged erythema, or crusting is abnormal and necessitates lowering the dose settings; darkening or crusting of lentigenes lasting 7–10 days, erythema lasting 2–3 days, and mild edema lasting 1 day are considered to be normal responses
If patient reports no complications, increase energy by 0.5 to 2.0 J/cm^2 per treatment; after initial two to three treatments at 4-week intervals, can do maintenance treatments at 6-month intervals for photoaging; stress importance of sunscreen

Adapted from Sadick NS, Weiss R. Intense pulsed-light photorejuvenation. Semin Cutan Med Surg 2002;21:280–28[8]

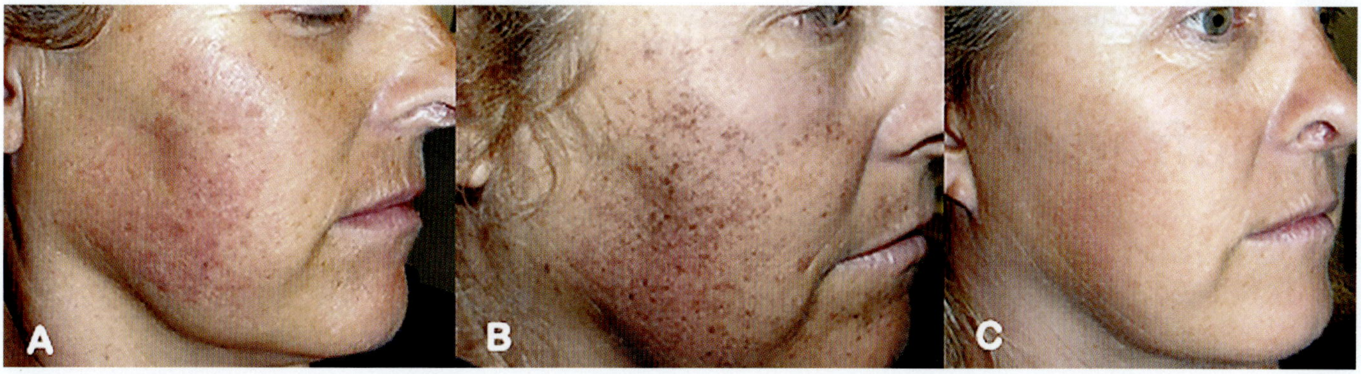

Figure 2–6 Sequence of events following intense pulsed light treatment. (**A**) Immediately after treatment. (**B**) Forty-eight hours after treatment. (**C**) Six weeks after treatment.

reaction that should be thoroughly explained to patients prior to treatment. As with telangiectasias, it may be necessary to pause treatment to view this endpoint after a series of test pulses before continuing treatment. Within 24 to 48 hours posttreatment, lentigines will take on a darker and crusty appearance. These remnants will spontaneously peel away over a 5- to 6-day posttreatment period (Fig. **2–6A–C**), or they can be removed by using microdermabrasion.

◆ Conclusion

Photorejuvenation has been described as a dynamic nonablative process involving the use of IPL in a low-fluence, nonablative manner to reduce mottled pigmentation and telangiectasias and smooth the textural surface of the skin[11] (Table **2–3**). Other than mild transient erythema, there are no other immediate visible signs of treatment, and patients may resume normal activities immediately.

References

1. Kligman AM. Early destructive effect of sunlight on human skin. JAMA 1969;210:2377–2380
2. Kang S, Fisher GJ, Voorhees JJ. Photoaging: pathogenesis, prevention, and treatment. Clin Geriatr Med 2001;17:643–659
3. Weiss RA, Weiss MA. Noncoherent light sources. In: Kauvar ANB, Hruza G, eds. Principles and Practices in Cutaneous Laser Surgery. New York: Marcel Dekker; 2000: 361–376
4. Goldberg DJ. New collagen formation after dermal remodeling with an intense pulsed light source. J Cutan Laser Ther 2000;2:59–61
5. Moody BR, McCarthy JE, Hruza GJ. Collagen remodeling after 585-nm pulsed dye laser irradiation: an ultrasonographic analysis. Dermatol Surg 2003;29:997–999
6. Nelson JS, Majaron B, Kelly KM. What is nonablative photorejuvenation of human skin? Semin Cutan Med Surg 2002; 21:238–250
7. Weiss RA, Weiss MA, Beasley KL. Rejuvenation of photoaged skin: 5 years results with intense pulsed light of the face, neck, and chest. Dermatol Surg 2002;28:1115–1119
8. Sadick NS, Weiss R. Intense pulsed-light photorejuvenation. Semin Cutan Med Surg 2002;21:280–287
9. Goldman MP. Intense pulsed light and nonablative approaches to photoaging. In Rigel DS, Weiss RA, Lim HW, et al, eds. Photoaging. New York: Marcel Dekker; 2004:165–183
10. Huang YL, Liao YL, Lee SH, Hong HS. Intense pulsed light for the treatment of facial freckles in Asian skin. Dermatol Surg 2002;28:1007–1012
11. Bitter PH. Noninvasive rejuvenation of photodamaged skin using serial, full-face intense pulsed light treatments. Dermatol Surg 2000;26:835–842

3

Radiofrequency Technology

Neil Scott Sadick

Thermal treatment using optical energy for various types of dermatologic problems has become very popular over the past 20 years. Light-based therapies with lasers and intense pulsed light (IPL) technologies have been increasingly used in aesthetic medicine for epilation, removal of vascular and pigmented lesions, reduction of fine wrinkles, and treatment of acne.[1] The fundamental principle behind the use of light-based therapies is based on the theory of selective photothermolysis, which encompasses the following three tenets[2,3]:

1. Optical energy penetrates deep enough to reach the treated target.
2. Optical energy is mostly absorbed by the target, although surrounding skin may be heated significantly.
3. Optical energy is strong enough to create thermal damage of the treated target.

In selective photothermolysis, a pulse of light set at the proper wavelength and proper duration is delivered to targeted sites. Although effective for a broad range of dermatologic indications, limitations have also been realized with light-based therapies.[4] One of the main limitations is that optical energy must penetrate the epidermis to reach the depth of the targeted site. Optical energy is absorbed by melanin chromophores in the epidermis and hair shafts, and hemoglobin in blood. In photoepilation, light-colored hair is particularly difficult to remove because it has low levels of melanin and therefore may not absorb enough energy to achieve thermal destruction of the hair follicle. Conversely, high pigmentation of the epidermis also poses a problem because it may absorb too much energy, potentially causing adverse effects such as burns and hyperpigmentation. Wrinkles respond poorly to treatment with optical energy because collagen fibers do not contain chromophores. These limitations have stimulated investigators to look for new forms of energy that satisfy the principle of selective thermolysis but are devoid of thc main disadvantage of optical energy for dermatologic applications; that is, a strong interdependence between treatment efficacy/safety and chromophore levels in the epidermis.

This chapter evaluates the use of an alternative source of energy—electrical current—for the selective treatment of different biological targets. Different from selective photothermolysis, the treatment using electrical current is termed selective electrothermolysis.

◆ Electrical Current in Medicine

Electrical current has been used in medicine for more than a century. Low frequency or direct current (DC) causes spasms of the muscles and is used at low intensity for biostimulation, such as cardioversion of atrial fibrillation.[5] High frequency current in the range of 0.3 to 10 megahertz (MHz), or radiofrequency (RF) current, produces a pure thermal effect on biological tissue that is dependent on the electrical properties of the tissue. The high efficiency of RF current for tissue heating has made it useful for electrosurgery and an attractive source of energy for various dermatologic applications.[6,7] The mechanism of tissue heating is based on generating Joules of heat by electrical current. Generated heat is described by Joule's law:

$$H = j^2/\sigma$$

where j is the density of electrical current and σ is electrical conductivity.[8] The value opposite to conductivity is named resistance or impedance (ρ). Distribution of electrical current can be calculated using the method described in the color section that follows.

Electrical conductivity depends on the frequency of the electrical current and the type and temperature of the tissue. The distribution of electrical current depends on the geometry of the electrodes. Two typical configurations are used in medicine: unipolar and bipolar. The major difference between the two systems is how the RF current is controlled and directed at the target. However, there is no difference in ultimate tissue effect at the same RF fluence.

Method for Calculating Distribution of Electrical Current σ

Distribution of electrical current is described by a continuity equation

$$div\, j = 0 \qquad (A1)$$

where j is density of the electrical current. The equation states that electrical current starts in one of the electrodes and has to reach the other electrode closing the electrical loop through the electrical circuit.

According to the Ohm equation the current density is higher when conductivity and electrical field are higher:

$$j = \sigma E \qquad (A2)$$

where σ is electrical conductivity of tissue and E is electrical field strength, which is described by following equation:

$$E = -grad\ \varphi \qquad (A3)$$

where φ is a potential of the electrical field.

Combining Equations (A1) through (A3) the following equation for potential of the electrical field can be obtained:

$$div\,(\sigma\, grad\ \varphi) = 0. \qquad (A4)$$

Electrical conductivity depends on frequency of the electrical current and the type of tissue and its temperature. For analyzing electrical current distribution Equation A4 is solved using numerical computerization with boundary conditions depending on geometry of electrodes.

Unipolar System

A unipolar or monopolar system delivers energy through one electrode with a relatively small contact point

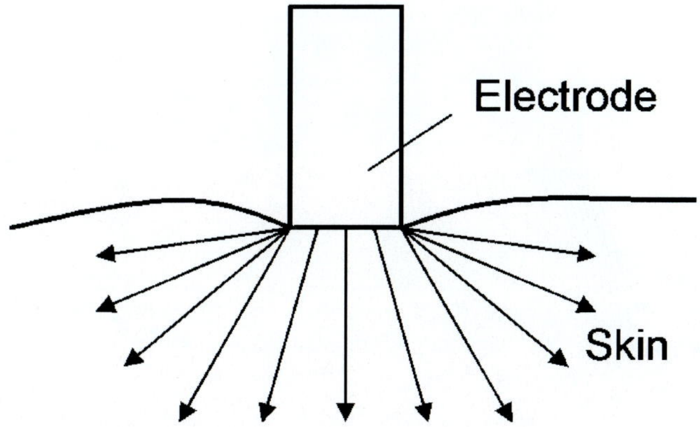

Figure 3–1 Schematic representation of the flow of electrical current through the epidermis using a cylindrical unipolar electrode.

applied to the treatment area while another large-size ground electrode is applied to the body at a distance far from the active electrode. A cylindrical electrode is applied to the skin surface, and the schematic flow of electrical current is depicted in Fig. **3–1.** Electrical energy is concentrated near the tip of the electrode and decreases rapidly with distance. Penetration depth of RF current can be estimated as half the electrode size. Therefore, a 10 mm unipolar electrode has a penetration depth of ~5 mm, which is deep enough to reach muscles.

The advantage of a unipolar system is its ability to create a high-power density on the surface of the electrode. This attribute makes it popular in electrosurgery where a small-size electrode is used. The disadvantage of a unipolar system is its unpredictable behavior as the current passes through the body to the grounding electrode. In aesthetic medicine, examples of a unipolar system include the Visage (ArthroCare Corp., Sunnyvale, California) and ThermaCool (Thermage Inc., Hayward, California).

Bipolar System

A bipolar system passes an electrical current between two electrodes at a fixed distance. Both electrodes are applied to the treated area, and electrical current propagation is limited by the area between electrodes. The behavior of electrical current in a bipolar system is depicted in Fig. **3–2.** Distribution of electrical current as a function of depth (calculated using the method described in the Equations section later in this chapter) for different distances between electrodes is presented in Fig. **3–3.** Using the same definition of penetration depth as used for the electromagnetic radiation and particularly the depth where density of value is decreased by factor $e = 2.72$. The penetration depth of electrical current can be estimated as half the distance between electrodes.

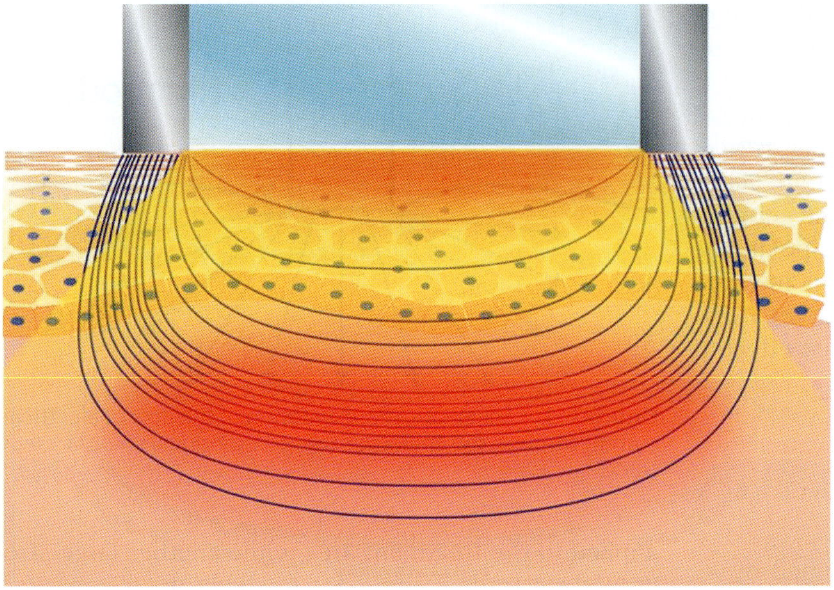

Figure 3–2 Schematic representation of the flow of electrical current through the epidermis using a bipolar system.

The main advantage of a bipolar system is the controlled distribution of RF current inside the tissue, which is limited by volume between the two electrodes. Therefore, the bipolar system is less suitable for electrosurgery but appropriate for hemostasis and controlled vessel contraction using an intravascular catheter. In aesthetic medicine, examples of bipolar systems include the Aurora™ and Polaris™ systems (Syneron Medical Ltd.; Yokneam, Israel).

◆ Electrical Conductivity of Different Tissue Types

Table **3–1** shows the electrical conductivity of different tissues at normal temperature and a frequency of electrical current at 1 MHz. Blood and parts of the body with high blood content have the highest electrical conductivity. Bone has very low electrical conductivity, and therefore, electrical current does not penetrate the

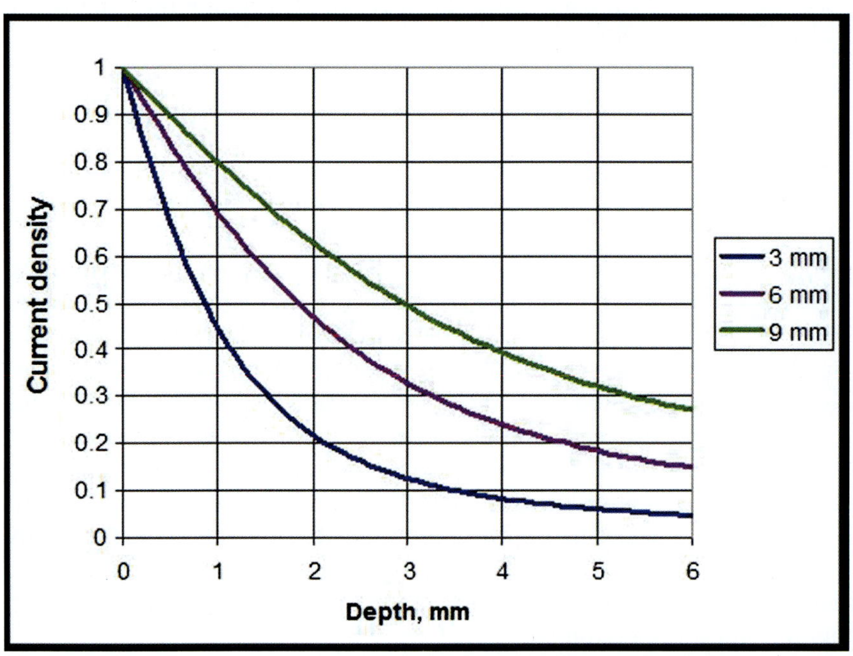

Figure 3–3 Normalized distribution of electrical current density as a function of the depth for different distances between electrodes in a bipolar system.

Table 3–1 Electrical Conductivity of Different Types of Tissue at 1 MHz

Tissue	Conductivity (S m m^{-1})
Blood	0.7
Bone	0.02
Fat	0.03
Dry skin	0.03
Wet skin	0.25

bone but rather flows around it. Dry skin is also resistant to electrical current and must be hydrated to permit passage of electrical current into the tissue. Conductivity of tissue increases proportionally with frequency. In Fig. **3–4,** the RF current from the electrodes penetrates the epidermis and concentrates in areas with high electrical conductivity. The pattern of distribution of electrical current demonstrates the possibility for selective treatment of blood vessels using conductive RF.

◆ Temperature Dependence of Electrical Conductivity

Tissue conductivity is significantly correlated with tissue temperature. The thermal coefficient (α) of skin conductivity is ~2% C^{-1}; that is, every 1°C increase in temperature lowers skin impedance by 2%.[9] Therefore, the distribution of electrical current can be controlled by precooling or preheating different parts of tissue. Fig. **3–5** describes the distribution of electrical current as a function of the depth of tissue with uniform temperature distribution for skin surface that has been precooled by 25°C. Surface cooling drives electrical current inside the tissue, increasing penetration depth. Likewise, preheating the target tissue increases conductivity and consequently selective heating by the RF current. Therefore, if the temperature of the target tissue is higher than that of the surrounding tissue, then the RF current will selectively focus to increase heating of the target tissue.

◆ Clinical Applications

In aesthetic medicine, the use of RF as an energy source for selective electrothermolysis is a relatively new concept. Systems that incorporate the RF current have been in development for several years but were introduced only recently. Studies using these new technologies have demonstrated utility in hair removal, skin rejuvenation, and wrinkle reduction.

Hair Removal

The effective removal of unwanted hair using optical energy has been essentially limited to black and dark and

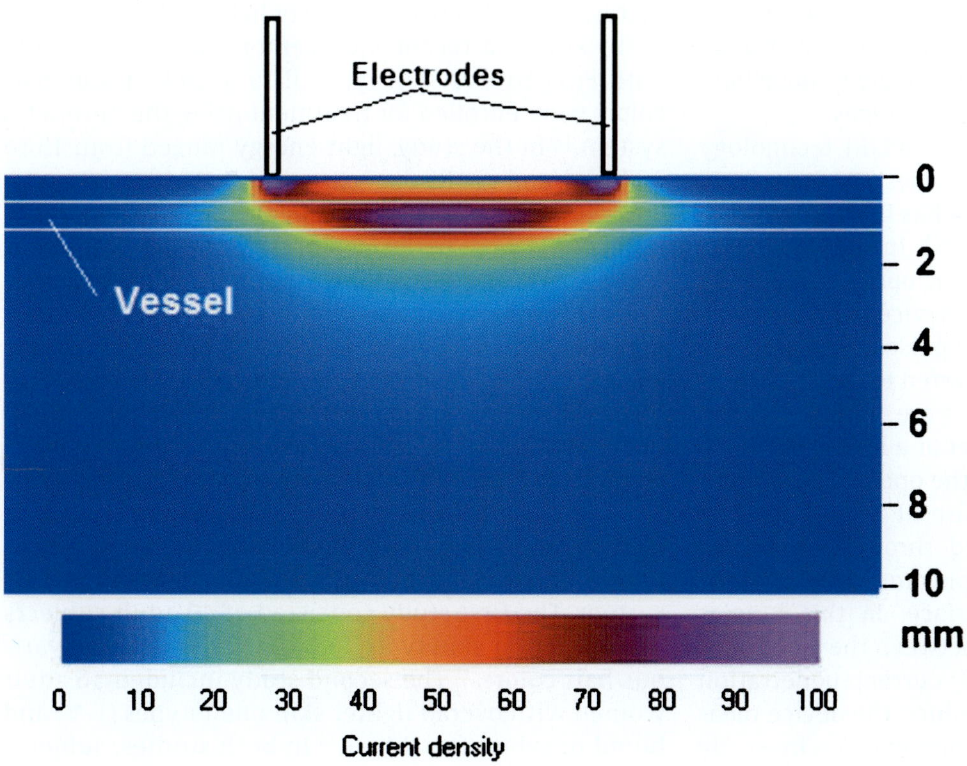

Figure 3–4 Normalized distribution of current density in tissue with blood vessel using a bipolar system.

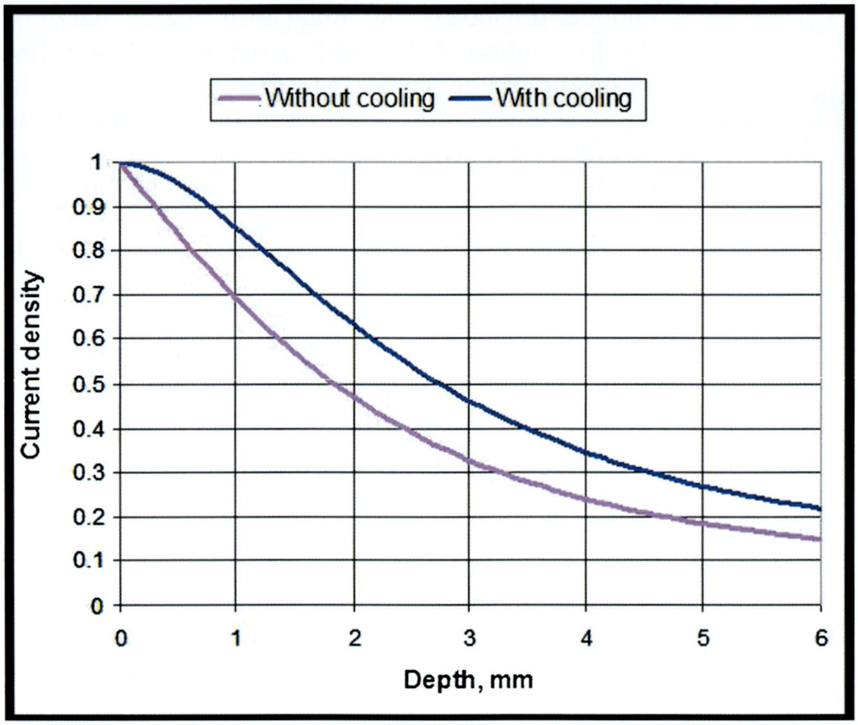

Figure 3–5 Normalized current density distribution as a function of the depth for precooled and normal skin.

medium tones of brown hair.[10] Treatment of light-colored hair has been particularly difficult because of the limited concentration of melanin chromophores in hair follicles. In addition, safety is a concern in dark skin types, who have an increased risk of blistering and dyschromia, even with longer-pulse lasers.[11] It would make sense that the combination of low levels of optical energy and electrical conducted RF current, the latter of which is not dependent on melanin for thermal absorption, may be able to effectively and safely remove hair, including light-colored hair, for all skin types.

A recently introduced combined IPL/RF technology integrates optical and electrical energies simultaneously applied to tissue. This technology has been referred to as electron-optical Syneron (ELOS). In the Aurora DS system, IPL (680–980 nm) producing optical energies as high as 30 J/cm^2 and a bipolar RF device that generates RF energy as high as 20 J/cm^3, and pulse durations up to 120 msec, are combined and delivered to targeted sites. Pulses of optical and RF energies are initiated at the same time, but the RF pulse is set at a longer duration than the optical pulse, enabling the optical component to preheat the target and increase RF selectivity. The conducted RF energy is applied through electrodes embedded in the system applicator and brought into contact with the skin surface. In this bipolar system, the shape and distance between the electrodes are optimized to provide an RF current penetration depth of 4 mm. During the procedure, the device measures changes in the skin impedance, which is inversely related to temperature and wavelength, and allows active dermal monitoring. Skin temperature is controlled and protected by the epidermal contact cooling maintained at ~5°C provided by the system.

The combined use of optical and RF energy for the hair removal system has shown efficacy where light-based therapies have not shown significant efficacy; that is, in the effective removal of light hair and safety in dark skin. In a recent multicenter study, 60 patients with Fitzpatrick's skin types II to V and various hair colors were enrolled for treatment using the Aurora DS system.[12] In the study, light energy ranged from 15 to 28 J/cm^2, and the RF energy ranged from 10 to 20 J/cm^3. Subjects received three treatments 6 to 8 weeks apart. Hair counts were performed prior to the first treatment and 3 months after the last treatment. Maximum hair reduction was observed at 2 to 8 weeks. At 3 months, hair clearance ranged from 64 to 84%, depending on the anatomical site. Treatment was most effective for hair in the axillae. In most cases, higher RF energy (15–20 J/cm^3) was used, and results indicate that efficacy is determined by the level of RF energy, not optical energy.

The primary author has conducted two studies to investigate the efficacy and safety of combined optical and RF energies for hair removal using the Aurora DS system. The first study consisted of 40 adult subjects with different skin types (Fitzpatrick's II–V) and various hair colors.[13] The second study included 36 adult women with overall lighter skin phenotypes (I–V) and blond or white facial hair.[14] In both studies, subjects received four treatments at 8- to 12-week intervals over a period of 9 to 12 months. Depending on skin and hair phenotypes, light energy ranged from 15 to 30 J/cm^3. Higher optical energy was used in lighter skin phenotypes and hair color. The RF current ranged from 10 to 20 J/cm^3, depending on the anatomical site; higher RF energy was used in facial regions (versus lower body regions). Results were monitored 18 months after the first treatment or 6 months after the last treatment.

In both studies, maximum hair reduction occurred 6 to 8 weeks following treatment, and hair density was observed to decrease progressively following each subsequent treatment. As observed in the first study, hair removal efficiency was greater in subjects with dark hair (mean clearance 80–85%). This is similar to that reported using other light-based technologies.[15a] Both studies showed that light hair phenotypes had hair clearances of between 40 and 60% (Table **3–2**). Results showed no significant dependence of treatment on skin color because light and dark skin types responded similarly to treatment. Side effects were minimal and transient. In the first study, 20% of subjects had mild erythema that resolved within 24 hours posttreatment. In the second study, 8% of subjects had transient hyperpigmentation that did not require therapy, and 14% had mild erythema, which resolved within 24 hours. Schroeter[15b] used the Aurora S to treat 28 women with hirsutism with an average of 6.6 treatments per site. The mean success rate in clearance was 73.5%. Results showed dependence on pulse times and age of patients but no dependence on skin type or hair color.

Potentially greater effectiveness may be obtained by optimizing treatment parameters and technique for combined optical and RF energies; for instance, manipulating optical and RF frequencies, increasing the number of passes, or increasing the number of treatments over a given time. These methods are currently being investigated.

Table 3–2 Mean Hair Removal Efficiency by Hair Color after Four Treatment Sessions (Month 18), Using Combined Intense Pulsed Light and Radiofrequency Energies with the Aurora DS System

	Study 1[13]		Study 2[14]	
Hair Color	*n*	Mean Clearance (%)	*n**	Mean Clearance (%)
Black	16	85	—	—
Brown	13	80	—	—
Blond	5	60	21	52
Red	3	60	—	—
White	3	40	20	44

*Number of subject treatment sites.

Skin Rejuvenation

Skin rejuvenation is a complex treatment that includes removing vascular and pigmented lesions, improving skin texture, and reducing fine facial wrinkles. Effective treatment of these indications typically entails multiple treatments and more than one light-based device.[16–18] IPL provides good results for vascular, pigmented lesions and skin texture, but wrinkle improvement is not significant.[17] Long-pulse neodymium:yttrium-aluminum-garnet (Nd:YAG) lasers provide improvement of fine wrinkles but are not effective for pigmented lesions because of low chromophore absorption and show variable results for vascular lesions.[18]

The efficacy and safety of combination optical and RF energies for skin rejuvenation have been recently reported.[19] Treatment of the face and upper neck was performed for 100 subjects with Fitzpatrick's skin types II to IV using the Aurora SR system. Most subjects had combined clinical indications that included pigmented and vascular lesions, skin laxity, or enlarged pores. Each treatment consisted of one to three passes over the face using various optical (580–980 nm with pulse durations up to 120 msec) and RF parameters that were determined by individual skin type. Subjects received three to five treatments, depending on lesion type. To determine treatment effect, subjects were interviewed after their last treatment about their satisfaction level.

Based on results, improvements were observed in erythema and telangiectasias (70%) and lentigines and other hyperpigmentations (78%), as determined by subject satisfaction levels (Table **3–3**). In addition, both physicians and patients observed significant improvements in fine and coarse perioral, periocular, and

Table 3–3 Patient Satisfaction in Skin Rejuvenation Study Using Aurora SR System[18]

	% Patients (*N* = 100)		
Lesion Type	Satisfied	Neutral	Not Satisfied
Solar lentigo	78	22	0
Rosacea/ telangiectasias	70	30	0
Fine lines	57	40	3
Plumpness	86	11	3
Skin laxity	58	37	5
Pores	63	24	13

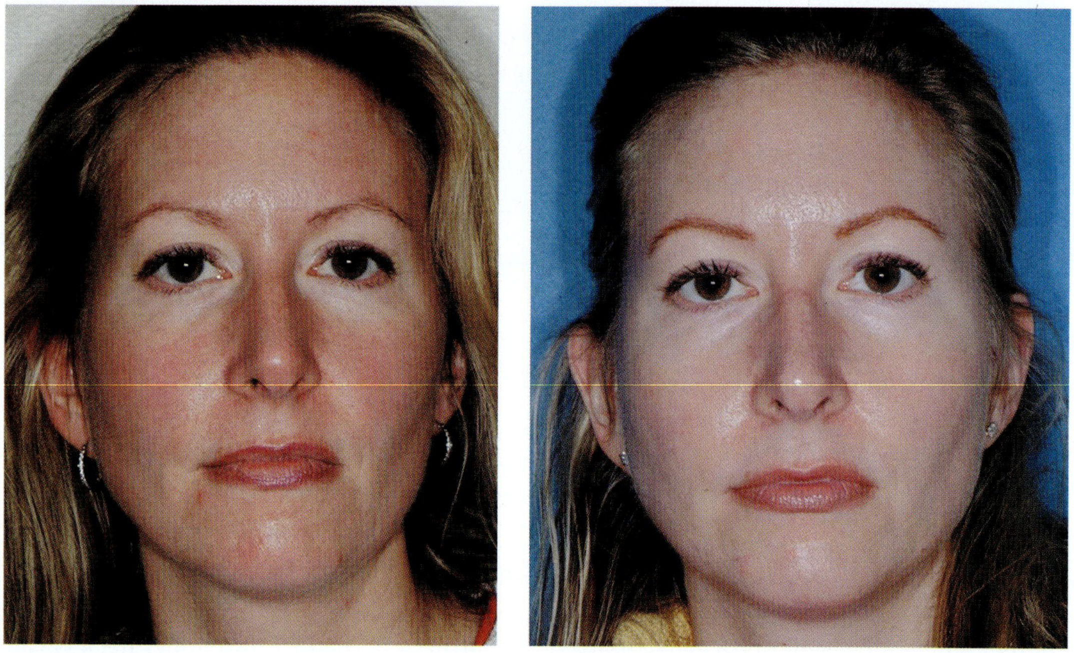

A B

Figure 3–6 (**A**) Pre combined intense pulsed light and radiofrequency (IPL + RF). (**B**) Post IPL + RF for three treatments (RF:20 J/cm^3/Light: 26 J/cm^2; 3 months).

forehead wrinkles. There was an average improvement of 60% in skin texture and fine wrinkles. The authors noted that wrinkle reduction with combined optical and RF energies was significantly greater than IPL alone (based on clinical experience) (Fig. **3–6A,B**). Moreover, subjects who had undergone both types of treatment reported a preference for the combined optical and RF procedure because of a greater degree of skin improvement, more rapid onset of effects, and slightly greater treatment comfort. Crusting of pigmented lesions was commonly observed the day following treatment. Small blood vessels vanished typically after two treatments. The typical number of treatment sessions required to get these results is presented in Table **3–4**. Only a small number of subjects (2.8%) were not satisfied with the level of skin texture improvement. The remaining 97.2% of subjects were satisfied with the results and opted to continue with treatment.[19]

Wrinkle Reduction

Nonablative treatment of deep wrinkles remains a difficult challenge in aesthetic medicine. Earlier carbon dioxide (CO_2) resurfacing techniques often caused long-lasting erythema ($\geq$3 months) and postinflammatory hyperpigmentation and required postoperative pain management. Introduction of the erbium:YAG (Er:YAG) lasers improved the safety and recovery profile of laser surgery; however, the application is limited primarily to the treatment of fine wrinkles and superficial defects.[6]

The first large prospective study to evaluate an RF resurfacing system for the treatment of wrinkles was published in 2000.[20] Ninety-five subjects (mean age, 52 years) with mild to severe photodamage (Fitzpatrick classes I–III) in the periorbital (75 treatment sites) or perioral (50 sites) regions were enrolled. Prior to treatment, subjects received nerve blocks and local infiltration anesthesia. The RF resurfacing device (Visage) was equipped with a multielectrode-tipped stylet to produce a low-heat process termed coblation (cold + ablation). The power setting for the RF resurfacing system was 125 to 139 V. A maximum of two passes were allowed for

Table 3–4 Typical Number of Sessions to Get Treatment Results in Skin Rejuvenation Study Using the Aurora SR System[18]

Lesion Type	Number of Treatments
Lentigos/freckles	1–3
Vascular lesions	2–3
Skin laxity	1–2
Fine lines	2–5
Pore closing	3–5
Acne scars	4–7

class I wrinkles and up to three passes for class II or III wrinkles. The stylet was applied continuously and evenly at a rate of ~1.0 to 1.5 cm per second, with overlap by ~30%. Subjects were examined postoperatively on days 2, 7, 14, and 28, and then at 2, 3, and 6 months. Photographs were taken at baseline and 6 months, and five independent panelists scored the improvement in wrinkles. All panel members scored a positive improvement in Fitzpatrick wrinkle score. Similarly, subjects and investigators noted an improvement in wrinkles. The degree of improvement correlated with the severity of wrinkles at baseline. Higher power settings and greater number of passes appeared to result in increased efficacy. All treatment sites were more than 90% reepithelialized within 7 days. Adverse effects included transient postinflammatory hyperpigmentation (26%) and hypertrophic scarring (4%). Erythema was uniformly present at week 1, and progressively resolved at each visit up to the 6-month follow-up examination. The authors concluded that RF resurfacing may be comparable in efficacy to laser resurfacing. With regard to safety, they indicated that RF resurfacing may provide more rapid healing and less pain and erythema than that seen following CO_2 laser, but comparable with that after short-pulsed Er:YAG laser (Fig. **3–7A,B**).

Another technology (ThermaCool) (Thermage Inc., Hayward, California), delivers RF energy for nonablative tissue tightening while cooling the skin with a cryogen spray. Heating of the dermis can lead to shrinkage of collagen fibrils, and thermal injury inflicted on tissue activates fibroblasts for tissue remodeling. A delayed effect of neocollagenesis is probably due to a wound-healing response. The resultant effect is collagen contraction and tissue tightening followed by new collagen production over time. The cryogen spray allows parallel cooling during the procedure to preserve the surface of the skin and prevent it from burn. However, a potential adverse effect of this system is pain accompanying the procedure as a result of a high depth of penetration. Two studies investigating the efficacy of this system for nonablative skin tightening have recently been published. In a preliminary study, Iyer et al[21] assessed the ThermaCool to treat the lower face and anterior neck of 40 subjects (age 35–70 years). Subjects received one to four treatment sessions at 6- to 8-week intervals. Energy fluence was ~100 J/cm^2. Response to treatment was gradual, with visible effects occurring 4 to 6 weeks after treatment. Subjects who received more than one treatment noticed further improvement after subsequent treatments. The procedure produced softer nasolabial folds, less visible jowls, sharper and tighter jaw line, and less wrinkles on the anterior neck. Treatment was reported to be moderately painful. Three subjects had superficial blisters, but these healed without scarring.

In the other study, Ruiz-Esparza and Gomez evaluated the ThermaCool for wrinkle treatment.[22] Fifteen subjects (age 41–68 years) were enrolled. Five subjects were treated with a 0.25 cm bipolar electrode; eight with a "window frame" electrode; and two with a 1 cm monopolar electrode. A thick layer of ELA*Max* (Ferndale

A 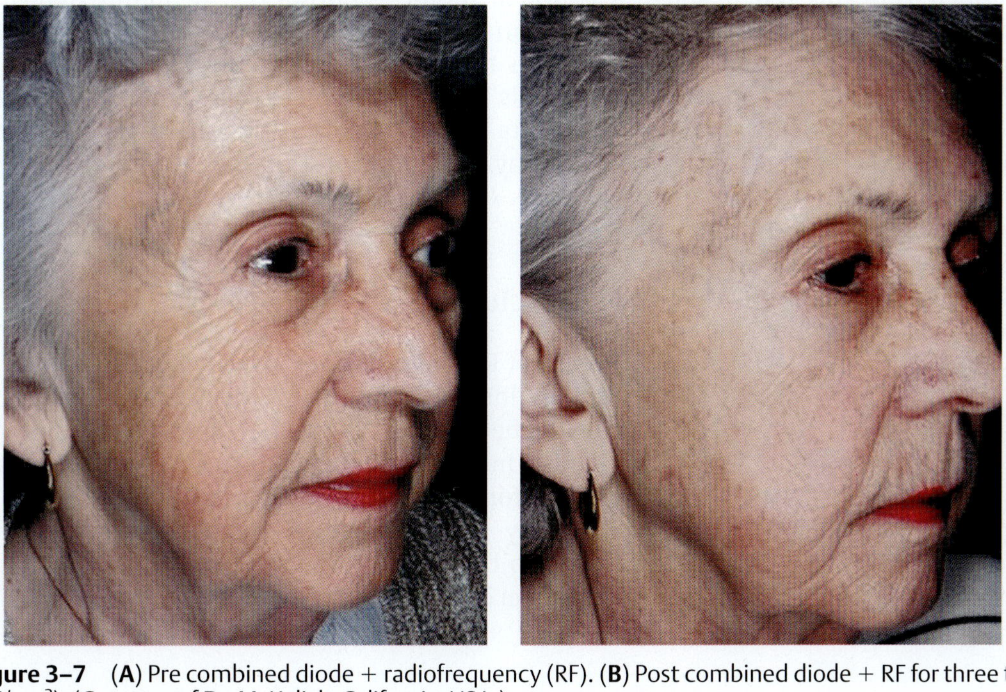 B

Figure 3–7 (**A**) Pre combined diode + radiofrequency (RF). (**B**) Post combined diode + RF for three treatments (RF: 80 J/cm^3/Light: 30J/cm^2). (Courtesy of Dr. M. Kulick, California, USA.)

Laboratories, Inc., Ferndale, Michigan) was used for topical anesthesia. Pain was used as a clinical indicator of the maximum tolerable energy delivered. The energy used was 52 J/cm^2; the average current was 0.447 A. Photographs were taken at baseline and at each week following treatment for up to 14 months. Four independent physicians outside of the study were asked to review and standardize photographs to evaluate results. In this study, 14 of the 15 patients obtained cosmetic improvement from facial skin tightening, with visible results occurring ~12 weeks after the treatment session. Subjects experienced minimal discomfort that required no postoperative care. Treatment was most effective in the preauricular regions and less effective in other areas of the face, such as the nasolabial folds and cheeks. Of note, these authors also studied this system for moderate to severe acne in 22 patients, with excellent response reported in 82%.[23]

A combination of diode laser energy and RF current may also have a role in the treatment of wrinkles. The premise is that RF energy will penetrate into the skin and cause heating of the deeper tissue with neocollagen formation whereas the laser energy will be synergistic with this effect and also address the more superficial problems of unwanted pigmentation and visible vascularity. In the Polaris WR™ system, the optical energy is produced by a diode laser with a wavelength of 900 nm and pulse duration as long as 150 msec that can generate fluence up to 50 J/cm^2; the system can generate RF energy levels as high as 100 J/cm^3 with pulse duration as long as 250 msec. Geometry of electrodes provides a penetration depth of ~2 mm. Two case reports have been described using this system and show promising results.[24] Both were women with significant wrinkling, undesirable vascularity, and hyperpigmentation of the skin. One was 80 years old; the other was 57 years old. Both subjects had significant reductions in the signs of aging. Following each treatment, both subjects had mild swelling for 1 to 2 days. Normal activities were not compromised. These preliminary data are encouraging. Studies are currently under way to optimize treatment parameters to improve results and treatment comfort, as well as examine the effect on all skin types.

◆ Summary

Current light-based therapies are limited by their dependence on chromophore levels in the epidermis or hair shaft for selective thermal destruction of targeted sites. This dependence on chromophore levels creates a window of efficacy and safety for the treatment of various dermatologic indications. In recent years, the use of an alternative source of energy—electrical—has become available through systems that use conducted RF current for selective electrothermolysis. RF current affects the dermis layer directly while reducing the risk of skin burns and other adverse effects associated with optical energy. Good effects have been obtained with the use of RF current for wrinkle reduction (Visage). Tissue contraction has also been achieved using a high energy RF device (ThermaCool), but the major limitation (because of its high depth of penetration) is a lack of improvement in pigmented and vascular lesions. Moderate to severe pain can also accompany the procedure. Studies have also shown significant improvements in the treatment of acne vulgaris.[23]

The latest technology, ELOS, combines RF with optical energies and may expand the efficiency of selective thermal treatment for all skin types. ELOS is based on the premise of a synergistic activity between the two forms of energy that occurs when the various treatment parameters are set optimally, depending on the hair color, skin type, or severity of the lesion. By combining RF and optical energies, lower levels of both energies can be used. This may reduce the risk of side effects associated with either RF or optical treatments alone. There are multiple potential uses, including the effective removal of unwanted hair and treatment of all aspects of aging, from pigmented and vascular lesions to texture improvement and wrinkle reduction. Studies using ELOS-based systems have demonstrated its effectiveness in hair removal (Aurora DS), including light hair and all skin types, and skin rejuvenation (Aurora SR) for skin types I to IV. Preliminary case reports evaluating the Polaris WR show promising results of combined treatments for wrinkle reduction. Further studies are under way to optimize treatment parameters and technique.

◆ Conclusion

The use of RF energy alone (Visage or Thermage) or in combination with optical energy (Aurora, Polaris) is likely to become an increasingly popular therapeutic direction in aesthetic medicine. Additional studies are required for quantitative measurement of the effect of RF energy on skin texture. Histological studies are needed to help understand the mechanism of dermal reaction on conducted RF influence.

References

1. Alster TS, Lupton JR. Lasers in dermatology: an overview of types and indications. Am J Clin Dermatol 2001;2:291–303
2. Anderson RR, Parish JA. Selective photothermolysis: precise microsurgery by selective absorption of pulsed radiation. Science 1983;220:524–527
3. Lask G, Elman M, Slatkine M, Waldman A, Rozenberg Z. Laser-assisted hair removal by selective photothermolysis: preliminary results. Dermatol Surg 1997;23:737–739
4. Ruiz-Esparza J. Medical applications of resurfacing lasers. Adv Dermatol 2000;16:453–474
5. Trohman RG, Parrillo JE. Direct current cardioversion: indications, techniques, and recent advances. Crit Care Med 2000;28:N170–N173
6. Carruthers A. Radiofrequency resurfacing: technique and clinical review. Facial Plast Surg Clin North Am 2001;9:311–319
7. Tasto JP, Ash SA. Current uses of radiofrequency in arthroscopic knee surgery. Am J Knee Surg 1999;12:186–191
8. Gabriel S, Lau RW, Gabriel C. The dielectric properties of biological tissues, III: Parametric models for the dielectric spectrum of tissues. Phys Med Biol 1996;41:2271–2293
9. Duck FA. Physical Properties of Tissue. New York: Academic; 1990:173
10. Ort RJ, Dierickx C. Laser hair removal. Semin Cutan Med Surg 2002;21:129–144
11. Nanni CA, Alster TS. Laser-assisted hair removal: side effects of Q-switched Nd:YAG, long-pulsed ruby, and alexandrite lasers. J Am Acad Dermatol 1999;41:165–171
12. Hair removal using a combination of electrical and optical energies: 3-month clinical study. Data on file. Yokneam, Israel: Syneron Medical Ltd.
13. Sadick NS. Hair removal using a combination of conducted RF and optical energies: an 18-month follow-up. J Cosmet Laser Ther 2004;6:21–26
14. Sadick NS, Laughlin SA. Effective epilation of white and blond hair using combined radiofrequency and optical energy. J Cosmet Laser Ther 2004;6:27–31

15a. Orf RJ, Dierickx C. Laser hair removal. Semin Cutan Med Surg 2002;21:129–144

15b. Schroeter CA, Groenewegen JS, Reineke T, Neumann HAM. Hair reduction using intense pulsed light source. Derm Surg 2004;30:168–173

16. Bjerring P, Clement M, Heickendorff L, Egevist H, Kiernan M. Selective nonablative wrinkle reduction by laser. J Cutan Laser Ther 2000;2:9–15
17. Goldberg D. Nonablative surface remodeling: clinical and histological evaluation of a 1320 nm Nd:YAG laser. J Cut Laser Ther 1999;1:153–157
18. Levy JL, Besson R, Mordon S. Determination of optimal parameters for laser for nonablative remodeling with a 1.54 μm Er:Glass laser: a dose response study. Dermatol Surg 2002;28:405–409
19. Bitter P Jr, Mulholland S. Report of a new technique for enhanced noninvasive skin rejuvenation using a dual mode pulsed light and radiofrequency energy source: selective radiothermolysis. J Cosmet Dermatol 2002;1:142–143
20. Grekin RC, Tope WD, Yarborough JM Jr, et al. Electrosurgical facial resurfacing. Arch Dermatol 2000;136:1309–1316
21. Iyer S, Suthamjariya K, Fitzpatrick RE. Using a radiofrequency energy device to treat the lower face: a treatment paradigm for a nonsurgical facelift. Cosmet Dermatol 2003;16: 37–40
22. Ruiz-Esparza J, Gomez JB. The medical face-lift: a noninvasive, nonsurgical approach to tissue tightening in facial skin using nonablative radiofrequency. Dermatol Surg 2003;29:325–332
23. Ruiz-Esparza J, Gomez JB. Nonablative radiofrequency for active acne vulgaris: the use of deep dermal heat in the treatment of moderate to severe active acne vulgaris (thermotherapy): a report of 22 patients. Dermatol Surg 2003;29:333–339
24. New approach to nonablative wrinkle treatment: combination of conducted RF and laser: case report. Data on file. Yokneam, Israel: Syneron Medical Ltd.

4

Chemical Peels: Superficial and Medium Depth

Marian Cantisano-Zilkha and Stephen Bosniak

Chemical peeling began in ancient Egypt over 5000 years ago. Only fruit acids and lactic acids were then available. By the end of the nineteenth century, physicians started using other peeling agents, such as salicylic acid, resorcinol, phenol, and trichloroacetic acid. Phenol was first used to remove acne scars. The advent of alpha hydroxy acids (AHAs) and trichloroacetic acid has made chemical peeling a safer and more popular procedure.[1]

Laser technology has evolved rapidly, giving cosmetic physicians and their staff a new spectrum of treatments for skin rejuvenation. But chemical peels, still an effective therapeutic option for reversing photoaging, should not be forgotten. Their simplicity—ease of performance and low cost—make them an essential element in every skin care regimen. Physicians working with their aestheticians can offer their patients a variety of alternatives to achieve the best results, while recognizing the possibilities and limitations.

Superficial peels are recommended to treat a variety of superficial conditions involving the epidermis and superficial dermis: mild actinic damage, superficial wrinkling and dyschromia, actinic keratoses, and active acne. Series of peels are recommended, over specified periods of time. They require minimal or no recovery time and are rarely associated with adverse reactions or complications. And they can be used on patients of any skin type, particularly if notable inflammatory responses are avoided. Patients with tendencies for facial telangiectasias may find that these superficial peels and microdermabrasion may exacerbate their broken capillaries and are best avoided.[2]

Although effective in any age group, patients in their midthirties with early dyspigmentation, fine wrinkles, and mild actinic keratoses will find these peels a satisfying introduction to noninvasive facial therapies. With these peels we can achieve an improved appearance of the skin with more uniform color and texture and less visible pores. The effects are cumulative with time—augmented with the use of homecare products—and require maintenance. Superficial peels work well in combination with the other selections on the noninvasive facial rejuvenation menu—injectable therapies, intense pulsed light (IPL), and nonablative lasers. With the exception of acne rosacea patients, most patients can benefit from this procedure.

We use medium-depth peels primarily to treat moderate to severe dyschromia and moderate rhytidosis. It is an excellent therapeutic option for treating moderately photoaged skin, where the epidermis is atrophic and the stratum corneum thickened, and there are histologic findings of epidermal dysplasia, collagen, and elastin degeneration, translated as moderate facial rhytids. Severe photoaging is more predictably managed with carbon dioxide (CO_2) laser resurfacing.

◆ Patient Selection

The following criteria must be considered when making the patient/peeling agent selection:

1. Fitzpatrick classification
2. Age of the patient (younger patients respond better)
3. Lifestyle (sun exposure, alcohol, drugs, smoking)

4. Current skin care regimen
5. Previous skin treatments (including other chemical peels, use of various lasers or other technology aimed at rejuvenation)
6. Previous facial cosmetic surgeries
7. Current medication
8. Vitamin supplementation
9. Previous history of herpes simplex (pre-treat with acyclovir or other antiviral agents)
10. Realistic expectations and healing time

Once these variables are fully understood by the physician and patient, the physician will make the best recommendation, according to the specific needs and desires of the patient. The patients who require minimum recovery after the peel will receive superficial peels at regular intervals. The results will arise gradually, be limited to the surface of the skin, and, when combined with a good home care regimen, will provide a noticeable improvement (Figs. **4–1A,B; 4–2A,B**). Patients that have severe epidermal damage extended to the superficial layer of the dermis and with coarse facial wrinkling are good candidates for medium-depth peels (Fig. **4–3A,B**). The results will be dramatic, but with significant postpeel downtime, requiring at least 4 to 5 days of recovery. Postpeel home care speeds up recovery and emphasizes the importance of maintenance to maximize the results.

In summary, understanding the final histologic response to superficial and medium depth peels, the histological changes that occur during healing, and how much discomfort and downtime the patient is willing to endure, will allow the physician to appropriately select a peeling agent. The use of a prepeel regimen (lotions with low concentration of AHAs, retinoids, bleaching agents, topical antioxidants, and sunscreen) is highly recommended for at least 2 weeks prior to the peel. It prepares the skin for the treatment and also allows the physician to gauge if that patient can follow instructions and what kind of commitment can be expected from the patient to prolong and maximize the effects of the peel.[3]

◆ Superficial Peels

AHAs are the agents most frequently used in superficial peels. Often called fruit acids, AHAs are a group of naturally occurring substances found in food and in particular in fruits (glycolic acid in sugarcane, malic acid in apples, citric acid in citrus fruit). They are recommended for a variety of skin conditions but particularly those characterized by hyperkeratinization (the fine wrinkling associated with photodamage and acne).

Glycolic acid is the most used AHA, and even though its mechanism of action is not totally understood, it has an effect in disrupting keratocyte cohesion and therefore correcting an abnormally thickened stratum corneum. By creating a thinning of the stratum corneum, AHA improves the general texture and uniformity of the skin, facilitating the penetration of other

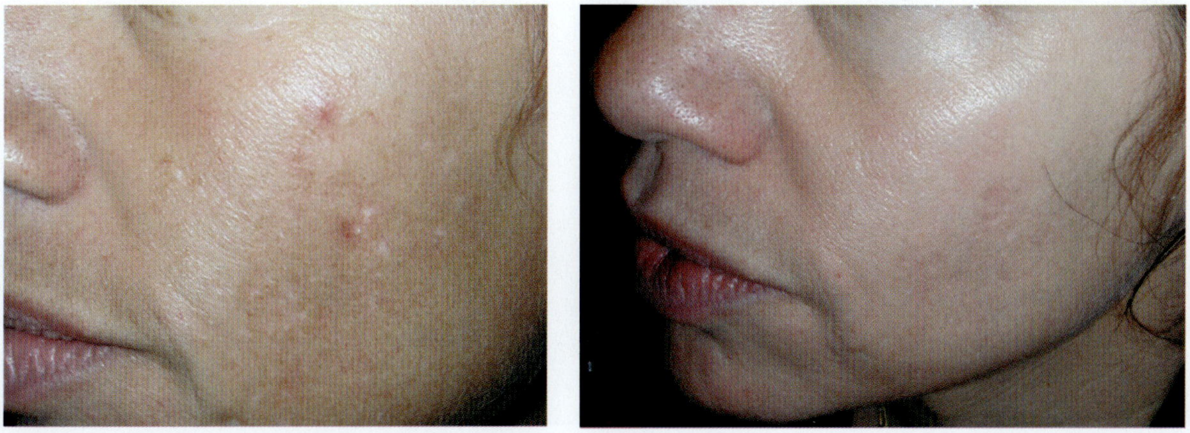

A B

Figure 4–1 (**A**) This patient exhibited superficial facial contour irregularities and irregular pigmentation. (**B**) After multiple series of alpha hydroxy acid (AHA) peels of increasing strength and daily use of home care products (containing AHA, retinoids, hydroquinone, vitamin C) there is a marked improvement in this patient's skin texture and pigmentation.

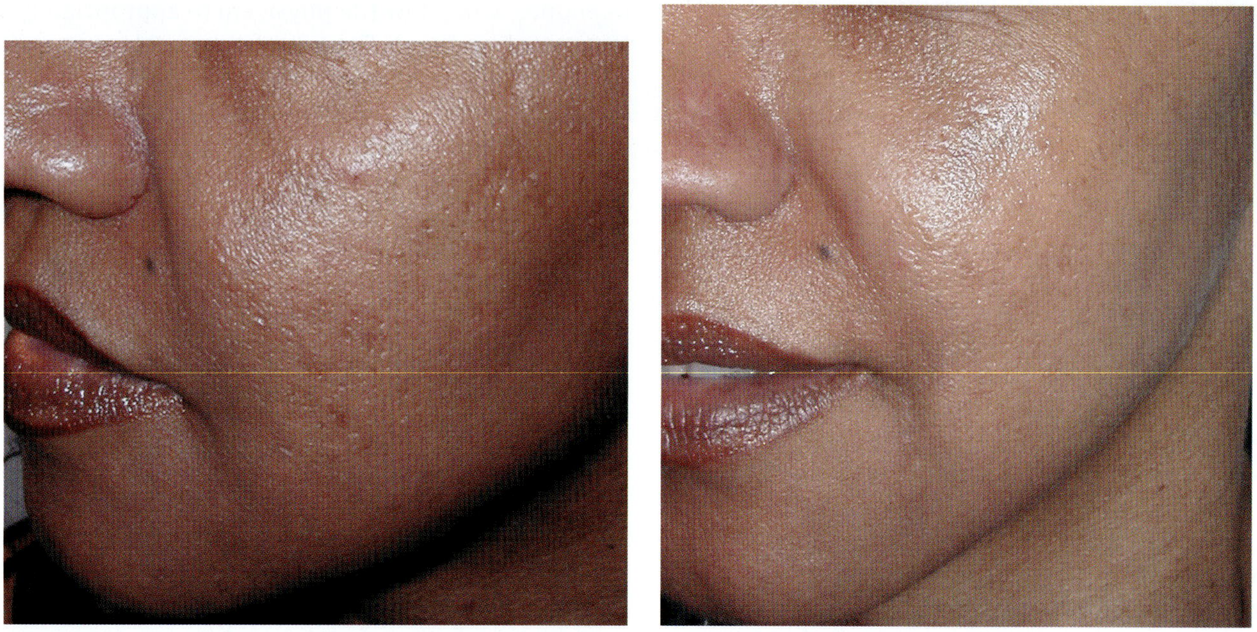

A B

Figure 4–2 Alpha hydroxy acid peels and homecare products can yield significant benefits in patients of all skin types. (**A**) This patient with skin type IV had superficial contour irregularities and irregular pigmentation. (**B**) She noted a significant improvement in her skin texture and pigmentation after treatment.

topical agents (such as Retin-A). Also, by increasing the hydration of the stratum corneum and stimulating synthesis of cellular ground substances (glycosoaminoglycans), AHAs reduce fine wrinkling.

As a peeling agent, AHAs can be found as a solution or as a gel, and are used in concentrations of 15 to 30% (by aestheticians) and 50 to 70% (by physicians). They are systemically safe, nontoxic acids, produce few complications, and offer instant gratification. They have to be neutralized to terminate their action, either by rinsing them off with water or by applying other neutralizing solutions.

Factors affecting the depth of penetration of a glycolic peel are the concentration, method of application, skin pretreatment, and duration of the acid in contact with the skin.

Other superficial peeling agents include trichloroacetic acid (TCA) in concentrations 10 to 20%; salicylic acid 50%; and Jessner's solution [resorcinol 14 g, salicylic acid 14 g, lactic acid 14 g, ethanol (95%) in 100 mL].

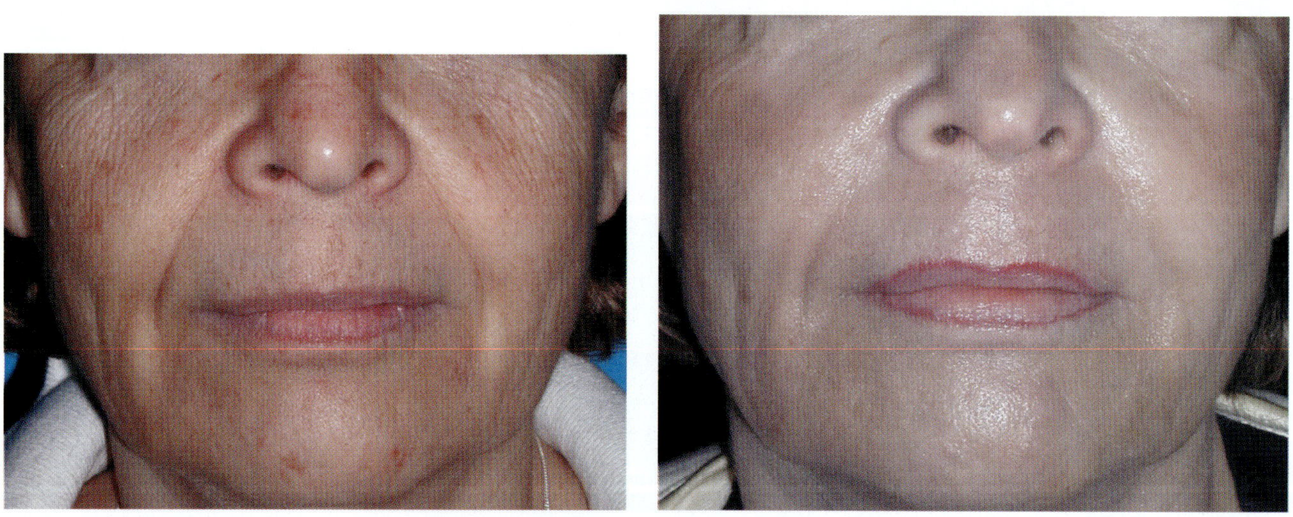

A B

Figure 4–3 (**A**) Although contemplating a rhytidectomy for facial skin redundancy, laxity, and rhytidosis, she pursued a noninvasive approach. (**B**) A medium-depth trichloroacetic acid (TCA) peel can improve rhytidosis and dyspigmentation more effectively than a superficial alpha hydroxy acid peel. This patient enjoyed the benefits of Thermage, Restylane, and Botox before receiving the TCA peel—the final element of her noninvasive facial rejuvenation.

Steps of Application

Skin Preparation

The use of AHA lotions and topical retinoids in a home care regimen begun at least 2 weeks prior to the peel will enhance the efficacy.

Room and Material

The room should have a sink with running water and a tray with the following items: brush, swab, gauze, timer, small cup, headband, and hand fan. The patient is asked to remove contact lenses and face makeup prior to the treatment.

Cleansing

For adequate penetration of the peeling agent, cleansing and degreasing the skin are essential steps. We use headbands to keep the hair away from the face. Remove all the makeup with makeup remover, use a toner to remove remaining debris from the skin and degrease the skin thoroughly with a folded 4×4 gauze pad moistened with alcohol or acetone. The fumes may be irritating and care must be taken not to drip the solutions in the eyes when degreasing the forehead. When cleaning the eyelids use cotton-tipped applicators.

Selection of Peel Strength

We begin our series of AHA peels using a 70% buffered gel. As soon as the patient becomes erythematous, we neutralize the peel. With each successive peel we increase the time until a maximum of 10 minutes is reached. Then the strength is gradually increased. Fifty percent unbuffered AHA is added to the 70% buffered in solution. At each new level of concentration, the time of application is also gradually increased at each session until 10 minutes is reached.

Application

The solutions can be applied to the face with a cotton-tipped applicator, brush, or gauze square. To reduce the possibility of dripping into the eyes, we prefer AHA gel as a peeling agent, and keep the head of the patient elevated. The applications begin on the forehead and then continue inferiorly, with quick and even strokes. The entire face should be covered in ~15 seconds. After the peel is applied and the timing begun, a small hand fan can be used to minimize the mild burning or tingling sensations. After 10 minutes, the endpoint should be a mild erythema. In areas with thinner stratum corneum (the eyelids) or deep folds where the gel can pool (nasolabial folds or oral commissures) the AHA may have to be neutralized before the rest of the face. Close observation of these patients during the peel, avoiding excessive erythema and contolling epidermolysis, is critical to limiting complications.[4]

Neutralization

The patient may rinse the face thoroughly with water to neutralize the AHA. Care should be taken to close the eyes tightly. Because the AHA is neutralized by water, if it gets in the patient's eyes it is unlikely that it will cause any serious injury; however, it will burn and may cause a mild conjunctivitis or keratitis.

Postpeel Care

Following AHA peels the patient typically feels slightly tight and very "clean," and on occasion may feel mild irritation when stronger concentrations of AHA are used. We recommend a bland moisturizer to be used three times daily for 2 days and then the patient should resume the home care routine. If there is any irritation, a mild topical steroid cream such as hyrocortisone 1% is recommended, and only after the inflammation is gone should AHAs and retinoids be resumed with the full daily regimen. If erythema persists, follow-up by the physician is indicated.

Complications and Management of Complications

Complications following AHA peels are rare and are related to the depth of the peel. They are listed on the AHA consent form (see Fig. **4–4**). They also include the following:

1. Herpes simplex. Patients with a previous history of herpes simplex should be pretreated prophylactically with acyclovir.
2. Erythema. High-strength peels may leave the patient erythematous. If this persists for more than 1 to 2 days, topical steroid cream is recommended, particularly in darker-skinned patients.
3. Pigmentary disturbances. In darker-skinned patients inflammation is avoided by using lower strengths of AHA. An inflammatory response following a peel in a darker-skinned patient most likely will cause at least a transient hyperpigmentation. Severe inflammatory responses potentially could cause either hypopigmentation or hyperpigmentation.
4. Crusting. In areas of epidermolysis, crusting is treated with topical antibiotics and zinc oxide (which is soothing and also a total sun block).
5. Infections. Although rare, infections may result from epidermolysis and poor wound care.
6. Scarring. Exceptionally rare, scarring is probably the result of epidermolysis, poor wound care, and infection.

Consent Form for Alpha Hydroxy Acid Peels

I understand that I am going to have a light glycolic acid (alpha hydroxy acid) peel. I understand that this is a superficial type of peel that normally creates, at most, only one or two days of mild redness with occasional areas of flaking skin.

I understand that if I have a history of cold sores, this peel can cause another breakout and I will need to take medication.

I understand that on rare occasions this peel can penetrate deeper in certain areas, causing a crusted scab to form. I understand that if this area is not treated appropriately it could become infected and possibly lead to the formation of a scar or change in skin pigmentation. It is my responsibility to contact the doctor's office if any crusted area forms or if my skin does not look and feel completely normal within three to four days after my peel.

I am undergoing this peel in an effort to improve my skin texture and color. I understand I may achieve some improvement in my fine wrinkles as well, but no guarantee has been made to me regarding my level of improvement from this peel. The doctor has explained to me that I may need several of these peels to achieve my best results.

______________________	______________
Patient Signature	Date
______________________	______________
Witness Signature	Date

Figure 4–4 Consent Form for Alpha Hydroxy Acid Peels.

If the peel is done in a very superficial fashion (minimal erythema), it can be repeated on a weekly basis. A series of five to six peels should be recommended until no further improvement is accomplished. Patients that show little or no improvement after the first peels, should be reevaluated and a different modality or a more aggressive peel should be offered.

◆ Medium-Depth Peels

TCA is the agent of choice to create a medium-depth peel. It can penetrate the basal layer of the epidermis, reach the papillary dermis, and even extend to the upper reticular dermis. The concentration will determine the depth of the peel. Concentrations of 10 to 20% function as superficial peels, primarily exfoliants, and affect the outside layer of the epidermis only. They could be recommended to treat mild actinic changes of the skin or for patients who do not desire to endure a longer recovery healing time. The chest and neck are areas that we recommend to be treated with these low concentrations of TCA.

TCA in concentrations from 30 up to 40%, are considered medium-depth peels and will affect the papillary dermis. Even though the concentration of the acid is the most important factor to determine the depth of the peel, other factors such as the patient's skin type, skin preparation, how it was applied, number of layers, how wet the applicator was, and pressure of the application all influence the final result.

Preparation

Patients with a history of herpes simplex should be pretreated with acyclovir 400 mg q.i.d. beginning 1 day preoperatively and continuing for 1 week following the peel. The skin should be primed with AHAs, retinoids, and bleaching agents, preferably 2 weeks prior to the peel, to expedite reepithelialization and reduce the risk of secondary postinflammatory dyspigmentation.

Steps of Application

Cleansing

When the skin has been adequately pretreated, the stratum corneum is thinner and TCA penetration is enhanced. A thorough cleansing, eliminating remaining debris with a toner, and then degreasing the skin with alcohol or acetone all facilitate the effectiveness of the procedure. Jessner's solution can be used before the application of TCA to enhance the depth of penetration of the TCA.

Application

The patient does not need to be sedated, but analgesics are highly recommended 30 minutes prior to the peel. Comfortable clothes are recommended, and a headband will keep the hair away from the face. We often use

Vaseline or other petrolatum-based emollients at the limits of the area to be peeled to avoid unwanted dripping of the solution down the neck, into the hairline, or into the ears. The head should be elevated to a 45 degree angle, and the peel is applied in a pattern with a 4 × 4 folded gauze pad or 2 small cotton-tipped applicators held together, beginning on the forehead, from the midline to the side, then to the other side, continuing down the nose, under the eyelid (2 or 3 mm below the lower lid margin), down the cheek, the other eyelid and cheek, and the perioral area. After several minutes a frosting will become apparent and the evenness of the application can be assessed. The decision can then be made as to where to apply additional TCA and if another full pass is warranted.

Technical Points to be Observed

1. The skin should be pulled tight in areas of deep wrinkling to allow the acid to get deep into the wrinkle.
2. Care is taken not to overlap applications because this can lead to unintended localized increased peel depth.
3. Extend the peel into the hairline and 1 cm below the jawline to avoid a visible demarcation line.
4. TCA peels are also technique dependent, and different variables will affect the outcome. Therefore, the same pressure should be used throughout the entire application, and changed in areas where a deeper penetration is desired. The skin preparation with retinoids, or the pretreatment with keratolytic agents such as Jessner's solution, will also increase the depth of the peel.

Determining the Depth of the Peel and Evaluating for Additional Coats

Level of Frosting

Frosting is due to the coagulation of proteins on the skin, and the intensity of the frosting will determine the level of the peel (Fig. **4–5A,B**).

No frosting or minimum frosting signifies a very superficial peel, limited to the stratum corneum.

Minimum frosting results in a mild erythema and scattered areas of frosting; the peel is limited to the superficial epidermis.

Mild frosting with erythema showing through signifies a full epidermal peel.

Total frosting is apparent when a peel penetrates from the epidermis to the papillary dermis. The skin assuming a grayish appearance is a dangerous sign that perhaps it has penetrated too deeply into the reticular dermis and could lead to scarring. The time between the application of the peel and the frosting is ~40 to 90 seconds. The physician should wait until the frosting is completely evident before evaluating the need for another coat. The second coat can be weaker in concentration than the first coat, if desired.

Time to Change from Frosting to Erythema

How fast the skin changes from frosting to erythema denotes the depth of the peel. When the peel is superficial (to the basal layer of the epidermis) the frosting fades to erythema in ~15 minutes. When the peel is medium in depth (to the papillary dermis) this skin change occurs in

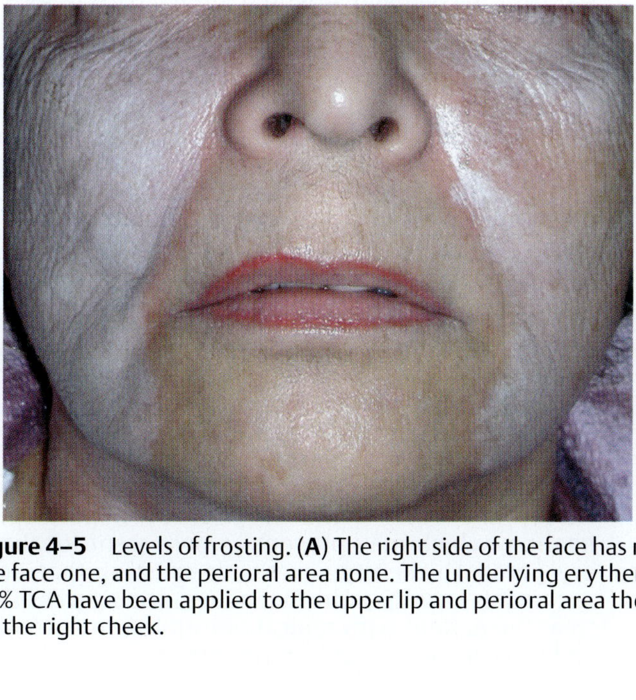
A

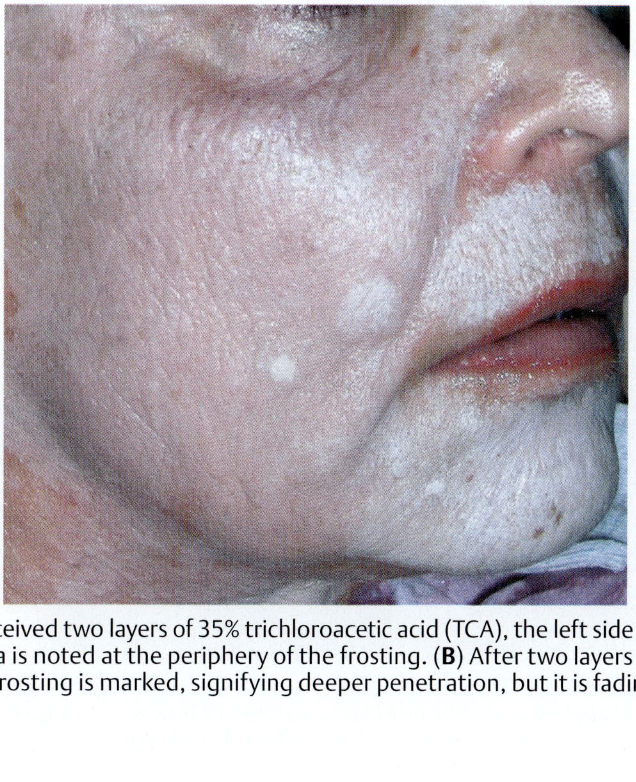
B

Figure 4–5 Levels of frosting. (**A**) The right side of the face has received two layers of 35% trichloroacetic acid (TCA), the left side of the face one, and the perioral area none. The underlying erythema is noted at the periphery of the frosting. (**B**) After two layers of 35% TCA have been applied to the upper lip and perioral area the frosting is marked, signifying deeper penetration, but it is fading on the right cheek.

~30 minutes. When the depth of the peel is deeper (to the reticular dermis) the frosting disappears in ~60 minutes.

Most patients do not need sedation for these peels, and some physicians like to apply cold compresses as soon as they reach the ideal level of penetration of the peel to ameliorate the symptoms of burning and pain. We find that the application of a full-face Natragel mask (Gel Concept, Whippany, New Jersey) following the application of TCA ameliorates the discomfort rapidly and profoundly. In an unpublished study we found that in 10 patients having full-face TCA peels, patients rated the discomfort level between 8 and 10 (on a scale of 10) and that after the application of the gel mask they rated the discomfort level between 2 and 4. Water does not neutralize TCA because it is an aqueous-based solution; but water can be used to dilute any excess TCA that remains on the skin, preventing further deepening of the peel.

◆ Postpeel Care

The healing time will depend on the depth of the peel. Superficial peels heal very fast (in 1 or 2 days) and only gentle cleanser and a moisturizer are required. Patients can resume their skin care routine with Retin-A, AHAs, and sunblocks in about 7 to 10 days.

Medium-depth peels require a longer time for healing. Initially the skin will acquire a leathery appearance and it will turn from light to dark brown within ~72 hours (Fig. **4–6**). The dark crusting will begin to flake off first in the areas with more muscular activity (around eyes and mouth and ultimately on the forehead). Within 4 to 5 days of the peel, most of the crusting is gone, revealing a smooth, radiant, and slightly erythematous skin (see Fig. **4–3B**). But the skin may remain sensitive for another week. Patients should wash their face with gentle cleansers and frequently apply bland emollients to the skin (Vaseline, Aquaphor, or CU3 copper peptide cream) to keep the skin from feeling dry and tight.[4] If the patient is disturbed by itching, 1% hydrocortisone can also be applied.

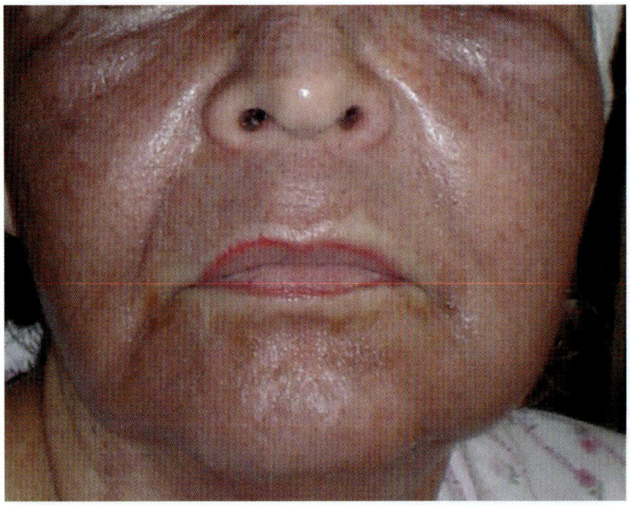

Figure 4–6 Three days following a 35% trichloroacetic acid peel applied with multiple layers, patches of brown crusting remain, and intense erythema and moderate edema persist.

Important Precautions

During the first few days following the peel, patients are advised to sleep on their back to avoid inadvertent maceration of their face. During the early recovery phase, sun avoidance is critical. A large-brimmed hat, sunglasses, sunblock, zinc oxide, and makeup will discourage secondary postinflammatory hyperpigmentation.

Patients are admonished not to pick off the brown crusts because this may leave an area that remains persistently erythematous and become secondarily hyperpigmented.

Complications

These are listed on the TCA peel consent form (see Fig. **4–7**).

1. Hyperpigmentation. Sun exposure or medication (birth control pills and anticonvulsive medications) can cause hyperpigmentation. The importance of sunblock at all times and the use of hats and sunglasses must be stressed. Treatment with Retin-A combined with hydroquinone or kojic acid, in general is useful as a pretreatment before the peel and is helpful in treating postpeel dyspigmentation.
2. Hypopigmentation. The occurrence of hypopigmentation is proportional to the depth of the peel. It is due to an inability of the melanocytes to recover after they have been affected or destroyed by the chemical agent. Lower-strength peels thus have less potential for causing hypopigmentation and are recommended when treating more pigmented patients. To prevent a demarcation line between face and neck, the peel should be feathered using a lower concentration on the adjoining areas. AHAs, retinoids, and bleaching agents can also be used on the more pigmented areas to reduce demarcation.
3. Herpes simplex. All patients with a history of herpes simplex are treated prophylactically with acyclovir.
4. Scarring. Although scarring is a rare occurrence, it may be secondary to excessive depth of the peel, infection, and trauma. Patients who have used Accutane within 1 year are not candidates for TCA peeling or laser resurfacing due to the friability of the skin and poor healing properties. Patients who undergo TCA peels should be carefully monitored, and if we detect any early signs of poor or hypertrophic healing, which may present as persistent localized erythema, thickening, excessive crusting that does not resolve with mild cleansing, we aggressively treat the patient with topical or intralesional steroids and topical and systemic antibiotics.[3]

Consent Form for Trichloroacetic Acid Facial Peel

A skin peel is not a "cure all" treatment, but for appropriate conditions, it can give you marked improvement. It is important that you have a thorough understanding of what the peel can and can't do for your particular condition.

I, ________________________, give my consent for Dr. ________________ to perform a skin peel on my face or other area of my body __________ to treat the following conditions:

I understand that this is a program of treatments and that I may need several peels to achieve my best results.

___ I understand that the degree of improvement I can expect to see depends on many variables and therefore cannot be guaranteed. Additionally, I understand that strict adherence to the doctor's instructions is necessary to ensure my best results.

___ I understand that Dr. ________________ has the right to discontinue my treatment at any stage if he or she thinks that I am not following instructions, or if he or she believes that no further improvement is possible.

___ I understand that the skin peel is an outpatient procedure done in the office, that consists of the application of medications to the skin. I understand that I can expect to have one to two minutes of stinging or burning sensations immediately after the medication has been applied, but this will then stop.

___ I understand that during healing from my peel, my skin will look darker and shiny and that I may be unable to work. My particular peel and its relationship to my ability to work have been discussed with me by Dr. ________________.

___ I consent to have my photographs taken before, during, and after my treatment. These may be used for educating future patients and in possible publications and promotions. My name will not be used.

___ Although complications are rare, they do occur. Prompt recognition and treatment of any complication is necessary to decrease its potential danger. It is extremely important that I follow doctor's instructions exactly and that I notify the office if I have any the following complications:

⇒ ☐ Skin infections—usually appearing as a red tender area, often with a scab
⇒ ☐ Cold sore on my lips or face
⇒ ☐ Allergic reaction to any medications I am using in conjunction with the peel
⇒ ☐ Appearance of thick scars or keloids in the areas of my peel
⇒ ☐ Prolonged sensitivity to the wind or sun
⇒ ☐ Persistent areas of increased or decreased pigmentation

________________________________ __________
Patient signature Date

________________________________ __________
Witness signature Date

Figure 4–7 Consent Form for Trichloroacetic Acid Facial Peel.

◆ Conclusion

AHA and TCA peels fit well into our menu of noninvasive therapies. They can minimize demarcation lines when patients have had segmental facial laser resurfacing. They enhance our regimen of home care products. TCA peels are most effective in diminishing dyspigmentation and improving skin texture and rhytidosis. AHA peels are an essential component in our skin maintenance program.

References

1. Matarasso, A. Non Operative Techniques for Facial Rejuvenation, Part I. Clin Plast Surg 2000;27:501–502
2. Pugliese, P. Physiology of the Skin II. Carol Stream, IL: Allured Publishing; 2001:300, 302
3. Thomas J, James M, Baker TM. Facial Skin Resurfacing. Boston: Quality Medical Publishing; 1998:chapts 4,5
4. Rubin, MG. Manual of Chemical Peels: Superficial and Medium Depth. Philadelphia: JB Lippincott; 1995:chapts 4,7, 8

5

Neuromodulation and Management of Facial Rhytidosis

Stephen Bosniak

The concept of relaxing facial muscles and diminishing their secondary wrinkle-producing effects has become a basic technique in facial rejuvenation. It is a foundation on which other noninvasive and surgical procedures can be built (see also Chapters 1, 4, 6, 9, 14, 15, and 16). In selected cases it can be used alone. In others it is an element in the menu of combined therapies. These techniques continue to evolve as new technologies are introduced and our experience with neuromodulating injectables increases.[1–9]

We instruct our patients and the physicians that we train that the endpoint of treatment is not complete immobilization of the treated muscle. Nor is it a completely flat, immovable surface. Our therapeutic goal is a natural, relaxed look: to soften and diminish lines and furrows. And it is in this regard that we choose to use the term *neuromodulation* and not *chemodenervation*. It is about aesthetically choosing a therapeutic endpoint.[10]

◆ Mechanisms of Action

Botulinum toxin type A binds to the nerve endplate and blocks the release of acetylcholine. This bond is permanent and acetylcholine release begins again when the nerve sprouts a new endplate.[11,12] The clinical effects after Botox injections begin in 3 to 5 days; the final effects are evident in 7 to 10 days and persist for 90 to 120 days. Our experience has been primarily with Botulinum toxin type A (Botox and Botox Cosmetic), but we have also used botulinum toxin type B (Myobloc) on occasion and have communicated with European physicians using Dysport. Myobloc has a more rapid onset of action than Botox (approximately 3–4 days), but also a shorter duration of action (~42 days). Fifty to 100 units of Myobloc are equivalent to 1 unit of Botox.[13,14] Dysport is also a type A botulinum toxin but has a more marked spreading effect and has a more complete ablation of dynamic rhytids. Patients have described its effect as "heavier" than Botox.[15,16] Three to five units of Dysport are equivalent to 1 unit of Botox.[17]

◆ Relevant Facial Anatomy

A thorough and intimate knowledge of facial anatomy is a prerequisite for understanding how to effectively employ neuromodulation as an adjunctive treatment in facial rejuvenation. Understanding the balance of facial musculature will allow the creative, effective, and safe use of this technique.[18]

The Forehead and Eyebrow

The broad, thin frontalis muscle elevates the forehead and eyebrows (Fig. **5–1**). This muscle and the transverse forehead wrinkles that it can produce should be treated with great care and only in the appropriate patients. Patients who have blepharoptosis or redundant upper eyelid folds that impair the visual axis or constrict their peripheral visual fields will unconsciously elevate their eyebrows, attempting to expand their peripheral vision. These patients will notice transverse forehead furrows and often will want them treated. Treating their forehead furrows with neuromodulating agents can reduce their ability to raise their eyebrows and expand their visual fields and can also unmask or accentuate their

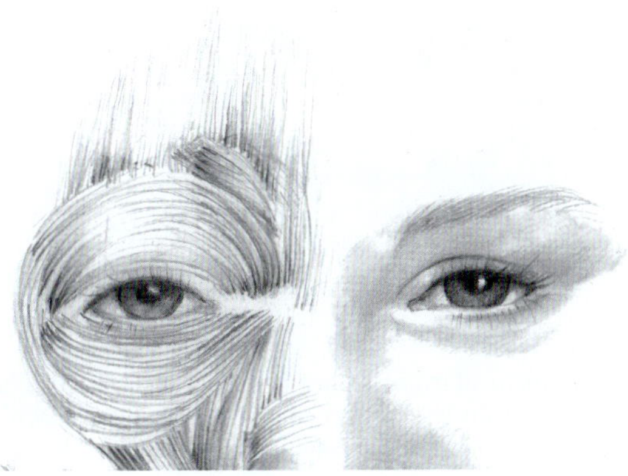

Figure 5–1 The broad, thin frontalis muscle elevates the forehead and eyebrow, and the orbicularis muscle depresses the eyebrow.

blepharoptosis or eyelid heaviness. Our current concept is to modify the level and contour of the eyebrow by treating the brow depressors first and then treating any residual forehead rhytidosis during a subsequent treatment.

The corrugator, procerus, and orbicularis muscles are brow depressors. Treating them with neuromodulation can elevate the eyebrows, diminish upper lid heaviness, and reduce forehead furrows. Corrugator and procerus relaxation will elevate the medial and central brow. Relaxing the superior, lateral orbicularis muscle will elevate the lateral brow.[19] These brow-elevating effects are best performed without treating the forehead itself. In this manner the frontalis can work to elevate the brow against the diminished activity of the brow depressors. Any residual forehead rhytidosis can be treated secondarily.

The Glabella

The powerful, paired corrugator muscles produce two deep vertical folds—the hallmark of intense frowning. At an early stage, neuromodulation can effectively relax these muscles and ablate these furrows. But when these muscles have been active for a long time and when the overlying skin has lost some of its turgor and elasticity, these furrows remain, even at rest. In these cases, combined filling and neuromodulation are necessary for a complete effect. The single, flat procerus muscle, when contracted, creates horizontal furrows on the bridge of the nose (Fig. **5–2**). It can conveniently be treated with the corrugator muscles.

The Eyebrow and the Upper Eyelid

The position of the eyebrow will determine the degree of redundancy of the upper lid fold. An elevated eyebrow will lessen upper lid fold redundancy and a ptotic

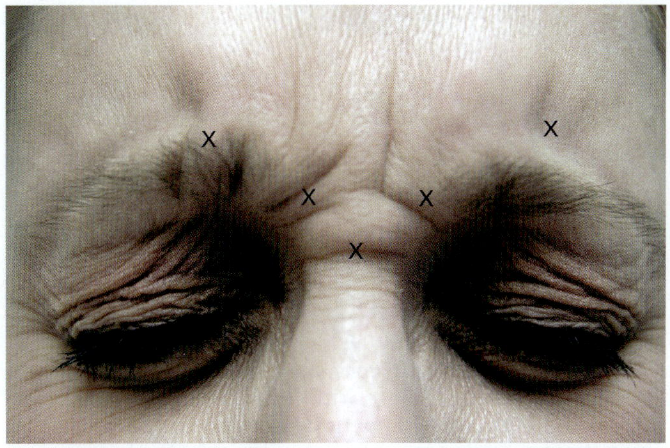

Figure 5–2 A hypertrophic, hyperactive corrugator muscle demonstrates prominent vertical furrowing and a broad insertion across the midline of the brow. A hypertrophic, hyperactive procerus muscle demonstrates marked horizontal furrowing of the glabella. Glabella injection sites (5.0 units per site) are noted.

eyebrow will accentuate it. A ptotic eyebrow can even obscure the superior sulcus. In mild cases neuromodulation can postpone surgical correction of the upper lids and brows, demonstrate possible surgical outcomes, and diminish asymmetric surgical results. Treating the superior lateral portion of the orbicularis can effectively reduce crow's feet and elevate the brow without risk of blepharoptosis. The eyebrow can be shaped with creative and intelligent neuromodulation. Treating the central portion of the superior orbicularis muscle will result in ptosis. This is often used effectively for temporary amelioration of corneal exposure and upper eyelid retraction.

The Lateral Canthus and Lower Eyelid

The inferior lateral portion of the orbicularis muscle can be treated lateral to the orbital rim to diminish crow's feet without risk of displacement of the lower lid margin or change in the shape and dimensions of the palpebral aperture. Lower eyelid wrinkles and hypertrophic pretarsal orbicularis muscles (Fig. **5–3**) can also be treated with neuromodulation provided that there is no lateral canthal or lower lid margin laxity. The lower lid pretarsal orbicularis can also be treated in younger patients wishing to widen their palpebral aperture. Completely eliminating a pretarsal orbicularis roll is not always indicated because it is considered to be a sign of youth. If there is preexisting laxity or lower lid retraction and the lower lid pretarsal orbicularis muscle is treated, lower lid retraction and inferior scleral show will be accentuated as will lower lid rhytidosis. This can be accompanied by premalar lymphedema. Aside from unmasking incipient lower lid laxity, neuromodulation of the lower lids may also

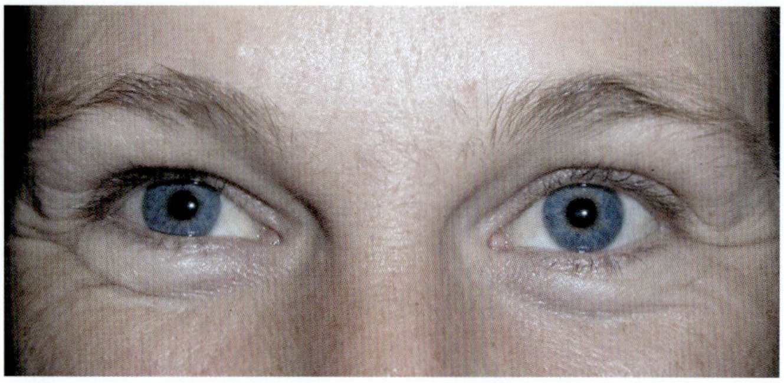

Figure 5–3 Hypertrophic, hyperactive pretarsal orbicularis oculi muscles create a transverse ridge on the lower lids. Patients may confuse these with lower lid "bags," but these ridges are located more superiorly than prolapsed orbital fat. This patient exhibits a lower lid Botox effect on the left. There is less of a pretarsal orbicularis muscle fold and a widened vertical palpebral aperture.

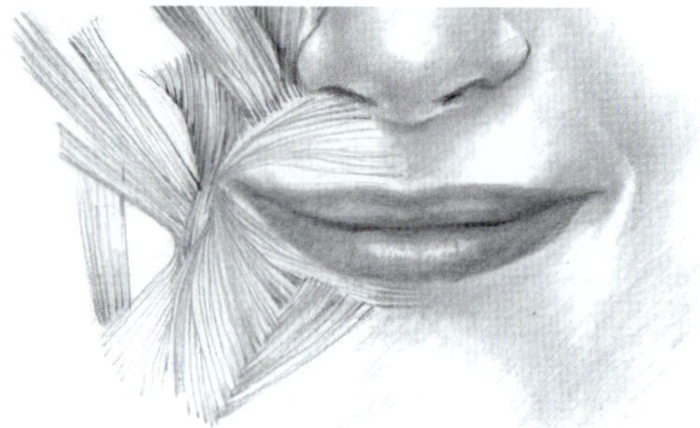

Figure 5–4 The perioral muscles are in delicate balance. The depressor anguli oris pulls the corner of the mouth down, while the zygomaticus major and minor pull it up.

reveal early lower lid fat herniation that the patient had not been previously aware of. This must be recognized, demonstrated, and explained to patients before they are injected.

The Orbicularis Oris, Depressor Oris Anguli, and Perioral Complex

These muscles function in a delicate balance. The orbicularis oris functions as a sphincter. Its overaction can cause vertical upper lip rhytids. The depressor anguli oris muscle arises from the border of the mandible and inserts at the lateral corners of the mouth. This muscle contributes to the depth of oral commissure (melomental fold or marionette lines). Relaxing the depressor anguli oris allows the zygomaticus major and minor to elevate the corner of the mouth without opposition, facilitating filling of the oral commissures. But treating these areas requires precision. Misplaced or overdosed treatments can upset this delicate balance. Understanding this balance will allow the treating physicans to treat patients with facial asymmetries following Bell's palsy (Figs. **5–4; 5–5A,B**).

The Platysma

This flat, broad muscle is also a lower lip depressor. It runs from the chin, at the oral commissures, to the deep subclavicular tissues. Neuromodulation of this muscle can assist in the amelioration of platysmal bands and concentric neck rings.[20] Pretreatment of the platysma may also enhance the effects of facial tightening procedures like Therma-Lifting (Thermage, Hayward, California).

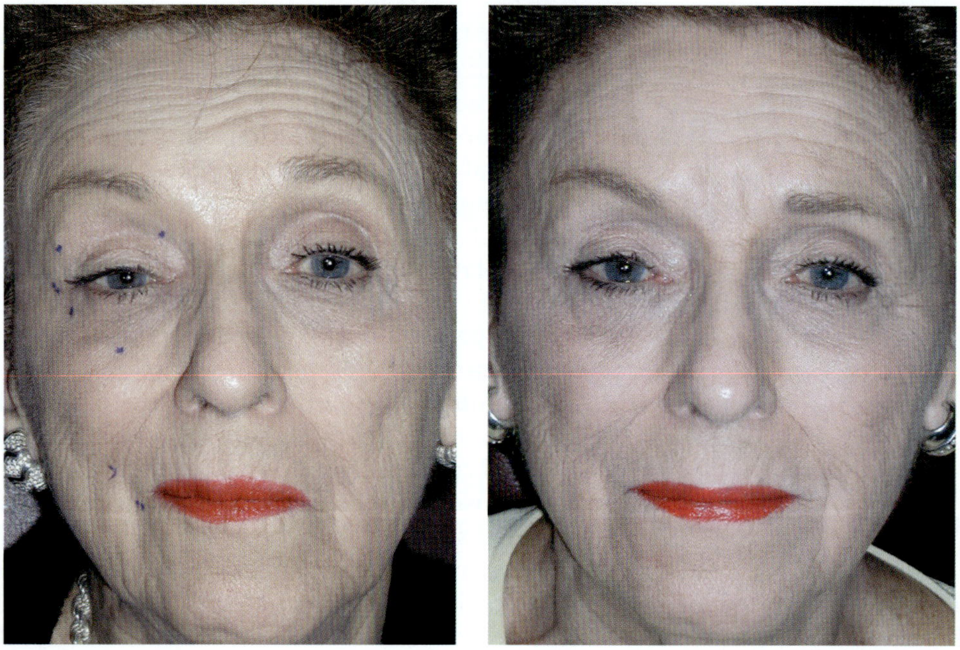

A B

Figure 5–5 (**A,B**) In repose and animation, this patient exhibits upper and lower facial asymmetry, which was significantly improved with Botox neuromodulation.

◆ Clinical Applications

One hundred units of Botox Cosmetic powder are freeze-dried in each vacuum-sealed glass vial. Different vials can be mixed to different strengths for different muscles. Although it is apparent that, once reconstituted, Botox Cosmetic can remain active (if refrigerated) for several weeks, we are not certain if there is any degradation in potency during that time. We prefer to use our Botox within the first 4 hours of mixing it. There is also some discussion about the use of preserved saline versus nonpreserved saline. Although it is claimed that the use of preserved saline diminishes discomfort during injection (there is less of a burning sensation) and that it lengthens the time that reconstituted refrigerated Botox can last, we continue to use nonpreserved saline for reconstituting Botox. We feel that it may be more potent and gives reproducible results.

The actual mixing of Botox also requires some attention. The vacuum seal must be broken with two needle punctures before instilling the saline to avoid an overexuberant mixing and a frothing of the Botox, which can affect potency. An alternative is to remove the cap completely. Although to date we have never had a bad Botox Cosmetic vial with insufficient vacuum, the vacuum should always be checked before removing the cap. The saline should be slowly added, angled against the side of the vial, avoiding frothing of the mixture.

Dosage

Dosage is of critical importance. Often patients will come to us claiming that Botox doesn't work on them. Adequate dosage for each muscle group treated is the key. An insufficient dose will yield an insufficient result. By the same token, we also avoid overtreating because this is also not a desired cosmetic result. We tell our patients that we can always add more. Because the patient may not begin to notice the clinical effect for at least 3 to 5 days, and the full effect may not be evident for 7 to 10 days, we request a revisit for a touch-up in 1 to 2 weeks following the initial treatment session. Following the patient's touch-up session, we do not re-treat before 3 months. The following are some general dosage parameters that are safe starting points for facial neuromodulation using Botox.

Summary of Botox by Anatomic Areas

Forehead: 10–15 units
Glabelar: 20–60 units
Crow's feet and brow depressors: 10–20 units
Lower eyelids: 1–2 units
Upper lip: 1–2 units
Melomental folds (marionette lines): 2–5 units
Platysma bands: 20–50 units

◆ Treatment Techniques

Patient Preparation

To avoid bruising and to decrease to possibility of downtime, this regimen is followed. Patients are given three *Arnica montana* C5 pellets sublingually immediately preceding their injections and asked to continue taking them q.i.d. for 2 to 3 days. If there is bruising, they are asked to continue taking them until the bruising is gone. The injection sites are cleaned with alcohol. Photocaine anesthetic cream (University Pharmacy, Salt Lake City, Utah) is then applied to these areas and covered with a soothing peppermint Natragel mask (Gel Concepts,

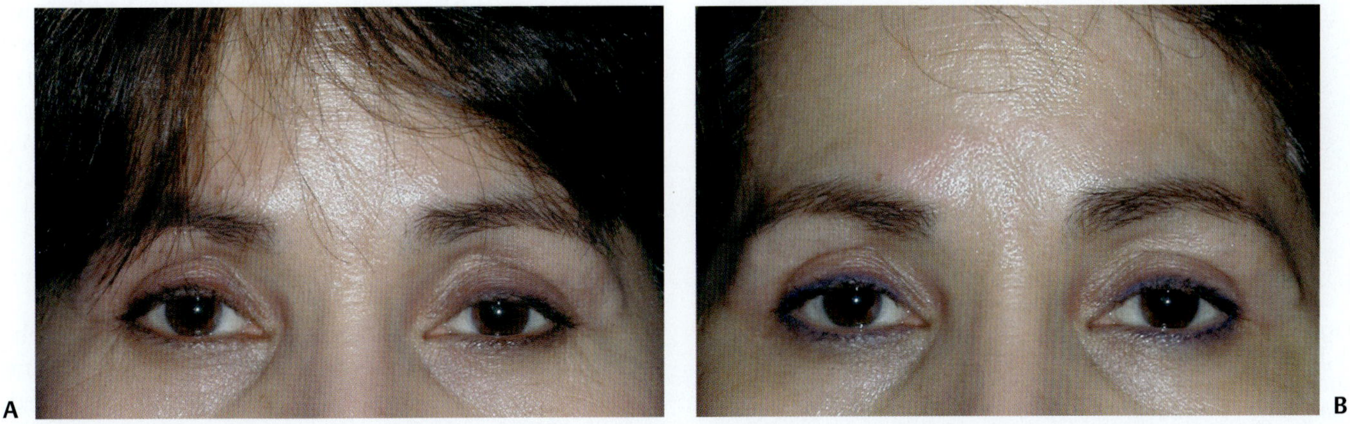

Figure 5–6 **(A,B)** After having occidentalizing surgery elsewhere, this patient was unhappy with her deep superior sulci. Botox neuromodulation of the frontalis muscle subtly lowered her brow levels and reduced the depth of her sulci.

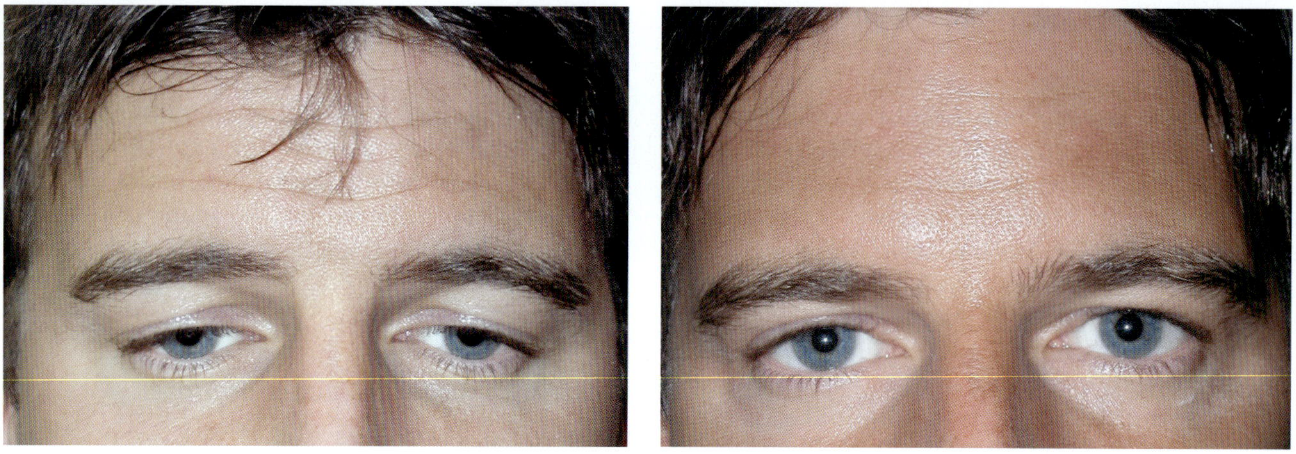

A B

Figure 5–7 (**A,B**) Central forehead furrows that persisted in repose improved following neuromodulation of the frontalis muscle.

Whippany, New Jersey) for 15 minutes. When there is sufficient skin blanching and anesthetic effect, the injection sites are further cooled with ice and then cleaned with alcohol. Following the injections, direct pressure is applied until there is no sign of oozing from the injection sites. This is followed by a 5-minute reapplication of the soothing mask.

Forehead

Before treatment, the brow level, contour, and symmetry are noted. The palpebral apertures, lid-crease fold complex, redundancy of the upper lid fold, and lid hooding are observed and noted. The transverse forehead creases are noted. The patient is asked to raise the eyebrows and the dynamic furrows are noted. Any adjustments of the brow level and contour are first performed with neuromodulation of the brow depressors (corrugator, procerus, and lateral orbicularis oculi muscles) (Fig. **5–6A,B**, page 35) and the patient is asked to return in 1 week for treatment of residual forehead creases (Fig. **5–7A,B**). Treatment of the forehead is avoided in patients who have blepharoptosis or who have redundant upper lid folds and are utilizing their frontalis muscle to maintain adequate palpebral apertures and a clear visual axis (Fig. **5–8**).

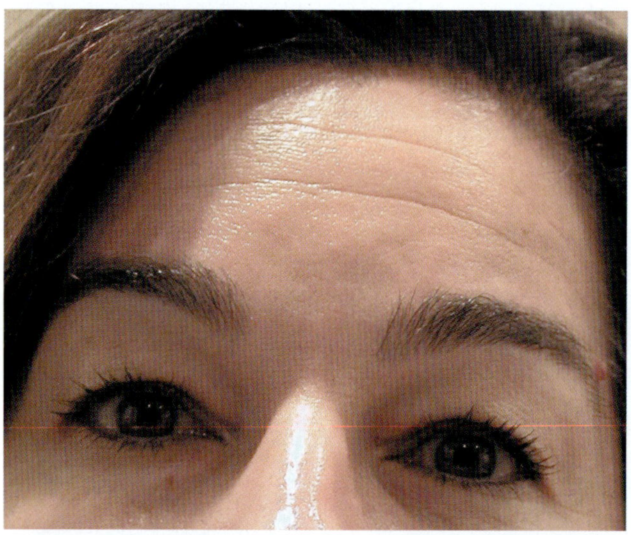

Figure 5–8 Patients with blepharoptosis or upper eyelid hooding are constantly using their frontalis muscles to keep their visual axis clear and their vertical palpebral apertures open maximally. Their brow depressors and central frontalis muscle can be treated, but neuromodulation of the entire forehead is contraindicated.

After we have decided to treat the frontalis muscle, we again observe the dynamic rhytidosis by asking the patient to elevate the brows. We can treat along the length of each horizontal furrow (at least 1 cm above the eyebrows). Beginning at the extreme lateral aspect of each rhytid 0.1 cc injections (2.5 units/0.1 cc; 100 units reconstituted in 4 cc) are spaced 1 to 2 cm apart. We can also treat segmentally achieving a further balance for eyebrow level and contour shaping. If, after brow depressor neuromodulation, there is segmental brow retraction, this can be corrected with 1 to 2 units injected into the wrinkle that is visible when the patient elevates the eyebrows (Fig. **5–9A,B**). We find that utilizing lower doses in the forehead yields a more natural result with an improved brow level and contour. We now typically limit our total dose in the frontalis muscle to 10 to 15 units.

Glabella and Brow Depressors

The patient is observed in repose. If a deep furrow is observed, it is filled with a filling agent, either Restylane (Medicis, Scottsdale, Arizona) or layered Perlane (Q-Med, Uppsala, Sweden) and Restylane (Figs. **5–10A,B; 5–11A,B, 6–2A,B**). We then ask the patient to frown, palpate the

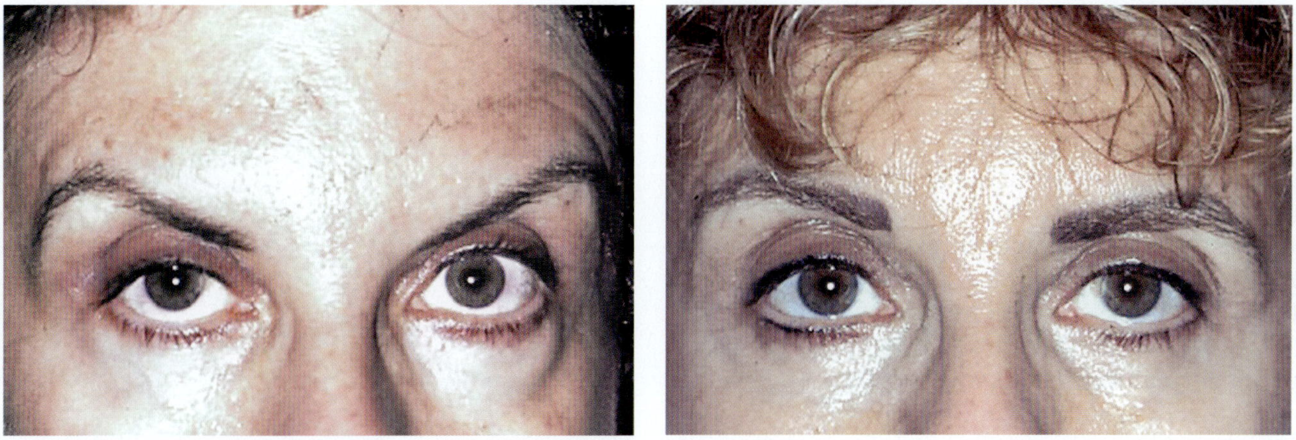

A B

Figure 5–9 (**A,B**) Lateral brow retraction can follow treatment of the lateral brow depressors. This can be ameliorated at the patient's 1-week follow-up appointment with 1 or 2 units of Botox injected in the areas of lateral forehead dimpling.

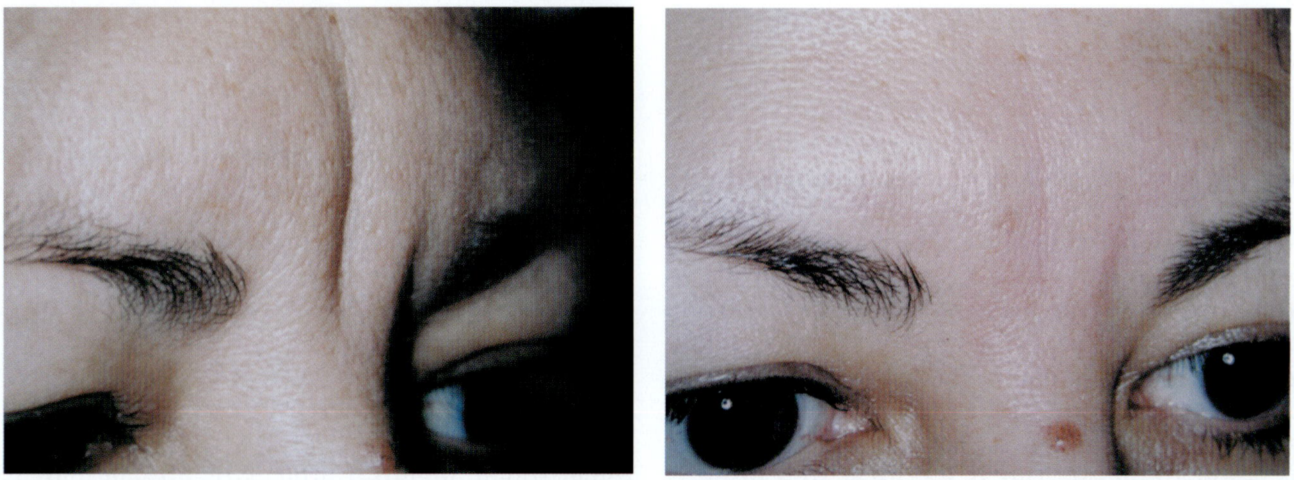

A B

Figure 5–10 (**A,B**) Deep glabellar furrows that are present in repose respond well to filling with layered Restylane on Perlane and neuromodulation of the corrugator and procerus muscles. The results of this combination therapy often last up to 1 year, and 20% of our patients who have been treated in this manner have only required Botox maintenance without repeat injections of filling agents.

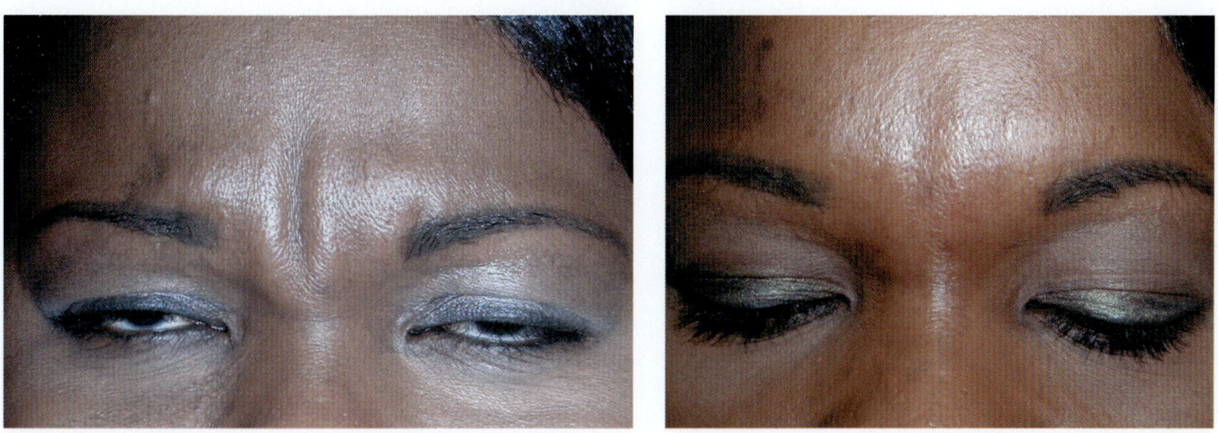

A B

Figure 5–11 (**A,B**) Botox neuromodulation is effective in patients of all skin types. Doses may vary with gender and race, however. This patient required 60 units for an acceptable result.

corrugator muscle, and give two 0.1 cc injections (5 units/0.1 cc; 100 units reconstituted in 2 cc) medial and lateral to each corrugator muscle insertion. This will also treat the medial brow depressors. One 0.1 cc injection (5 units/0.1 cc; 100 units reconstituted in 2 cc) is then given on the bridge of the nose, over the procerus muscle insertion. These muscles are brow depressors. When they are relaxed and the elevating action of the frontalis muscle is unopposed, a brow elevation can be achieved. Often these injections will have to be repeated in 7 days because the average dose to relax the corrugator muscles is 40 units.[21] And on occasion some corrugator hyperactivity may be seen and palpated more laterally requiring additional injections of 5 units per site (Fig. **5–2**). However, our treatment protocols avoid overtreatment and brow ptosis. Residual fine lines or frank rhytidosis will require further filling to complete rhytid ablation.

Crow's Feet and Orbicularis Muscle

Asking the patient to smile will delineate the extent and depth of crow's feet rhytidosis and thus determine the number of injection sites (Figs. **5–12; 5–13A,B**). Three to four 0.1 cc injections per side (2.5 units/0.1 cc; 100 units reconstituted in 4 cc), spaced equidistantly lateral to the orbital rim will usually be sufficient to soften crow's feet rhytidosis and to avoid exacerbation of lower lid laxity or retraction. An injection 1 to 2 mm medial to the lateral orbital rim and 1 mm inferior to the lateral brow will segmentally relax the lateral and superior orbicularis muscle and will elevate the tail of the brow. This is a critical step in brow shaping.

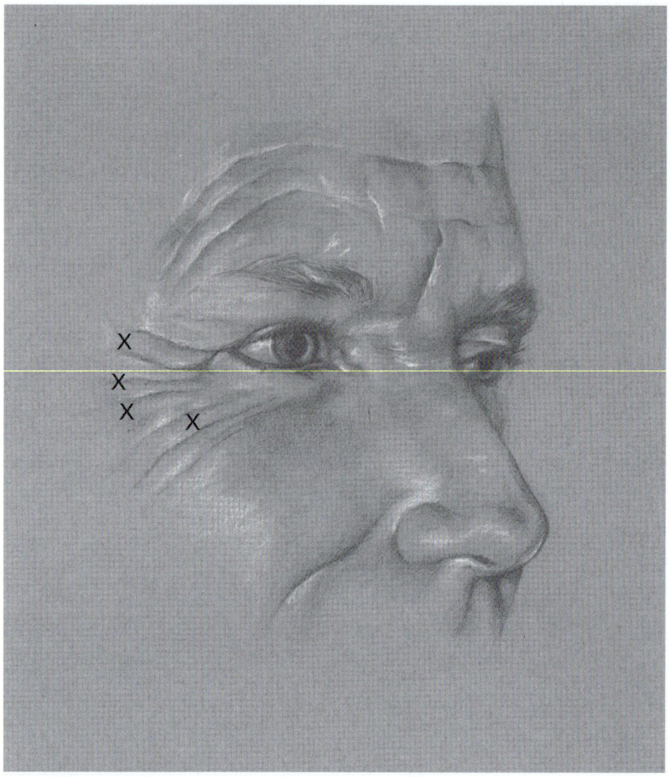

Figure 5–12 Crow's feet are softened with three to four injections of 2.5 units (per site) of Botox lateral to the lateral orbital rim. Care is taken to avoid injecting lateral rhytids inferior to the inferior orbital rim, as this may affect smiling.

Lower Eyelids

Hypertrophic pretarsal orbicularis muscle folds that create a ridge in the pretarsal area can be softened with

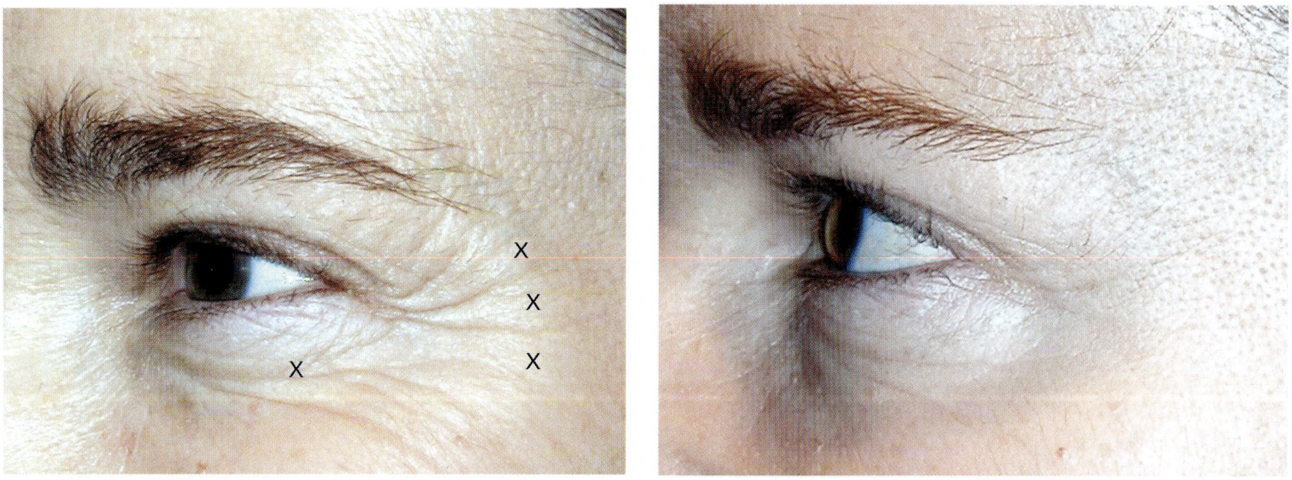

A

B

Figure 5–13 **(A,B)** Crow's feet, lateral upper and lower eyelid rhytidosis, pretarsal orbicularis muscle are treated with 2.5 units per injection site. The patient is asked to smile and the rhytids are identified. Injection sites are marked.

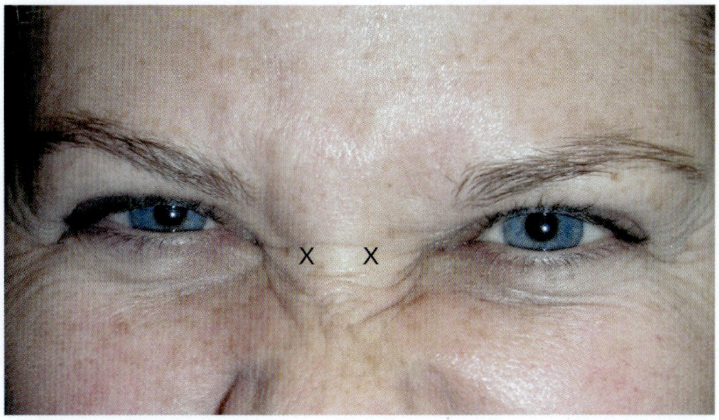

Figure 5–14 "Bunny lines"—animated transverse rhytids at the lateral aspect of the nasal bridge—are treated with 2.5 units to each side.

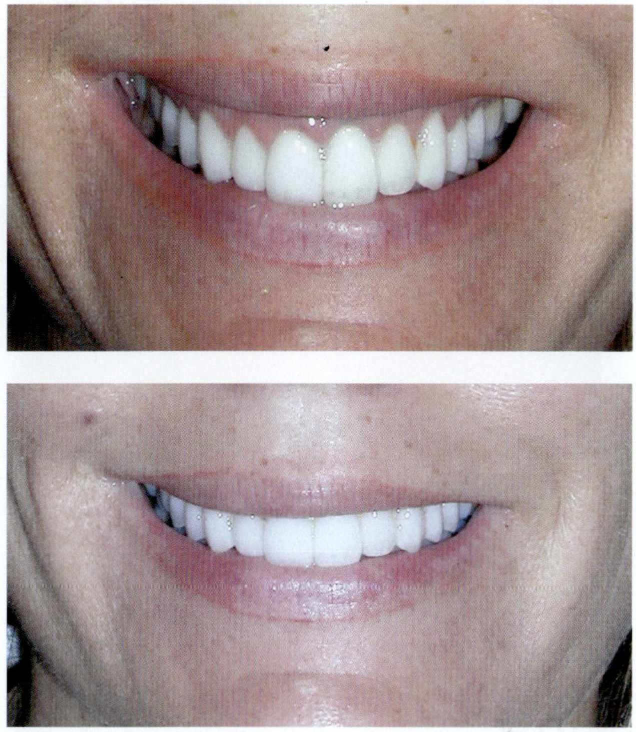

A

B

Figure 5–15 (**A,B**) The "gummy smile" corrected with 2 units to each levator labii superioris alaeque nasi muscle.

2.5 units given in one or two locations, provided that there is no preexisting lid margin or lateral canthal tendon laxity or lower lid retraction.[22,23] On occasion, lower lid rhytidosis may persist or even be accentuated following crow's feet injections. They may be the result of recruitment of opposing muscles (levator labii), when muscles not normally involved in smiling become overactive following neuromodulation of the orbicularis oculi. This process may also be visible on the bridge of the nose, producing "bunny lines" (nasalis muscle) (Fig. **5–14**). A trial of one or two 0.1 cc injections (1.25 units/0.1 cc; 100 reconstituted in 8 cc) equidistantly placed into the dynamic rhytid is worthwhile. In general we most frequently perform Botox neuromodulation of the lower eyelids as a pretreatment for resurfacing.

Nasolabial Folds

Using Botox to treat the nasolabial groove is a distinct area of controversy. We prefer to fill the groove (Restylane, Perlane, New Fill) or, in patients with marked redundancy of the fold, to tighten the fold (with Thermage or laser resurfacing) and then fill in the residual fold (Restylane, Perlane, New Fill). Nonetheless Michael Kane[24] has made some compelling arguments for treating these patients with neuromodulation of their levator labii superioris alaeque nasi muscles if they have canine or gummy canine smiles as well[25,26] (Figs. **5–15A,B**).

Vertical Upper Lip Rhytids

These may be cautiously treated with 1 to 2 units for each side of the lip, spaced 1 cm from the midline, 1 cm apart. If overtreated, the patient will have an asymmetric smile. Because of the small doses used, successful outcomes rarely last longer than 2 months. However, this technique works well in combination with the use of fillers (Restylane, Restylane Fine Lines) and as a pretreatment for laser resurfacing.

Melomental Folds (Marionette Lines, Oral Commissures) and Cobble Chin

This multicontoured area is difficult to treat completely with any single modality. A combination of neuromodulation to the depressor oris angulii will subtly elevate the corners of the mouth and allow more efficient filling of the residual depression (Figs. **5–16A,B**). When patients are asked to show the doctor their lower teeth, the depressor angulii oris can often be palpated. If this is not possible, the injection site can be identified by extending a straight line from the nasolabial fold to the border of the mandible. One or two units are injected on each side. If the injection is given too medially, the lower lip retractors may be injected and patients may have difficulty lowering their lower lip. If the injection is given too superiorly, the orbicularis oris may be injected, resulting in incompetence of the lower lip. Cobble chin, a relatively uncommon condition caused by hyperactivity of the mentalis muscle, can be treated

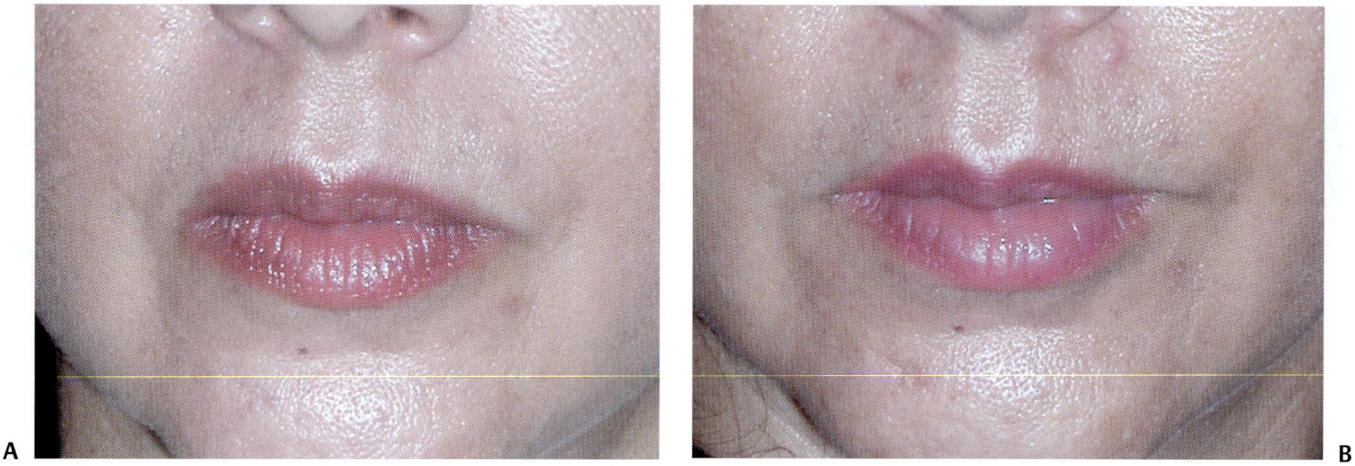

Figure 5–16 (A,B) Neuromodulation of the depressor anguli oris muscles will subtly elevate the corners of the mouth.

with one or two units of Botox into the areas of dimpling (Figs. **5–17A,B**).

Platysma

When platysmal bands are evident, they are grasped between the physician's fingers, and 2.5 units per site are injected 1 cm apart along the entire length of the band (Fig. **5–18**). We do not exceed 50 units during one treatment session (see Chapter 8).

◆ Combination Therapies

There are several areas where neuromodulation yields improved and longer-lasting results when combined with other modalities.

With Fillers to Treat the Glabella

In patients with deep static furrows that persist even at rest, filling them gives immediate improvement that is accentuated after the Botox effect is evident. The improvement lasts longer (6–12 months) than when either modality is used alone[27,28] (see Chapter 6).

With Fillers to Treat the Melomental Grooves (Marionette Lines, Oral Commissures)

Filling agents ameliorate these grooves, but often this improvement does not entirely satisfy the patient or the treating physician. Neuromodulation of the depressor angulii oris muscles elevates the corners of the mouth and diminishes the muscular ridge descending from the corner of the mouth[29] (see Chapter 14).

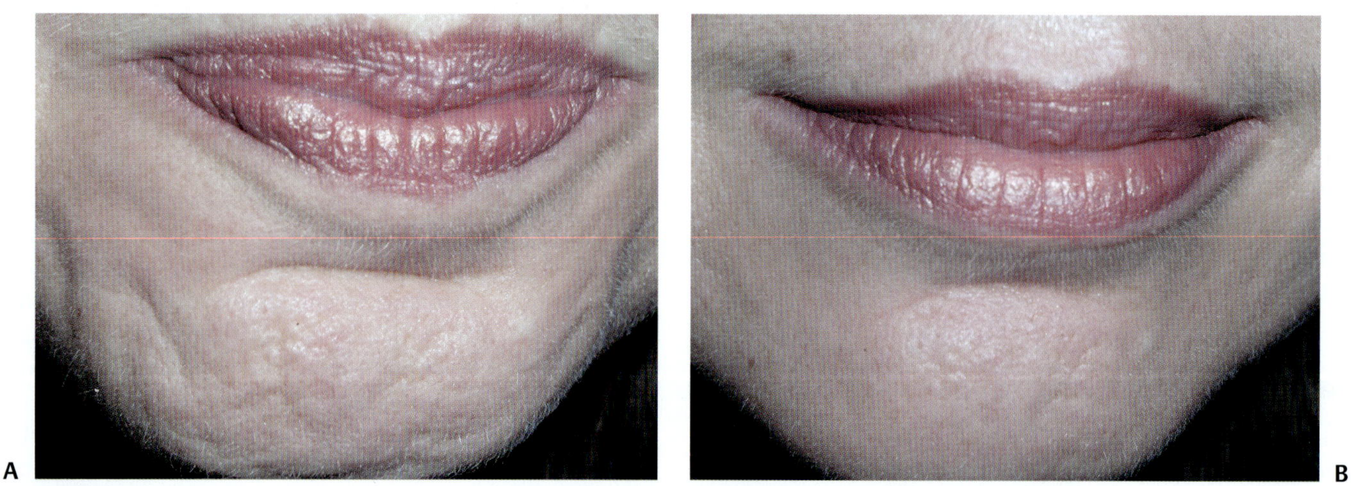

Figure 5–17 (A,B) The "cobblestone chin" can be relaxed with neuromodulation of the mentalis muscle.

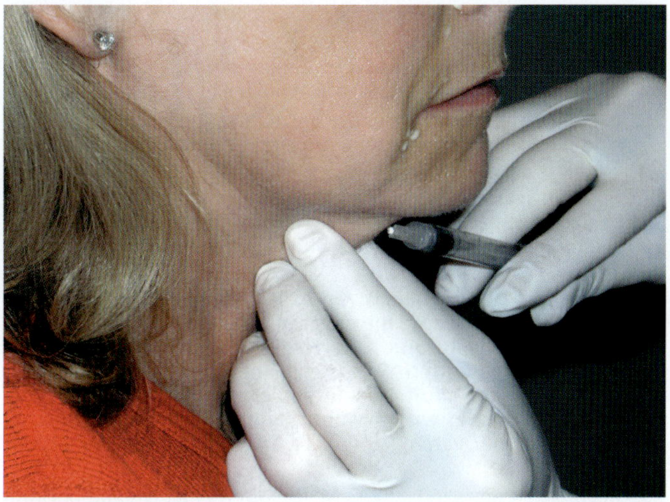

Figure 5–18 The platysmal band is grasped between the injecting physician's fingers.

Pretreatment for Intense Pulsed Light, Nonablative Laser, and Photomodulation Therapies

Intense pulsed light is an effective treatment for telangiectasias, diffuse erythema, acne rosacea, and pigment mottling. Although it is not its primary function, in addition, it can improve skin texture. It is apparent that any treatment that improves the quality and texture of the skin will make the neuromodulation effect more striking. However, there may be a secondary Botox effect that results in improvement greater than that achieved by either modality individually[30] (see Chapter 1). Similarly, neuromodulation appears to enhance the skin texture improvement achieved with nonablative lasers (1064 and 1320 nm). In all likelihood it will also augment the effects of nonthermal, nonablative photomodulation utilizing light-emitting diodes (LEDs).

Pretreatment for Laser Resurfacing

Neuromodulation has become standard procedure in our laser resurfacing protocol (see Chapter 9). Its effect is crucial during the period of collagen remodeling.[31] Under ideal circumstances we treat the patients 2 weeks prior to the laser resurfacing procedure. This gives us ample opportunity for additional preoperative touch-up injections when necessary.

Pretreatment for Thermage

Pretreating the submental platysma and vertical platysmal bands of facial Thermage patients 2 weeks before their treatment sets the stage for a more efficient effect, in theory lessening the resistance to the tightening of facial collagen fibers (see Chapter 1).

◆ Conclusion

Neuromodulation has evolved from a localized standalone therapeutic miracle that magically diminished dynamic lines, furrows, and wrinkles from patients' faces to an integral preparatory and potentiating step for all facial rejuvenation techniques. As we explore the intimate and delicate relationships and balance of the facial musculature, more indications for potential use will emerge.

References

1. Carruthers A, Carruthers J. Clinical indications and injection techniques for cosmetic use of botulinum A exotoxin. Dermatol Surg 1998;24:1189–1194
2. Carruthers J, Carruthers A. The adjunctive uses of botulinum toxin. Dermatol Surg 1998;24:1244–1247
3. Bosniak S, Cantisano-Zilkha M. Botulinum type A neurotoxin for upper facial rejuvenjation. Operative Techniques in Oculoplastic, Orbital, and Reconstructive Surgery 1999;2:164–167
4. Bosniak S, Cantisano-Zilkha M. Total eyelid rejuvenation. Operative Techniques in Oculoplastic, Orbital, and Reconstructive Surgery 1999;2:198–202
5. Fagien S. Botox for the treatment of dynamic and hyperkinetic facial lines and furrows: adjunctive use in facial aesthetic surgery. Plast Reconstr Surg 1999;103:701–713
6. Carruthers J, Carruthers A, Zelichowska A. The power of combined therapies: Botox and ablative facial laser resurfacing. Am J Cosmet Surg 2000;17:129–131
7. Bosniak S, Cantisano-Zilkha M. Botox: a 22-year experience. Operative Techniques in Oculoplastic, Orbital, and Reconstructive Surgery 2001;4:74–80
8. Bosniak S, Cantisano-Zilkha M. A combined approach to non-invasive facial rejuvenation: home care, peels, neuromodulation, and laser-assisted sub-surface collagen remodeling. Operative Techniques in Oculoplastic, Orbital, and Reconstructive Surgery 2001;4:65–68
9. Hexsel D, Trindade de Almeida A. Uso Cosmetico da Toxina Botulina. Porto Alegre, Brazil: Leandro do Santos Lima; 2002
10. Bosniak S. The uses of botox in ophthalmic plastic surgery. Keynote Presentation to the 28th Congress of the Brazilian Ophthalmologic Society. Salvador, Bahia, September 5, 1995
11. Holds JS, Alderson K, Fogg SG, et al. Terminal nerve and motor end plate changes in human orbicularis muscle following botulinum A exotoxin injection. Invest Ophthalmol Vis Sci 1990;31:178–181
12. Coffield JA, Considine RV, Simpson LL. The Site and Mechanism of Action of Botulinum Neurotoxin. New York: Marcel Dekker; 1994:3–13
13. Flynn TC, Clark RE. Botulinum toxin type B (Myobloc) versus botulinum toxin type A (Botox) frontalis study: rate of onset and radius of diffusion. Dermatol Surg 2003;29:519–522

14. Matarasso SL. Comparison of botulinum toxin types A and B: bilateral and double-blind randomized evaluation in the treatment of canthal rhytides. Dermatol Surg 2003;29:7–13
15. Moriarty KC. Indications and limitations of cosmetic botulinum toxin type A. Operative Techniques in Oculoplastic, Orbital, and Reconstructive Surgery 2001;4:81–88
16. Coleman-Moriarty K. Botulinum Toxin in Facial Rejuvenation. St. Louis: Mosby; 2003
17. Hechmann M, Breil S, Ceballos-Bauman A, Schaller M, Plewig G. Side-controlled intradermal injections of botulinum toxin A in recalcitrant axillary hyperhidrosis. J Am Acad Dermatol 1999;41:987–990
18. Larabee WF Jr, Makielski KH, Henderson JL. Surgical Anatomy of the Face. 2nd ed. Philadelphia: Lippincott Williams and Wilkins; 2004
19. Huilgol S, Carruthers JA, Carruthers JDA. Raising eyebrows with botulinum toxin. Dermatol Surg 1999;25:373–376
20. Matarasso SA, Matarasso SL, Brandt FS. Botulinum A exotoxin for the management of platysmal bands. Plast Reconstr Surg 1999;103:645–652
21. Carruthers JD, Lowe NJ, Menter MA, Gibson J, Eadie N, Botox Glabellar Lines II Study Group. Double-blind, placebo-controlled study of the safety and efficacy of botulinum toxin type A for patients with glabellar lines. Plast Reconstr Surg 2003;112:1089–1098
22. Flynn TC, Carruthers JA, Carruthers JA, Clark RE II. Botulinum A toxin (Botox) in the lower eyelid: dose-finding study. Dermatol Surg 2003;29:943–951
23. Flynn TC, Carruthers JA, Carruthers JA. Botulinum-A toxin treatment of the lower eyelid improves infraorbital rhytides and widens the eye. Dermatol Surg 2001;27:703–708
24. Kane M. First Annual National Education Faculty Training Meeting. Miami, FL, 2004
25. Rubin LR. The anatomy of a smile: its importance in the treatment of facial paralysis. Plast Reconstr Surg 1974;53:384–387
26. Pessa JE. Improving the acute nasolabial angle and medial nasolabial fold by levator alae muscle resection. Ann Plast Surg 1992;29:23–30
27. Bosniak S, Cantisano-Zilkha M. Hyaluronic acid gel injections for facial rejuvenation: a 3-year clinical experience. Operative Techniques in Oculopastic, Orbital, and Reconstructive Surgery 1999;2:177–181
28. Carruthers J, Carruthers A. A prospective, randomized, parallel group study analyzing the effect of BTX-A (Botox) and nonanimal sourced hyaluronic acid (NASHA, Restylane) in combination compared with NASHA (Restylane) alone in severe glabellar rhytides in adult female subjects: treatment of severe glabellar rhytides with a hyaluronic acid derivative compared with the derivative and BTX-A. Dermatol Surg 2003; 29:802–809
29. Bosniak S, Cantisano-Zilkha M, Rinaldi P, et al. Lip and perioral rejuvenation: a multidisciplinary approach. Operative Techniques in Oculoplastic, Orbital, and Reconstructive Surgery 2001;4:104–108
30. Carruthers J, Carruthers A. The effect of full-face broadband light treatments alone and in combination with bilateral crow's feet botulinum toxin type A chemodenervation. Dermatol Surg 2004;30:355–366
31. Bosniak S, Cantisano-Zilkha M. Cosmetic Blepharoplasty and Facial Rejuvenation. Philadelphia; Lippincott-Raven Publishers; 1999

6

Injectable Fillers

Stephen Bosniak, Marian Cantisano-Zilkha, and Ioannis P. Glavas

New insights into the facial aging process—subcutaneous tissue loss and osseoerosion—and the evolution of safer, longer-lasting, and more convenient, readily available materials for adding volume to facial structures have added a new dimension to noninvasive facial rejuvenation. The ease of performance, lack of downtime, and infrequency of complications have increased the popularity and patient acceptance of these procedures. Now alternatives to bovine collagen are readily available. These techniques fit in well with the menu of combination therapies—neuromodulation, nonablative and ablative lasers, intense pulsed light (IPL), and light-emitting diode (LED) therapies.

There have been many discussions theorizing the attributes of the perfect filling agent. The distillate is simple. We want a product that can be administered safely, conveniently, rapidly, and painlessly and without leaving any traces that it has been injected. We want a product that does not result in any complications and that lasts a long time (forever would be preferable if we didn't have to sacrifice safety for longevity). The ideal substance should be "biocompatible, nonimmunogenic, nonresorbable, nonpyogenic, noncarcinogenic, inexpensive, and nonmigratory, with the ability to be stored, shaped, removed, and sterilized easily."[1] We have not achieved filler nirvana, but the nonanimal-derived, stabilized hyaluronic acid products are the current state of the art, fulfilling much of our desired criteria.

Hyaluronic acid is a versatile macromolecule. It is a polysaccharide first isolated from bovine vitreous in 1934. It has been found in all tissues and in all vertebrates. It is a universal component of the extracellular space, where the molecule has multiple properties to constitute a matrix that supports the normal function of cells and tissues.[2] Non-animal stabilized hyaluronic acid (NASHA) is patented and produced by Q-Med AB, Uppsala, Sweden. We have used these products extensively since 1996 as an adjunct to our facial rejuvenation surgical procedures and as a stand-alone technique for adding volume to facial structures and for ablating rhytids.[3–7] Others have had similar experience with this product.[8–11] Hyaluronic acid derived from rooster combs (Biomatrix, San Tropez, France) has been used for almost 3 decades by ophthalmic surgeons during intraocular procedures. One of the authors (S.B.) participated in its early development to enhance and replace volume in the reconstructive and cosmetic arenas,[12,13] (unpublished Hylan B [Biomatrix] monkey studies in 1990–1995). Both of these products can be used without prior skin testing.

For the last 2 decades, the most widely available and widely used substance for filling in facial rhytids has been bovine collagen.[14] Collagen is a major structural protein in vertebrates, including humans. Approximately 25% of the protein in the human body and 75% in the skin is collagen. Injectable bovine collagen has been used extensively for facial rejuvenation since the 1980s.[15–21] It requires skin testing before it can be used as filler. The second generation, derived from human fibroblast cell culture, can be used without prior skin testing.[22] We will discuss this in greater detail later in this chapter.

The use of autogenous fat as a filling agent is somewhat more complicated. It has the advantages of potential permanence after implantation and unlimited volume available for implantation. But this technique has the disadvantage of requiring an additional procedure for harvesting and a degree of unpredictability after implantation. This discussion will be continued in Chapter 7.

The search for permanent synthetic fillers has been fraught with controversy. Materials that appear to give satisfying results in the short term may ultimately lead to complications after several years. With the exception of the silicone microdroplet technique, which can be useful when used in small quantities,[23] at this time we do not use filling agents that claim to be permanent. The dictum that permanent filler may give rise to a permanent problem seems reasonable. The theory that the use of permanent filler is acceptable if it can be removed easily if the need arises is also not realistic in most cases. Solid materials that are implanted surgically do, however, fall into this category, and are discussed with regard to midface lifting and cheek augmentation in Chapters 11 and 12. We do not use solid implants in the lips.

◆ Indications

Static Rhytids

Wrinkles, grooves, crevices, furrows, and fine lines that are the result of aging, sun exposure, and loss of skin and muscle turgor and elasticity can be filled, creating a smoother cutaneous surface and an illusion of a more youthful face. Facial animation (squinting, smoking) and a variety of facial expressions (smiling, frowning, crying, surprise) accentuate the static rhytids and will have to be treated concurrently.

Although theoretically any facial area can be filled, some areas typically require filling and other areas can only be partially filled or are filled with difficulty. We will discuss the filling of facial rhytids starting with the most cephalad areas, from the hairline, and work caudally, to the neck.

Tranverse forehead creases respond well to neuromodulation and usually do not require filling, except in cases of scarring and atrophic indentations following cutaneous steroid injections (Fig. **6–1A,B**). Within the 1 cm "no Botox" zone above the eyebrows, however, rhytid filling works well to supplement neuromodulation of the forehead.

The glabellar area is managed well with neuromodulation when the vertical furrows are apparent only during frowning. However, static furrows that persistent at rest will require combined filling and neuromodulation, which are effectively and efficiently performed during one session (Fig. **6–2A,B**). The depressions are filled and then the appropriate neuromodulating injections to the corrugator muscle insertions are given. In this manner the area can be filled most accurately. It is apparent that this combined therapeutic approach yields more complete and longer-lasting results than when either modality is used alone. The transverse crease over the bridge of the nose that is not completely effaced after neuromodulation of the procerus muscle can be filled in with satisfying results (Fig. **6–3A,B**).

Vertical creases in the lateral aspect of the upper eyelid are sometimes visible after neuromodulation of

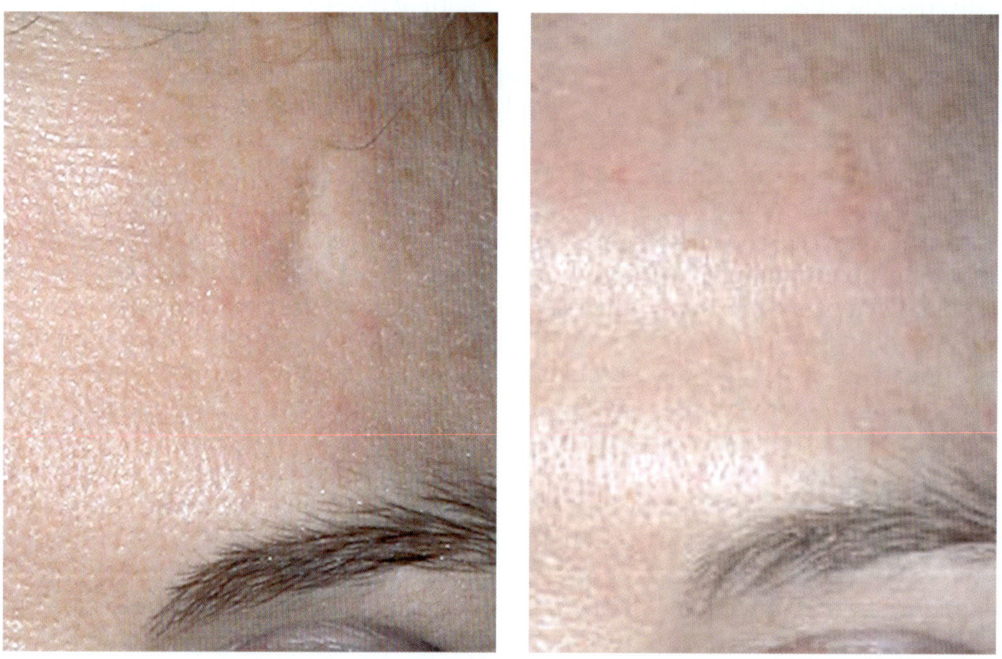

A B

Figure 6–1 (**A**) Acutaneous depression of the forehead followed Triamcinalone injections of a forehead scar. (**B**) Restylane was used to fill in cutaneous atrophic depressions following triamcinolone injections to reduce a scar.

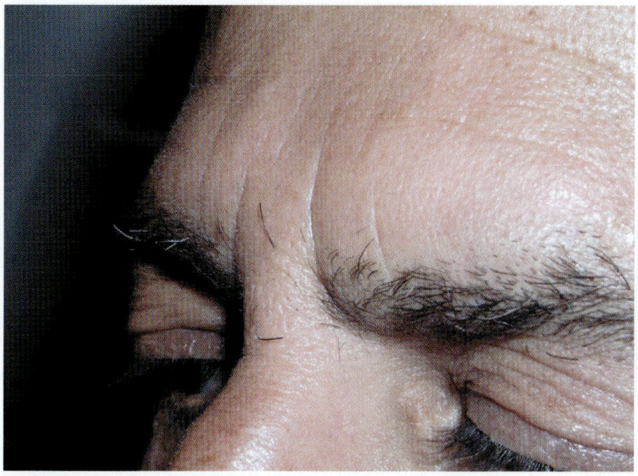
A

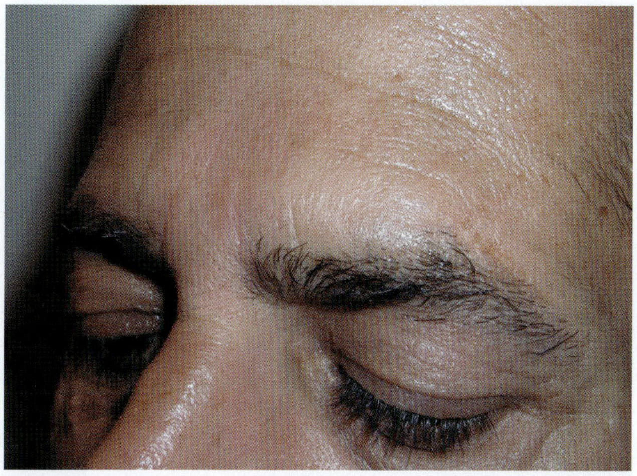
B

Figure 6–2 (**A**), Deep glabellar furrows evident at rest require more than neuromadulation alone for complete correction. (**B**) These deep glabellar furrows were filled with Restylane layered on Perlane and concomittantly treated with Botox neuromodulation (40 units).

the crow's feet and lateral canthal areas. In patients with upper eyelid redundant folds, upper lid laser-assisted blepharoplasty and laser resurfacing constitute the most effective treatment. But for patients who are not emotionally or financially ready for this procedure, filling agents can work remarkably well as a temporizing maneuver.

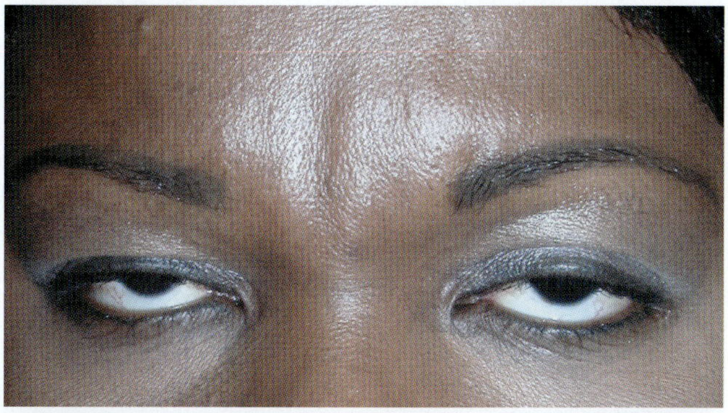
A

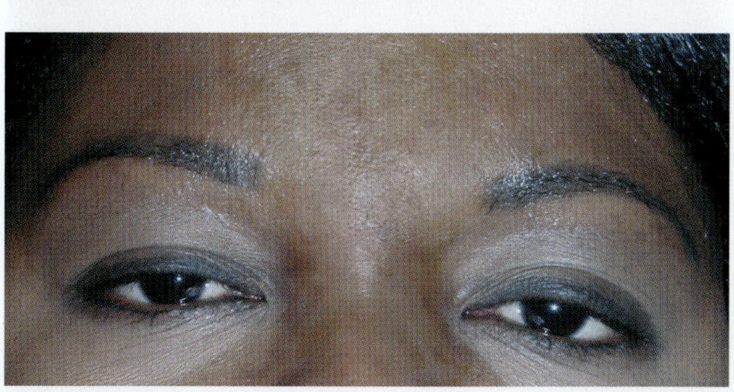
B

Figure 6–3 (**A,B**) After Botox neuromodulation of the patient's corrugator and procerus muscles (60 units of Botox), her residual furrows and the bridge of her nose were recontoured with Perlane.

We do not recommend filling of crow's feet creases or even deeper furrows in the lateral canthal area as a primary treatment. The skin is too fine and the muscle activity too rapid and repetitive. This area is much more efficiently managed with neuromodulation.

Meticulously applied, understated filling can be utilized for subtle lower eyelid contour irregularities. In thicker-skinned individuals with less translucent skin, tear trough deformities and hollowed, oversculpted lower lid contours can be filled in. When correcting tear trough deformities, the filling agent should be applied in the suborbicularis, supraperiosteal space. Even a pretarsal orbicularis muscle ridge can be re-created when desired.

Nasolabial grooves are prime regions for filling to camouflage midfacial laxity. A combination of layered thicker and thinner materials can be used for an enhanced effect (Figs. **6–4A,B; 6–5A,B**). The end results can be further accentuated with noninvasive skin tightening procedures utilizing radiofrequency or laser energy. Even following surgical midface lifting or nonsurgical tightening procedures, the application of filling agents to the nasolabial grooves may be necessary for the final effect.

Melomental grooves have been called by the unflattering name of marionette lines, or more clinically, oral commissures. These multicontoured facial cutaneous depressions can be ameliorated with filling agents, but more complete correction can be attained with concomitant neuromodulation of the depressor oris angulii muscles (the "dolphin shot") and midface tightening procedures when necessary (see Chapters 14–16). Using a layered technique of thicker more deeply injected fillers and more superficially injected thinner fillers is helpful. This combination technique can also be used to support the corners of the mouth.

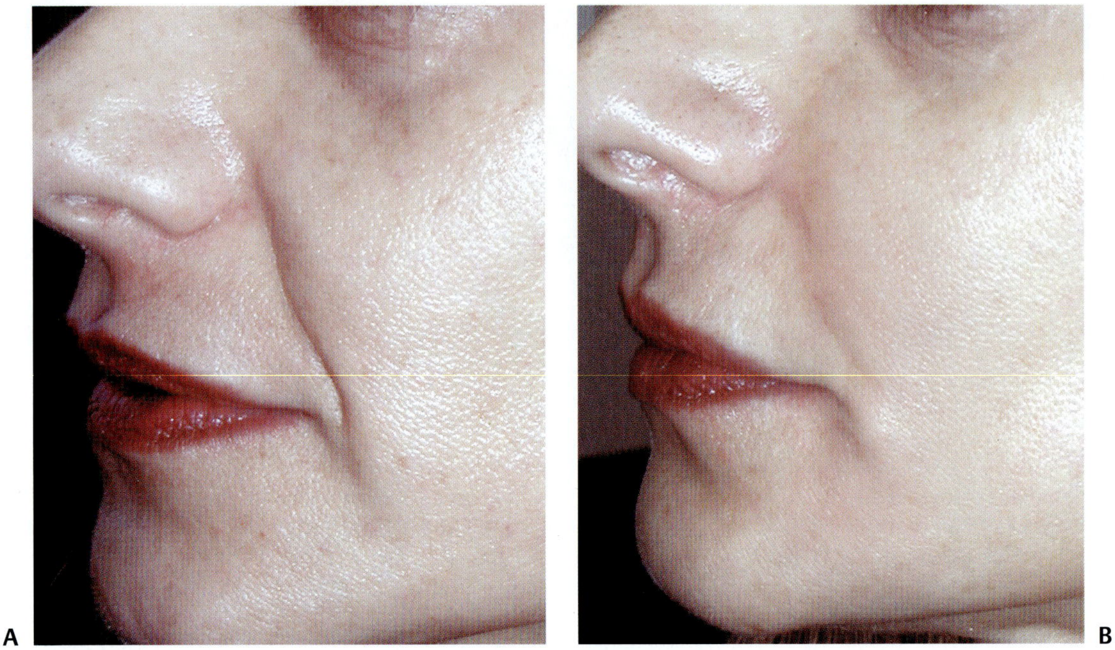

Figure 6–4 (A,B) Nasolabial folds were diminished with Restylane layered on Perlane.

Lips can be augmented and recontoured effectively with a combination of hyaluronic acid products of different viscosities, (see Chapter 14). The upper lip border can be accentuated and vertical rhytids softened with less viscous materials (Fig. **6–6A,B**), whereas the body of the lip is more efficiently filled with more viscous products (Fig. **6–7A,B**).

Recontouring of the facial bony contours (cheek bones, chin, jawline, nasal deformities) can be achieved with thicker fillers injected in a supraperiosteal plane (Fig. **6–8A,B**). This can give a satisfying result and can also have a temporizing effect so patients can see if they like their new facial contour before they have a definitive surgical procedure.

Soft tissue defects can be improved utilizing a variety of agents. Small, distensible traumatic and acne scars can be filled over time with multiple sessions, using hyaluronic acid gel or silicone (Fig. **6–9A,B**). Broad, ill-defined areas of scarring or atrophy will require thicker material that is available in larger quantities—fat, polylactic acid. Ice-pick scars are difficult to fill and are better managed with a biopsy punch, suturing, and nonablative laser collagen stimulation or 50% TCA focally applied with a tooth pick into the scar.

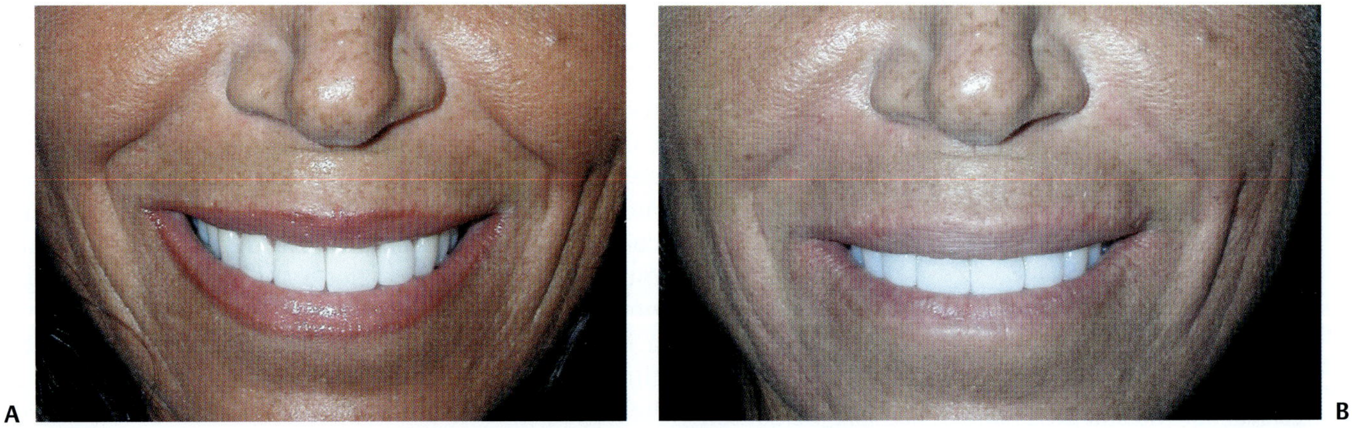

Figure 6–5 (A,B) Perlane was used to soften this animated patient's nasolabial folds.

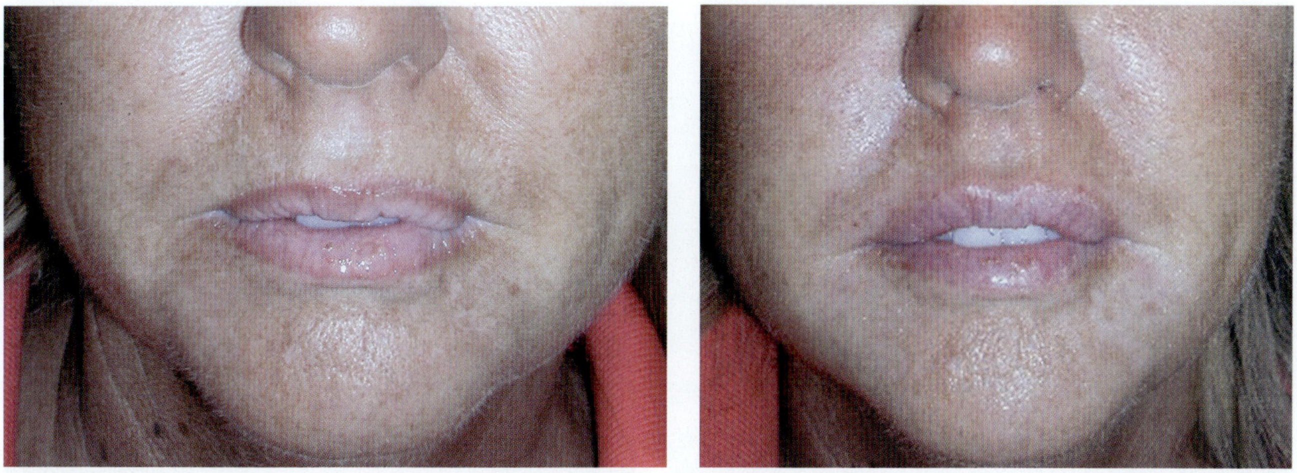

A B

Figure 6–6 (**A**) This patient desired treatment of her upper lip rhytids and augmentation of her lips and chin. (**B**) The perioral area has been rejuvenated with Botox neuromodulation of the depressor anguli oris muscles, Cosmoplast and Restylane to accentuate the upper lip border, and Perlane to fill the body of the lip, to support the corners of the mouth, soften the oral commissures, and augment the chin.

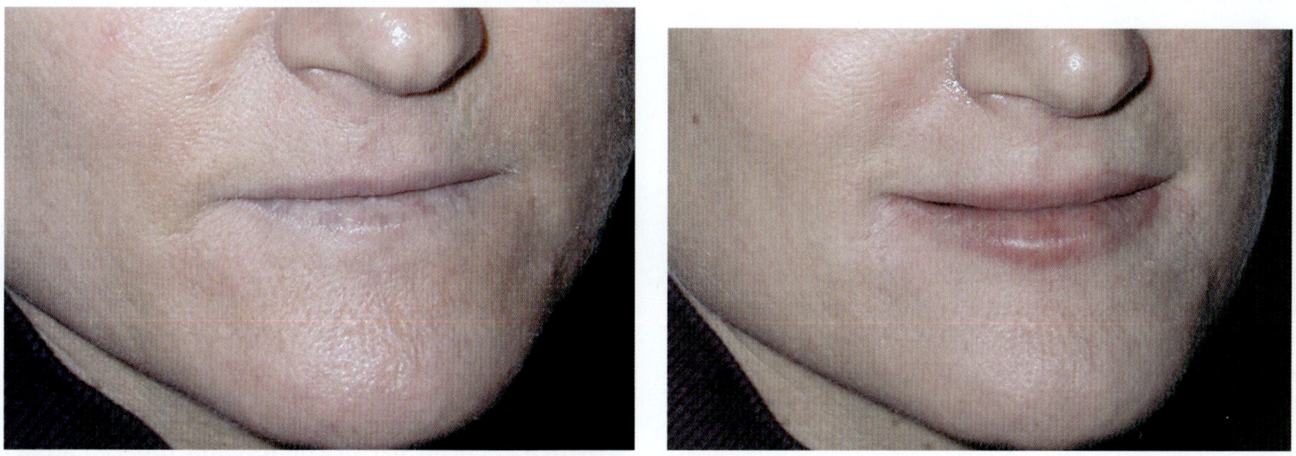

A B

Figure 6–7 (**A,B**) Perlane was used to create visible upper and lower lips.

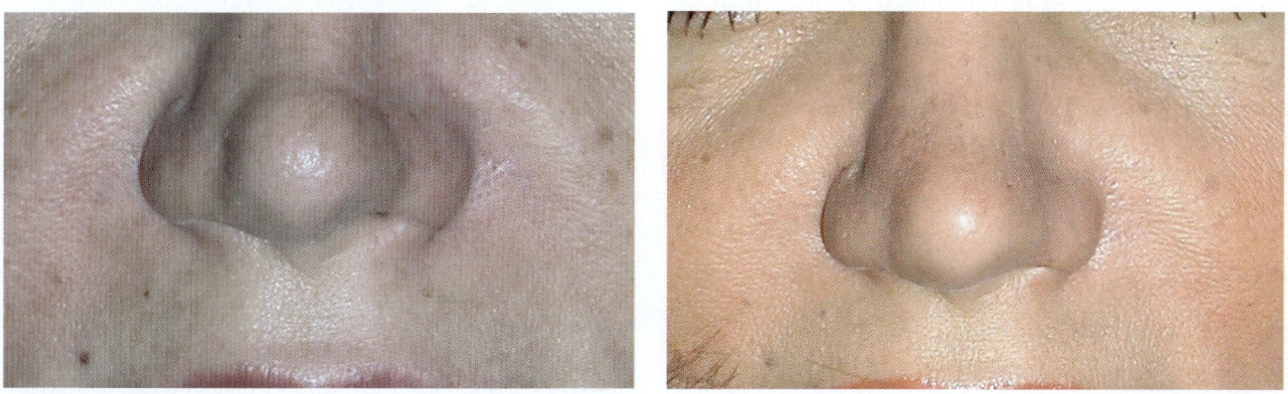

A B

Figure 6–8 (**A,B**) Perlane was used to correct these nasal deformities while the patient was contemplating corrective surgery.

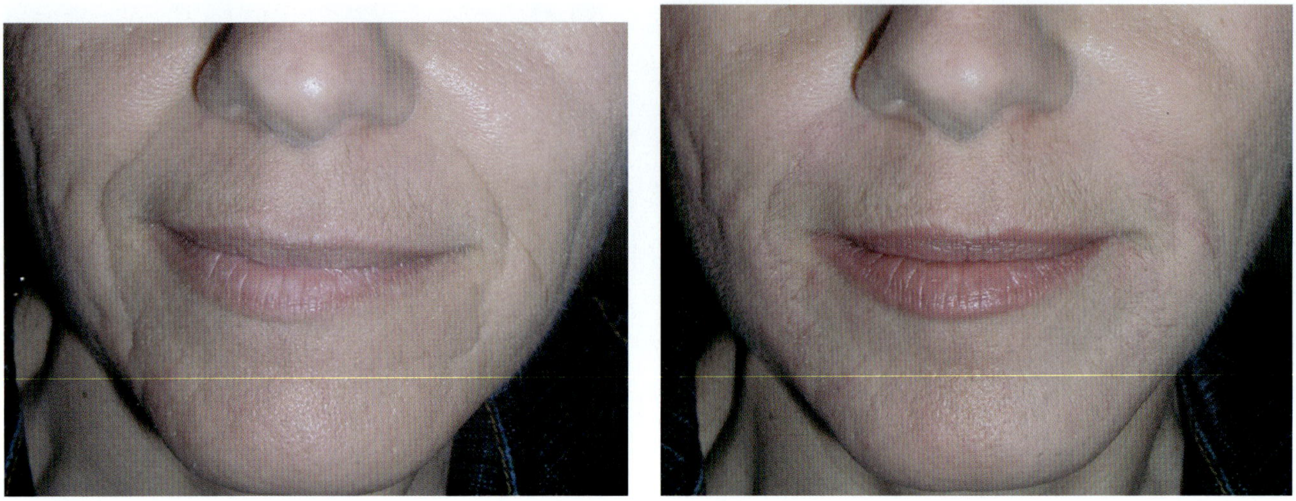

Figure 6–9 (**A,B**) Restylane layered on Perlane made a significant improvement in the correction of this patient's acne scarring.

◆ Choice of Materials

Permanent Filling Agents

Injectable filling materials can be classified as either permanent or temporary. As already stated, we do not in general use permanent filling agents. Silicone is a permanent filler. Fat is potentially permanent, but its duration after implantation can be unpredictable. Fat implantation is discussed in detail in Chapter 7.

Silicone in its liquid injectable form has been used since the 1940s. However, it has been misused during the subsequent decades. Excessive volumes and adulterated forms have been injected, causing subsequent complications and controversy. Two U.S. Food and Drug Administration (FDA)-approved medical-grade liquid injectable silicones are available today. Adatosil (Escalon Medical Corp., Chicago, Illinois) and Silikon (Alcon Laboratories, Fort Worth, Texas) are approved for the tamponade of retinal detachments. The FDA's Modernization Act (1997) allows for their off-label use for soft tissue augmentation.[23]

Silicone is inert and lighter than water and human tissue. Following microdroplet liquid silicone injection, there is a transient, mild inflammatory response for about the first 2 weeks, followed by a fibroblastic response beginning at 1 month and accompanied by collagen deposition.[24] Eleven to 14 months after implantation there is intense fibrosis. This may cause some hardening of the tissues injected, and thus silicone is best injected into areas of denser, less mobile tissue.

Temporary Filling Agents

Hyaluronic Acid and Hyaluron

Although hyaluronic acid is found in the highest concentrations in connective tissues, 56% is found in human skin. Because it is a uniform, unbranched linear polysaccharide, hyaluronic acid has a simple chemical structure that is identical in all species and tissues (only the length of the molecular chain varies), and it can be considered an ideal biomaterial.[2] It is composed of hydrophilic disaccharide units containing glucuronic acid and N-acetylglucosamine. Pure hyaluronic acid is inherently biocompatible. It is the impurities in the hyaluronic acid raw material, especially of animal origin, that can affect biocompatibility. The following products produce longer lasting results and fewer hypersensitivity reactions than collagen products.[10] No pretreatment skin testing is required.

Restylane (Q-Med, Uppsala, Sweden), FDA approved December 12, 2002, has 20 mg/mL of hyaluronic acid with a gel bead size of 250 μm and 100,000 units per mL. It has 0.5 to 1% cross linking.

Hylaform (INAMED, Santa Barbara, California), FDA approved April 2004, has 5.5 mg/mL of hyaluronic acid and 20% cross linking.

Perlane (Q-Med, Uppsala, Sweden), not approved in the United States, has 20 mg/mL of hyaluronic acid with a gel bead size of 1000 μm and 10,000 units per mL and less than 1% cross linking.

Hylaform Plus (INAMED, Santa Barbara, California), FDA approved October 13, 2004, has 5.5 mg/mL of hyaluronic acid, and has a larger gel particle size and is more viscous than hyaluronic acid. It has 20% cross linking.

Restylane Touch (Q-Med, Uppsala, Sweden), not approved in the United States, has 20 mg/mL of hyaluronic acid with a gel bead size of 100 μm and 250,000 units per mL.

Restylane, Perlane, and Restylane Touch (formerly Restylane Fine Lines) are NASHA products, biosynthesized from a nonanimal source and stabilized with relatively few cross links to minimize the probability of protein impurities bound to the entangled hyaluronic acid network. They are stabilized materials in a continuous three-dimensional molecular network: a gel that can take any form or shape.

The residence time of NASHA is dependent on the size of the gel particle, the concentration, and the existence of inflammation in the area. In healthy tissue, the extracellular capacity to degrade hyaluronic acid (into carbon dioxide and water) is very low. NASHA gels will stay approximately the same size and shape as injected despite continuous degradation because the molecule is extremely hydrophilic and the amount of hyaluronic acid in a NASHA gel bead is about five times larger than what is needed to maintain its volume; the excess material allows the gel bead to last longer. This process is called isovolemic degradation. Because there is limited cross linking, there is significant hydroscopic pressure-ability to absorb water and maintain volume.

We have used Restylane for fine lines and moderate rhytids and furrows with significant success since 1996. A sterile glass syringe with 0.7 mL of Restylane, a Luer lock and sterile 30-gauge needle are supplied. It does not have to be refrigerated. It is injected into the mid-dermis. In our hands the clinical effect lasts an average of 9 months (glabellar and nasolabial fold corrections last longer than lip body and oral commissure corrections). The residual material, still in place at the previous injection sites, acts as a foundation for subsequent injections. We have found that these secondary injections provide enhanced and longer-lasting corrections.

We have utilized Perlane (not yet available in the United States) since 2000 to effectively fill in deep furrows and contour irregularities. Because it is thicker, it can distend subcutaneous cicatrixes, allowing more effective filling. And because it is thicker, it will last longer than Restylane. Restylane can be layered over a foundation of Perlane for correction of residual superficial irregularities. Perlane is injected into the deep dermis or into the subcutaneous tissue. Perlane has a longer residence time than Restylane, lasting longer than 9 months. Perlane is also supplied in a sterile glass syringe containing 0.7 mL with a needle locking attachment and a sterile 27-gauge needle. It does not have to refrigerated.

We have used Restylane Touch (not available in the United States) since 2000 for correction of delicate upper lip rhytids. Because it is used in smaller quantities and is less viscous, it has a shorter residence time, averaging 3 to 4 months.

Hylaform and Hylaform Plus, are sterile, nonpyrogenic, viscoelastic, clear, colorless, transparent gel implants composed of cross-linked molecules of hyaluronan. Hyaluronan is a naturally occurring polysaccharide of the intercellular matrix in human tissues, including skin. Hyaluronan is chemically, physically, and biologically identical in the tissues of all species. These products are extracted from minced rooster combs (and may contain avian protein).

Theoretically, this tissue extraction technique could subject these avian-derived products to a higher level of impurities or contaminants. Hylaform (less viscous) is used in similar fashion to Restylane, and Hylaform Plus (more viscous) is used in a similar fashion to Perlane. Hylaform and Hylaform Plus differ from Restylane and Perlane in their method of production (avian versus biosynthesis). The thicker compounds are also produced differently. Perlane has larger hyaluronic acid bead sizes, and Hylaform Plus has more cross linking. More cross linking may affect the amount of possible contaminants as well as the longevity of the product. More cross linking will yield less hydroscopic pressure and less residence time.

Hylaform is injected intradermally for correction of superficial skin contour irregularities, folds, and wrinkles as a viscoelastic supplement to the intercellular matrix. Hylaform Plus, with additional cross linking, is more viscous and is injected subcutaneously for correction of deeper folds and broader surface irregularities.

Depending on the type of skin and lesion, best results are obtained in areas where these defects are readily distensible and where the correction can be visualized by manual manipulation (stretching) of the skin. No long-term studies are available describing the residence time of these products. In our experience Hylaform does not last as long as Restylane, and Hylaform Plus does not last as long as Perlane.

Hylaform is supplied in a 0.75 mL volume in a single-use 0.9 mL glass syringe assembled in a protective sleeve with a needle-locking device and packaged with two sterile 30-gauge needles. Contents of the syringe are sterile and nonpyrogenic.

Hylaform Plus is supplied in a 0.75 mL volume in a single-use 0.9 mL glass syringe with two 27-gauge needles.

Collagen

There are a variety of collagen products available. Although we don't utilize bovine collagen products in our practices, there are physicians who have used them for extended periods of time and are satisfied with their results. The average longevity of correction with these products is about 3 months, although longer persistence of results has been reported.[25–27] Because the products are liquid and not viscous, they may be easier to inject in certain facial areas (lip borders). Because they are mixed with anesthetic, they may be somewhat less painful for the patient, but over- and undercorrections must be gauged. Collagen fillers produced from bovine sources have a risk of inducing allergic reactions in patients with a history of severe allergies and known allergy to bovine products. Sensitivity skin tests prior to treatment are recommended for bovine derived collagen but not for human-derived fibroblast collagen products.

Zyderm 1 (INAMED Corporation, Santa Barbara, California) is highly purified bovine dermal collagen (35 mg/mL) dispersed in phosphate-buffered physiological saline. Zyderm 2 (INAMED) contains highly purified bovine dermal collagen with a concentration of 65 mg/mL dispersed in phosphate buffered physiological saline. Both contain 0.3% lidocaine (3 mg/mL) to provide local anesthesia at the time of the injection. The FDA approved Zyderm 1 in 1981, and Zyderm 2 was approved in 1983. They are provided in sterile disposable syringes ready for use and should be kept refrigerated until usage. Each syringe should only be used once. Because they are produced from animal sources skin sensitivity tests should be performed at 8 and 4 weeks prior to treatment to identify patients with sensitivity to the implant. The safety of use of more than 30 mL of Zyderm 1 over a 1-year period has not been established. It is recommended for fine lines and wrinkles. The safety of use of more than 15 mL of Zyderm 2 over a 1-year period has not been established. Because Zyderm 2 has twice the viscosity of Zyderm 1, it is recommended for deeper lines and furrows.

Zyplast (INAMED) contains purified bovine dermal glutaraldehyde cross-linked collagen with a concentration of 35 mg/mL similar to Zyderm 1 dispersed in phosphate-buffered physiological saline. Its cross linkage with glutaraldehyde made the collagen fibers stronger. Thus its indication is for correction of deeper skin wrinkles and deformities. Also the filling result lasts longer because the agent doesn't dehydrate at the same rate as non-cross-linked collagen. The FDA approved it in 1985. Skin sensitivity tests should be performed at 8 and 4 weeks prior to treatment to identify patients with sensitivity to the bovine collagen. The safety of use of more than 30 mL of Zyplast over a 1-year period has not been established.

Cosmoderm (INAMED) is purified collagen from human fibroblast cell culture that is grown under controlled conditions. It is dispersed in phosphate-buffered physiological saline and contains 0.3% lidocaine as local anesthetic. This is the second generation of injectable collagen fillers; the FDA approved it on March 11, 2003. They do not require a pretreatment skin test. As injectable fillers placed in the papillary dermis Cosmoderm 1 and Cosmoderm 2 have the same indications as their predecessors Zyderm 1 and Zyderm 2. They are not recommended to individuals with severe allergies that include history of anaphylaxis to bovine or collagen products. The safety of use of more than 30 mL and 15 mL of Cosmoderm 1 and Cosmoderm 2, respectively, over a 1-year period has not been yet established. The persistence of results using these produces is described as comparable to the bovine-derived products.

Cosmoplast (INAMED) is also derived from human fibroblast cell culture grown under controlled conditions, is cross linked with glutaraldehyde, and contains 0.3% lidocaine as local anesthetic. It is recommended for the same indications as Zyplast; that is, correction of deeper dermal folds such as nasolabial folds and marionette lines. Similar to Zyplast, no more than 30 mL total volume injection in one patient is recommended over a 1-year period; their longevities are also comparable.

Because of the flow characteristics and lidocaine content of the cell culture collagen products, there may be some practical advantages to using these products with hyaluronic acid products. For instance, using Cosmoplast to first outline upper lip borders may facilitate augmentation of the body of the lip with Perlane.

Several autologous and allogenic collagen products have been intermittently available. We have found that they require multiple injection sessions initially to attain an acceptable result and that the residence time is limited. Dermalogen (Collagenesis, Beverly, Massachusetts) is an injectable human dermal implant material made from a suspension of pooled human cadaver collagen.[28] Autologen (Collagenesis) is an injectable autologous human tissue matrix, primarily composed of intact collagen fibrils. The patient's skin is harvested during blepharoplasty or rhytidectomy and is processed.[28] The volume of skin harvested will limit the amount of human tissue matrix that will be available as a filling agent.

Isolagen (Isolagen Technologies, Paramus, New Jersey) is pending FDA approval. It is composed of injectable autolgous fibroblasts cultured for 4 to 6 weeks from a 3 mm punch biopsy taken from postauricular skin.[29]

Other Temporary Products

New Fill (Aventis Pharma, France) has been renamed **Sculptra** (Dermik Laboratories, Berwyn, Pennsylvania). It is synthetic polylactic acid powder that has to be mixed and put into suspension in sterile water and lidocaine. Each bottle contains 0.15 g of powder that has to

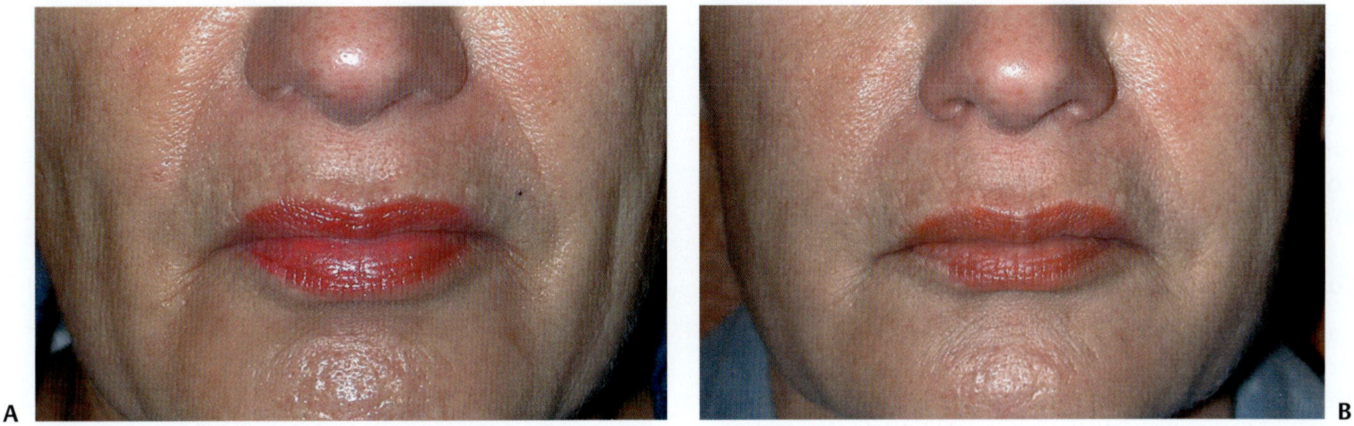

Figure 6–10 (A,B) New Fill filled out this patient's lower face and ablated her furrows and folds. (Courtesy of Dr. Anne-Lisse Lauffenburger, Switzerland.)

be mixed thoroughly to create a suspension injected with a 26-gauge needle (supplied with product). Six mL of diluents (4 cc sterile water and 2cc lidocaine) provide a sufficiently liquid suspension for easy injection and decrease the incidence of granuloma formation (pers. comm., Dr. Anne-Lise Lauffenburger, Switzerland, 2003; pers. comm., Boris Sommer, Germany, 2004). This product works well to fill in broad irregular areas (Fig. **6–10A,B**). It must be injected subdermally. Because the amount of correction improves with time, inciting a mild subcutaneous inflammatory response and secondary collagen production, a gradual filling in the contour defect is recommended. Rather than aiming for complete correction in one session, partial correction is augmented in 3- to 4-month intervals.

We will limit our discussion of collagen and hyaluronic acid products with suspended alloplastic microspheres to their use in patients with extreme soft tissue atrophy. We have found other applications of their use to yield untoward complications (granulomas, cutaneous ulcerations) too frequently. We have also heard of two cases of secondary central retinal vein occlusion following their periorbital use.[30]

Artefill (Artes Medical, San Diego, California) is composed of uniform polymethylmethacrylate (PMMA) beads (30–42 μm in diameter) suspended in collagen. It is not FDA-approved in the United States. The collagen acts as a temporary filler, and the microspheres create an inflammatory response with secondary collagen production and a longer lasting effect. Because is contains bovine collagen, it requires skin testing before use.

Matridex (BioPolymer GmbH, Germany) is hypromellose, dextranomere DEAE suspended in hyaluronic acid and cross-linked hyaluronic acid. The hyaluronic acid provides temporary filling without the need for pretreatment skin testing and the hypromellose and dextranomere DEAE (positively charged microparticles) promote fibroblast formation and collagen neogenesis, inducing a longer lasting effect (pers. comm., Stein Tveten, Oberstdorf, Germany, 2004). It is not approved in the United States.

Alloderm (Lifecell Corporation, Branchburg, New Jersey) is a solid acellular biological implant that is useful in eyelid and lip reconstruction and for repairing large facial contour deformities. Human dermal tissue is harvested from cadavers. The cells, which are targets for the immune response, are removed without altering the collagen and extracellular matrix of the dermis. The resulting dermal matrix is immunologically inert and serves as a framework to support revascularization and cellular repopulation. **Cymetra** (Lifecell Corporation) is its micronized, injectable form. It is supplied as a cryofractured, dried, acellular, particulate dermal matrix. When refrigerated, it has a shelf life of 2 years. A 5 mL syringe contains 330 mg of this material and it is reconstituted with 1 mL of lidocaine when prepared for use. We have found that when it is injected for lip augmentation considerable swelling and rapid resorption are the rule.

◆ Treatment Techniques

Patient Preparation

Regardless of the product to be used, each patient is prepped with alcohol and treated while sitting in an upright position. The patient is given three sublingual *Arnica montana* C5 pellets (Boiron, Newtown Square, Pennsylvania) immediately before the injections and asked to continue taking them four times daily for 3 days. Soothing Natragel masks (Gel Concepts, Whippany,

New Jersey) are applied to the areas to be injected to enhance cutaneous blanching and to augment topical anesthetic when applied. We use the topical anesthetic Photocaine (University Pharmacy, Salt Lake City, Utah) on every patient and rarely use regional blocks. The application of the topical anesthetic is monitored by the patient to insure that their areas of concern are addressed.

Collagen Products

Collagen products contain lidocaine. The area to be injected is cleaned with alcohol. Zyderm and Cosmoderm are used to ablate fine lines and augment lip borders utilizing linear threading and serial puncture techniques into the superficial or mid-dermis. A 30-gauge needle, with the bevel facing superficially, is used. Zyplast and Cosmoplast are injected into the deep dermis with a 27-gauge needle, bevel facing superficially, utilizing linear threading, serial puncture, fanning, and cross-hatching techniques to fill in deep contour irregularities and folds. Because 20% of the injected volume is anesthetic agent, at least 20% overcorrection is the desired endpoint of the treatment. These patients may be pretreated with Natragel masks (Gel Concepts) impregnated with menthol to cool and blanch the cutaneous surface as well as soothe and calm the patient.

Hyaluronic Acid Products

Hyaluronic acid products: Restylane, Perlane, Hylaform, and Hylaform Plus do not contain anesthetic agents. The area must be cleaned with alcohol and anesthetized with topical agents. We prefer Photocaine (University Pharmacy), applied in a thick layer, occluded with a Natragel mask (Gel Concepts). The Natragel mask impregnated with menthol is exceptionally soothing. It enhances the anesthetic effect of the Photocaine and gives the patient a sense of well-being. The mask and anesthetic cream are left in place for 20 minutes. After removal of the mask and cream and cleansing the skin again with alcohol, Restylane or Hylaform are used to treat fine and moderately deep lines and lip borders utilizing linear threading and serial puncture techniques. They are applied to the superficial and mid-dermis with a 30-gauge needle. Applications that are too superficial, especially in thin-skinned patients, will appear gray through the translucent skin. Perlane and Hylaform Plus are injected with a 27-gauge needle into the deep dermis or subcutaneously to fill in broader and deeper irregularities, utilizing linear threading, serial puncture, fanning, and cross-hatching techniques. No overcorrection is necessary. After injection, gentle massage may be performed to achieve a smooth and continuous contour with the surrounding tissue. Repeat injection may be performed at 1-week intervals until the final correction is achieved (Fig. **6–11**).

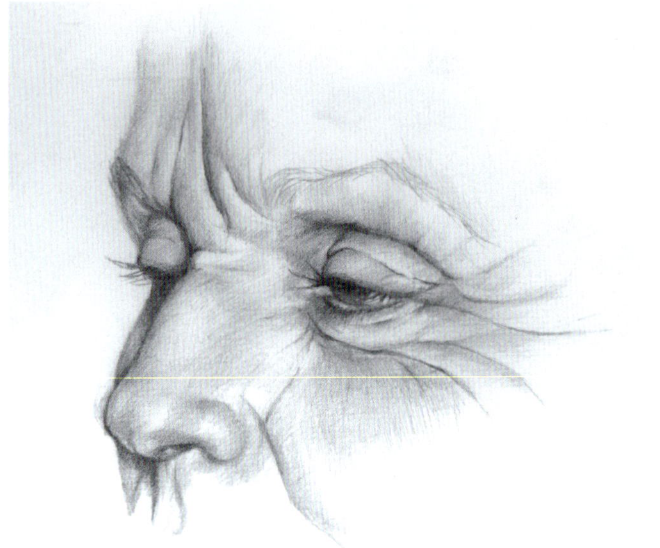

Figure 6–11 Deep glabellar furrows are filled with layered Restylane and Perlane. Botox neuromodulation of the procerus and corrugator muscles allows for collagen remodeling and a more complete, longer-lasting effect.

Polylactic Acid

Utilizing a 26-gauge needle, polylactic acid injections are given subdermally, using a linear threading, fanning, or cross-hatching technique after application of a topical anesthetic. Small amounts (1–2 mL) are injected over a 6-month period and are repeated every 4 weeks until a satisfactory correction is achieved.

Liquid Injectable Silicone

Microdroplet liquid injectable silicone (LIS) using a serial puncture technique is the safest and most efficacious use of LIS. For silicone of 350 centistokes viscosity, a 4 mm 30-gauge needle on a 1 mL Luer locking syringe will allow small volumes (0.005–0.02 mL) to be injected in a uniform fashion.[31–33] The desired plane of injections is either the deep dermis or the superficial subcutaneous tissue. The angle of the needle will determine the depth of the injection. The goal of this technique is to undercorrect initially, using small-volume injections and at each subsequent treatment session, in 1- to 3-month intervals, to augment until the final result is obtained. More viscous (1000 centistokes) silicone is injected with a 27-gauge needle.

◆ Results

Each of the temporary products used has its own inherent breakdown time or longevity. In addition, the greater the volume used and the less mobile the tissue into which it is implanted, the longer it will last.

Concomitant therapies such as neuromodulation will increase the persistence of the desired filling effect. Other skin therapies, although they may not increase the longevity of the final result, will certainly improve the final result.[10]

Generalizing our experience in the broad categories, collagen products last an average of 2 to 3 months. Hyaluronic acid products last an average of 6 months (the nasolabial furrows lasting slightly longer whereas the melomental depressions and lips slightly less). Products with suspended microspheres and polylactic acid may last for several years after being applied in a series of applications to achieve the final result. Filling glabellar furrows with hyaluronic acid products while concomitantly performing chemoneuromodulation of the procerus and corrugator muscles can yield satisfactory smoothing of the glabellar furrows for 9 to 12 months.

◆ Complications and Complication Avoidance

Localized bruising and puncture marks at the injection sites are accepted reluctantly by patients. They can be minimized with the use of topical vasoconstricting anesthetic agents, cutaneous preinjection and postinjection cooling with Natragel masks and ice, and postinjection pressure application.

Hyaluronic Acid

Mild transient localized erythema is the exception rather than the rule following hyaluronic acid implantation. Local areas of induration and gel aggregation can often be palpated for several days at the injection sites. Although they are rarely visible, the patient should be told that this is not unusual and will become less apparent with time. Following lip augmentation, superficial injections can leave more visible lumps. Because the product is very hydrophilic, any localized irritation and increased secondary edema will increase their prominence. This can be avoided if the patients are instructed not to continue rubbing the areas with the tongue. In areas of superficial implantation or translucent skin, the gel may be visualized as a gray shadow through the skin. Most female patients prefer the correction of the cutaneous depression and do not object to the grayish shadow. However, we give them the choice before the treatment. Localized edema following implantation is usually not problematic and may even accentuate the correction. We instruct our patients that if the correction is less evident in 5 to 7 days, this is not because the gel has dissipated but, rather, because they need more volume implanted. We ask the patients to return in 7 to 10 days for a possible touch-up. During 1996 and 1997, we saw two cases of sterile, suppurating granulomas with onsets 10 to 14 days following their initial injections. One required incision and drainage, the other was self-limited with complete resolution after 16 days. We have seen no other similar reactions with Restylane or Perlane since 1997.[6,7] Delayed reaction to Hylaform or Hylaform Plus may be somewhat different because they are cross-linked products of avian origin.

In areas where there has been an overfilling or where the implantation of hyaluronic acid has been too superficial, patients may not want to wait for the naturally occurring breakdown. These areas can be injected with hyaluronidase. Hyaluronidase is no longer commercially available, but it is still utilized on occasion during cataract surgery and can be ordered from compounding pharmacies.

Collagen

Bovine collagen requires two skin tests before use because the first skin test may function as a sensitization. Even patients with two negative skin tests may eventually exhibit an inflammatory response following implantation, requiring corticosteroid injections; these patients may develop localized atrophy at the injection sites. Many patients who have long histories of implantation develop subcutaneous cicatrization. This becomes evident when other products are used for volume augmentation at a later date. There has also been some controversy regarding sequential collagen implantation and the development or exacerbation of autoimmune and collagen-vascular diseases.[34–38]

Although patients with known inflammatory responses to collagen are discouraged from undergoing further treatments with human fibroblast derived collagen, it is hoped that these products will produce less inflammatory responses in fewer patients.

Microspheres

Products containing PMMA microspheres should not be used in the periorbital area because there is the possibility of a retrograde venous injection and central retinal vein occlusion with secondary blindness. Although the exact percentage has not been published, many of these patients develop granulomas. We have seen several patients who have been referred from Europe who have developed skin ulcerations. The products using bovine collagen to suspend the microspheres will also have complications secondary to bovine collagen use. Products containing hyaluronic acid may have complications secondary to its use (and its source).

Polylactic Acid

This product has to be reconstituted and mixed very well before use. If it is not mixed thoroughly enough or not sufficiently diluted, there may be an increased incidence of granuloma formation. If it is not used immediately upon mixing, it will clog the needle and require frequent needle changes. If it is not sufficiently diluted, there may be an increased likelihood of irregularity (pers. comm., Anne-Lise Lauffenburger, Switzerland, and Stephan Bessler).

Silicone

Microdroplet usage of ultrapurified silicone in properly selected patients may avoid the extreme and often unrepairable complications secondary to its abuse. Large volumes that have been injected will migrate with time. Because of the adjacent inflammatory reaction, these masses of silicone will be difficult or impossible to resect without leaving significant soft tissue deformities.

◆ The Future

New injectable tissue augmentation materials are already in the pipeline. Restylane is being used in Europe for facial contouring. It is more viscous and longer lasting than Perlane, lasting approximately 1 year. In Sweden, Q-Med Sweden's new product Macrolane,[2] much more viscous than Perlane and lasting 2 years, is undergoing clinical trials as an injectable breast implant. This product may also be valuable as an orbital implant. An existing Q-Med product, Deflux, is currently FDA approved for urinary incontinence alleviation.[2] It contains dextranomers and can last more than 2 years. Because it creates a gray cast to the skin, however, Q-Med Sweden discourages its subcutaneous use. This product however, may also be useful as an orbital implant.

Products containing a combination of hyaluronic acid and dextranomers may eventually be the key to longer lasting corrections of facial surface and contour irregularities. Also, there clearly will be great potential for stem cell implantation in the future.

References

1. Ellis DA, Makdesssian AS, Brown DJ. Survey of future injectables. Facial Plast Surg Clin North Am 2001;9:405–411
2. Agerup B, Wik O. NASHA: The Monograph. Uppsala, Sweden: Q-Med; 2001
3. Bosniak S. Superior sulcus deformities: a new solution to an old problem. Mexico City Association Para Evitar La Ceguera En Mexico, Mexico City, September 8, 1995
4. Bosniak S. The injectable orbital implant. American Academy of Ophthalmology, Joint Session with American Society of Ocularists, Atlanta Georgia, October 29, 1995
5. Cantisano-Zilkha M, Bosniak S. Hyaluronic acid gel injections for facial rejuvenation: a three-year clinical experience. Operative Techniques in Oculoplastic, Orbital, and Reconstructive Surgery. 1999;2:177–181
6. Bosniak S, Cantisano-Zilkha M. Restylane hyaluronic acid gel for facial rejuvenation: a $4^1/_2$ year experience. J Cosmet Laser Ther 2001;3:192–193
7. Bosniak S, Cantisano-Zilkha M, Glavas IP. Non-animal stabilized hyaluronic acid for lip augmentation and facial rhytid ablation. Arch Facial Plast Surg 2004;6:379–383
8. Olenius M. The first clinical study using a new biodegradable implant for the treatment of lips, wrinkles, and folds. Aesthetic Plast Surg 1998;22:97–101
9. Bousquet MT, Agerup B. Restylane lip implantation: European experience. Operative Techniques in Oculoplastic, Orbital, and Reconstructive Surgery. 1999;2:171–176
10. Narins RS, Brandt F, Leyden J, Lorenc ZP, Rubin M, Smith S. A randomized, double blind, multicenter comparison of the efficacy and tolerability of Restylane versus Zyplast for the correction of nasolabial folds. Dermatol Surg 2003;29:588–595
11. Carruthers J, Carruthers A. A prospective, randomized, parallel group study analyzing the effect of BTX-A (Botox) and nonanimal sourced hyaluronic acid (NASHA, Restylane) in combination compared with NASHA (Restylane) alone in severe glabellar rhytides in adult female subjects: treatment of severe glabellar rhytides with a hyaluronic acid derivative compared with the derivative and BTX-A. Dermatol Surg 2003;29:802–809
12. Larsen NE, Bosniak SL, Miller K. Evaluation (in vivo) of Hylan B (Hylan gel) soft tissue implants. Transactions of the Society for Biomaterials, March 1995
13. Larsen NE, Bosniak SL. Evaluation of Hylan B gel soft tissue implants. J Progressive Clin Insights 1995;3:10
14. Knapp TR, Kaplan EN, Daniels JR. Injectable collagen for soft tissue augmentation. Plast Reconstr Surg 1977;60:398–405
15. Yarborough JM. The treatment of soft tissue defects with injectable collagen. Am J Med Sci 1985;290:28–31
16. Castrow FF II, Krull EA. Injectable collagen implant: update. J Am Acad Dermatol 1983;9:889–893
17. Fagien S. Autologous collagen injections to treat deep glabellar furrows. Plast Reconstr Surg 1994;93:642
18. Knapp TR, Vistnes LM. The augmentation of soft tissue with injectable collagen. Clin Plast Surg 1985;12:221–225
19. Klein AW. Implantation technics for injectable collagen: two and one-half years of personal clinical experience. J Am Acad Dermatol 1983;9:224–228
20. Elson ML. Clinical assessment of Zyplast implant: a year of experience for soft tissue contour correction. J Am Acad Dermatol 1988;18(4 pt 1):707–713
21. Webster RC, Kattner MD, Smith RC. Injectable collagen for augmentation of facial areas. Arch Otolaryngol 1984;110: 652–656
22. Belange G, Elbaz JS. The role of an immunologic survey prior to using collagen implants: theoretical aspects and practical methods [in French]. Ann Chir Plast Esthet 1989;34:69–72
23. Hexsel DM, Hexsel CL, Iyengar V. Liquid injectable silicone: history, mechanism of action, indications, technique, and complications. Semin Cutan Med Surg 2003;22:107–114
24. Naoum C, Dasiou-Plakida D, Pantelidaki K, et al. A histological and immunohistochemical study of medical-grade fluid silicone. Dermatol Surg 1998;24:867–870

25. Matti BA, Nicolle FV. Clinical use of Zyplast in correction of age- and disease-related contour deficiencies of the face. Aesthetic Plast Surg 1990;14:227–234
26. Stegman SJ, Chu S, Bensch K, Armstrong R. A light and electron microscopic evaluation of Zyderm collagen and Zyplast implants in aging human facial skin: a pilot study. Arch Dermatol 1987;123:1644–1649
27. Lemperle G, Morhenn V, Charrier U. Human histology and persistence of various injectable filler substances for soft tissue augmentation. Aesthetic Plast Surg 2003;27:354–367
28. Fagien S. Facial soft tissue augmentation with injectable autologous and allogenic human tissue collagen matrix (autologen and dermalogen). Plast Reconstr Surg 2000;105:362–373
29. West T, Alser T. Autologous human collagen and dermal fibroblasts for soft tissue augmentation. Dermatol Surg 1998;24:510–512
30. Goncalves de Lucen a Filho, E. Estou te enviando o caso, a presentado no congresso brasileiro de retina e vitreov de 2004. Presented of the 29th Brazilian Congress of Retina and Vitreo, Florianopolis, Santa Catarina, Brazil, April 1–3, 2004
31. Orentreich DS, Orentreich N. Injectable fluid silicone. In Roenigk R, Roenigk HH, eds. Dermatologic Surgery: Principles and Practice. New York: Marcel Dekker; 1989:1349–1395
32. Polack SV. Silicone, fibrel, and collagen implantation for facial lines and wrinkles. J Dermatol Surg Oncol 1990;16:957–961
33. Alkek DS. Lip augmentation with silicone. J Dermatol Surg Oncol 1991;17:747–748
34. Keefe J, Wauk L, Chu S, DeLustro F. Clinical use of injectable bovine collagen: a decade of experience. Clin Mater 1992; 9:155–162
35. Hanke CW, Higley HR, Jolivette DM, Swanson NA, Stegman SJ. Abscess formation and local necrosis after treatment with Zyderm or Zyplast collagen implant. J Am Acad Dermatol 1991;25(2 pt 1):319–326
36. Moscona RR, Bergman R, Friedman-Birnbaum R. An unusual late reaction to Zyderm 1 injections: a challenge for treatment. Plast Reconstr Surg 1993;92:331–334
37. Cukier J, Beauchamp RA, Spindler JS, Spindler S, Lorenzo C, Trentham DE. Association between bovine collagen dermal implants and a dermatomyositis or a polymyositis-like syndrome. Ann Intern Med 1993;118:920–928
38. Trautinger F, Kokoschka EM, Menzel EJ. Antibody formation against human collagen and C1q in response to a bovine collagen implant. Arch Dermatol Res 1991;283:395–399

7

Facial Rejuvenation with Autologous Fat Injections

Roxanne Stambuk Panicacci and Karyn Grossman

Natural-appearing rejuvenation should be one of the overall goals of facial aesthetic surgery. For many years, the focus of surgical procedures has been on lifting lax skin, fat, and muscle. The face ages not only with ptosis, however, but also with fat atrophy. To correct these atrophic changes, filling materials are used. Although the search for the perfect filler material continues, fat is clearly coming to the forefront as a safe, noninflammatory, autologous material that plays a significant role in facial rejuvenation. This chapter reviews the history of fat transfer, our approach to fat transfer, and the controversies surrounding fat transfer to provide the cosmetic surgeon with a comprehensive review of this helpful technique of rejuvenation.

Neuber, who transplanted fat grafts from the arm to correct a facial soft tissue defect in 1893, presented the initial concept of autologous fat transfer.[1] He noted some success to transferring en bloc fat grafts to sites as long as they were smaller than an almond in size. Advances have been refined over the years from transferring bulk parcels of excised fat tissue from one site to another site to transferring liposuctioned fat strands to precise locations in 1 to 2 mL amounts. The history of fat transfer is reviewed excellently in many articles.[2–7] Bruning implemented fat injection to correct postrhinoplasty defects.[8] Peer helped to determine that ~50% of fat remained present after fat transplant.[9] In 1976, Fischer and Fischer performed fat extraction with a cellusuctiotome.[10] More recent historical contributions in fat transfer to the skin come from Illouz, who refined the technique of liposuction and reinjected fat from liposuction procedures to correct surgical soft tissue defects.[11,12] Fournier also made a key contribution by demonstrating "microlipoinjection" fat harvesting with 13-gauge needles attached to syringes combined with subcutaneous injections.[13] With the innovation of Klein's introduction of tumescent anesthesia,[14] infiltration of fat with large amounts of dilute anesthesia facilitated fat harvesting. Many authors have subsequently made key refinements in fat harvesting and injection techniques and optimization to promote fat injection survivability.[4,15–20]

In addition to facial rejuvenation, fat transfer has been used to solve the problems of unequal distribution of fat in facial hemiatrophy and lipodystrophy.[21] Many specialties including ophthalmology, neurosurgery, orthopedics, otolaryngology, and urology have used fat transfer techniques as a resource to restore structure and function to their respective areas of practice.[22–24]

There are many different techniques of fat transfer and supportive theories for these techniques. This has led to some confusion for many in regard to this procedure. Techniques range from the injection of only fresh fat, to the injection of only frozen fat, or a combination of both. Different authors also disagree on fat injection techniques, including fat preparation, instrumentation, and the method by which it is injected. Due to these wide variables, it is often difficult to compare different results in the literature. In the technique described here, fresh fat is injected on the initial visit, and frozen fat is injected on follow-up appointments.

To understand where to enhance the aging face with fat injection, one must first understand typical aging patterns of the face. Wrinkles, laxity, ptosis, fat atrophy, and fat hypertrophy tend to occur over time. Wrinkles, dyschromia, and telangiectasia are well treated with various procedures including ablative and nonablative laser treatments and botulinum toxin injections. Laxity and ptosis, which are usually related to intrinsic aging, manifest as brow ptosis, malar ptosis, jowl formation, and neck aging. These have typically been corrected with procedures including brow lifts, face and neck lifts, blepharoplasty, and treatments with a nonablative radiofrequency device (ThermaCool, Thermage Inc., Hayward, California). Although these procedures are adept at controlling laxity, patients often complain that they appear drawn or gaunt. The patient loses a perceived fullness in the face after these areas are lifted. After the lift, the remaining fat atrophy is more evident with hollowness in the buccal fat area, nasolabial or melolabial folds, mental area, lips, temporal fossa, and periorbital tissues. The lower two thirds of the face require volume replacement to restore the roundness and softness of the originally younger face. Volume can also be used in the upper face to create a more youthful contour of the forehead and ocular areas. Occasionally, areas of fat hypertrophy, which tend to occur in the submental region, the infraorbital fat pads, and jowling along the jawline, may require fat removal to re-create the soft fluid lines of a younger face. The progression of facial aging may be delayed through the usage of fat as a filler to structurally augment the supporting framework. The option of rejuvenation through fat injection is especially helpful for the younger generation, which may not need the lifting correction of a conventional surgical facelift. Thus fat injections are used in both younger and older patients to restore a youthful, fuller facial appearance.

Many of these indications can be corrected with various filler substances. When evaluating a filler substance, one wants to look for several characteristics. The substance ideally provides persistent and predictable correction via a reproducible technique. It is easily obtainable or fabricated, noninflammatory, noncarcinogenic, nonmigratory, multipurpose, biodegradable, and cost effective. There are quite a few available filler substances to restore the face, and many of them meet, to varying degrees, the properties of the ideal filler substance. However, fat is the only autologous long-lasting, noninflammatory product available. Although controversy exists as to the length that fat lasts, it is still an outstanding filler substance. The main limitations to fat injections are the inability to inject fat into small, superficial rhytids as well as a lack of donor site fat in certain individuals.

◆ Indications for Lipotransfer

Indications for autologous fat transfer include aging-related changes of the face, scars, and nonfacial changes. When approaching fat as a filler substance, it can be used to correct the nasolabial folds and oral commissures. It can also be fanned into areas to correct atrophy of the chin, buccal fat loss, and temporal wasting. Fat can also be placed into the infrabrow area to re-create upper lid fullness, which is associated with the perception of youth. Fat may also be used in the infraorbital area and nasojugal groove, but with caution, because these areas have a tendency to resorb unevenly, leaving small bumps. Correction of malar pouches can be accomplished by using fat to fill this area, as well as laterally to augment the cheekbones. Fat is also helpful for lip augmentation. Scarring indications include distensible acne scarring, trauma-related scarring, and atrophic congenital or acquired defects. Other enhanceable areas include the hands,[25] and other body contour defects.

◆ Patient Selection and Preoperative Evaluation

Any patient with the appropriate indications and sufficient donor fat can be a good candidate for this surgical procedure. Because this particular technique is performed with local anesthesia, an ideal candidate should not have extreme concerns in regard to being awake. In such instances, this procedure can be performed with intravenous sedation. Preoperative evaluation includes the benefits of the procedure for the patient, as well as a detailed discussion of the inherent risks. It is important that patients understand the filling nature of this procedure, and the slow building process that ensues. Routine preoperative laboratories and other indicated tests and medical clearance are performed. Antibiotics are started on the morning of the procedure and are continued for 5 days.

◆ Lipoharvesting

These authors prefer to use either outer thigh or hip lipocytes because these areas are usually the easiest to obtain and thus less traumatic for the patient. The authors use abdominal fat as a second choice because this fat tends to be more fibrous and, thus, more difficult to reinject. Overall, the site is dictated by where a sufficient quantity of donor material is obtainable. The selected site is demarcated with a surgical pen while the patient is standing to ensure a smooth contour. Most patients appreciate preoperative relaxation with oral valium dosages of 5 to 10 mg and/or one oral Vicodin.

Fat harvesting is accomplished while the patient is recumbent with the maintenance of sterile technique in an accredited surgical suite. After the patient is prepped and draped, a small wheal of 1% lidocaine is injected at the sites of insertion of the cannula. Approximately 120 mL of the tumescent solution (Table **7–1**) are injected into each donor site utilizing 60 mL syringes and a Luer locking syringe 20 cm, 2 mm radial injection

Table 7–1 Tumescent Anesthetic Solution (5 mg/kg lidocaine for 50 kg patient)

225 mL	Intravenous normal saline
12.5 mL	2% lidocaine (250 mg)
1 mL	Adrenaline 1:1000

cannula. The tumescent anesthesia is injected with a fanning radial motion into the donor site. Within 15 minutes, the tumescent solution has distributed to provide adequate anesthesia and vasoconstriction to minimize bleeding. Harvesting is performed with a blunt-tipped triport aperture microcannula 17 cm in length with a 2 or 3 mm aperture attached to a 60 mL syringe with a snapper device to maintain suction. A fanning radial motion with the dominant hand is used to remove 35 to 60 mL of fat cells per site (Fig. **7–1**). The syringe is capped and gravity is used to separate the fat cells, the supernatant, from the serosanguinous infranatant and intervening triglyceride layer. The infranatant and triglyceride layers are then discarded. If there are large quantities of heme, the remaining fat is washed with sterile saline and allowed to separate with gravity again. No centrifugation is performed. This supernatant fat is transferred via female–female transfer Luer locks to 3 mL syringes labeled with the patient's name, Social Security number, and procedure date. The harvested fat is stored in a centrally alarmed freezer at −20°C for 12 to 18 months.

◆ Lipoinjection Technique

The areas to be injected for facial rejuvenation are reviewed and marked as shown (Fig. **7–2**). For the initial injection of the freshly harvested tissue, either or both

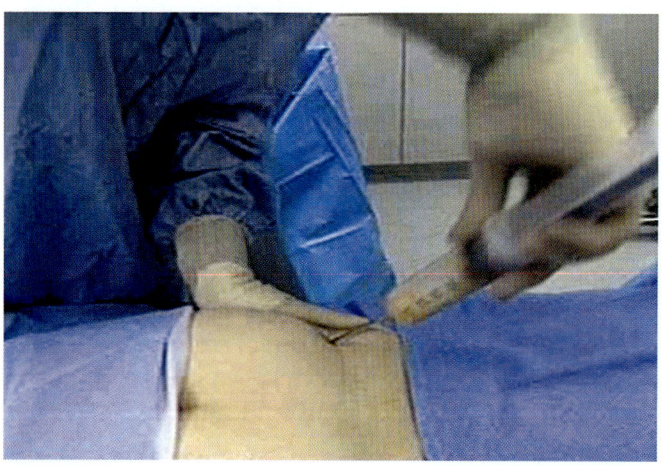

Figure 7–1 Lipoharvesting technique. A fanning radial motion with a 60 mL syringe with snapper device removes 35 to 60 mL of fat cells from the outer thigh.

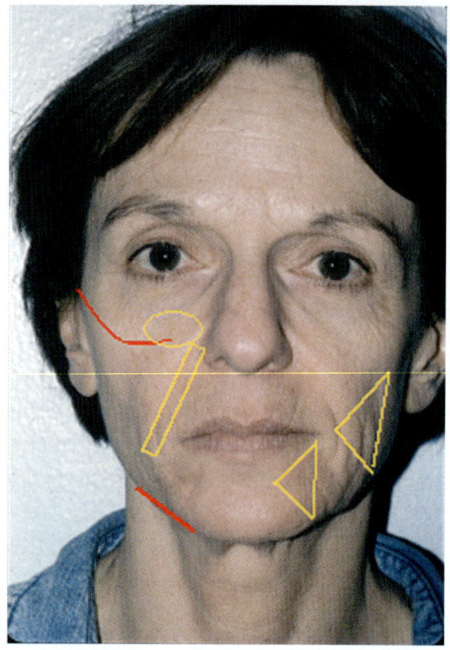

Figure 7–2 Injection areas. The cheek, nasolabial, malar cheek, and chin areas outlined in yellow are injected with autologous fat to provide filling and fullness in those areas. The cheekbone and jaw areas outlined in red are injected to provide structural augmentation.

local and regional anesthetic blocks are performed. The 3 mL syringe is attached to an 18-gauge, 2-inch, blunt-tipped, side-port microcannula. An 18-gauge needle is used to make initial puncture sites. The microcannula is placed into the deep subcutaneous plane parallel to the surface of the skin (Fig. **7–3**). This placement may be

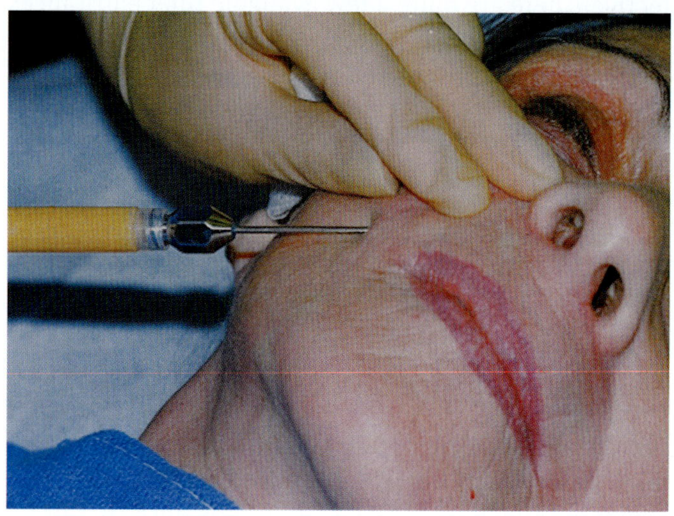

Figure 7–3 Lipoinjection technique. After local anesthesia or regional blocks (lips), and passage of fresh fat once through a Luer–Luer transfer adapter, fat is injected into the nasolabial folds through 18-gauge needle puncture sites via an 18-gauge, 2-inch, blunt-tipped, side-port microcannula.

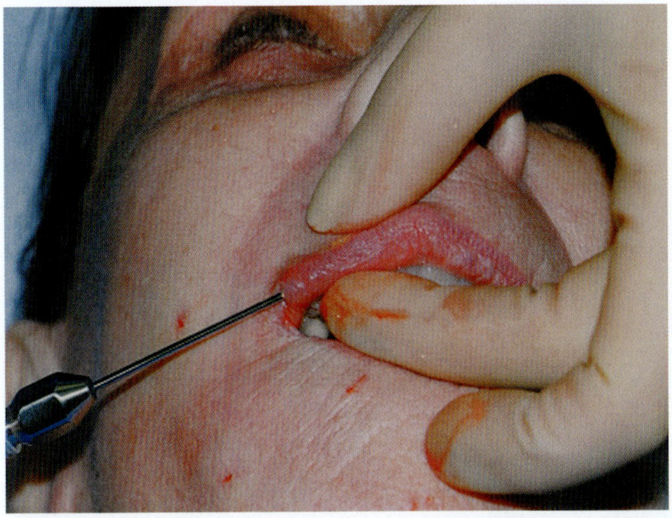

Figure 7–4 Lipoinjection technique. The microcannula is placed into the deep subcutaneous plane parallel to the surface of the skin, and the fat is injected on slow withdrawal in a retrograde fashion. The cannula may be repositioned in more superficial planes, and additional injections may be performed. Gentle compression with the fingers is used to mold the injected fat. With fresh fat, the goal is a 15 to 35% overcorrection.

either into the muscle tissue or into the subcutaneous fat layer. The fat is then injected on slow withdrawal in a retrograde fashion. The cannula is repositioned, either in a more superficial plane as in the nasolabial folds, or more laterally as in the cheek and chin area, and more fat is injected. Gentle compression is used to mold the fat (Fig. **7–4**). Enough fat is injected to achieve a 15 to 35% overcorrection. Injections into the lip can be into the vermilion border to define the lip or into the body of the lip to augment the size. Ice packs are applied to minimize swelling and discomfort.

◆ Follow-up Injections of Frozen Fat

Follow-up injections of frozen fat are repeated at 4- to 6-week intervals. To avoid specimen error, the patient's name and Social Security number are checked and initialed by the physician and assistant. The patient thaws the syringe of fat under the axilla or hands. Any small bit of watery infranatant is decanted. The fat is passed through a Luer–Luer transfer adapter and the syringe is attached to a 20-gauge, 1.5-inch needle for injection. Typically, no anesthesia is used except for blocks when the lips are injected. The frozen fat is injected in a similar manner to fresh fat lipoinjection already explained. No overcorrection is obtained, however. Ice packs are applied to decrease swelling and discomfort.

◆ Adverse Sequelae and Complications

Patients will typically experience minimal discomfort, mild edema for 2 to 3 days, and small scabbing at the cannula insertion sites with the initial injections. Other mild sequelae may include ecchymosis and, more rarely, hematoma formation. Patients may experience a sense of fullness and complain of temporary palpable but not visible lumping. If present, this will typically resolve over 2 to 5 days. Fat does not necessarily reabsorb evenly. Thus follow-up injections will be used to correct any initial asymmetry or asymmetric resorption. Erythema may occasionally occur over the injected areas.

The most concerning complications are vascular occlusions. Presumably fat that is either lodged against a blood vessel or placed within the lumen causes decreased blood flow to a given area. This occurrence becomes apparent when the skin initially blanches and then develops a gray-blue hue. If insufficient collateral blood flow is present, subsequent tissue necrosis and scar formation will result. Rapid treatment with topical nitropaste, aspirin, massage, heat, prophylactic antibiotics, and antivirals may help to avert permanent sequelae. Some have advocated hospitalization with heparinization in severe cases. There are several reports of blindness associated with periorbital glabellar correction,[26] and vision loss after injection into the nasolabial groove.[27] These presumably occur via reverse flow of fatty material through branches of the carotid arteries.[28] Some attribute increased risk of this complication to injection with a sharp-tipped instrument,[29] whereas others attribute it to injection with higher-pressure syringes greater than 1 mL.[30] Other complications include punctate scarring or pigmentation at the needle injection site, fat migration, and periorbital ridging. Uneven resorption or lumpiness associated with superficial fat placement as well as lipomatous cyst formation may respond to steroid, ultrasound, or microliposuction.[31] Rarely, infections with *Staphylococcus, Enterococcus, Streptococcus,* or *Mycobacterium* species may develop.[3,31] Marginal mandibular nerve injury, dysethesia, and parotitis are additional possible sequelae.[29]

◆ Clinical Examples

To demonstrate the ranges of improvements in facial rejuvenation with this technique of autologous fat injection, we have included some clinical examples. Fat injection around the mouth can achieve generalized softening, roundness, and filling of the nasolabial folds. When autologous fat is injected around the orbital rim and under the brow, the pupil appears larger and the supratarsal crease is less apparent. Overall, this

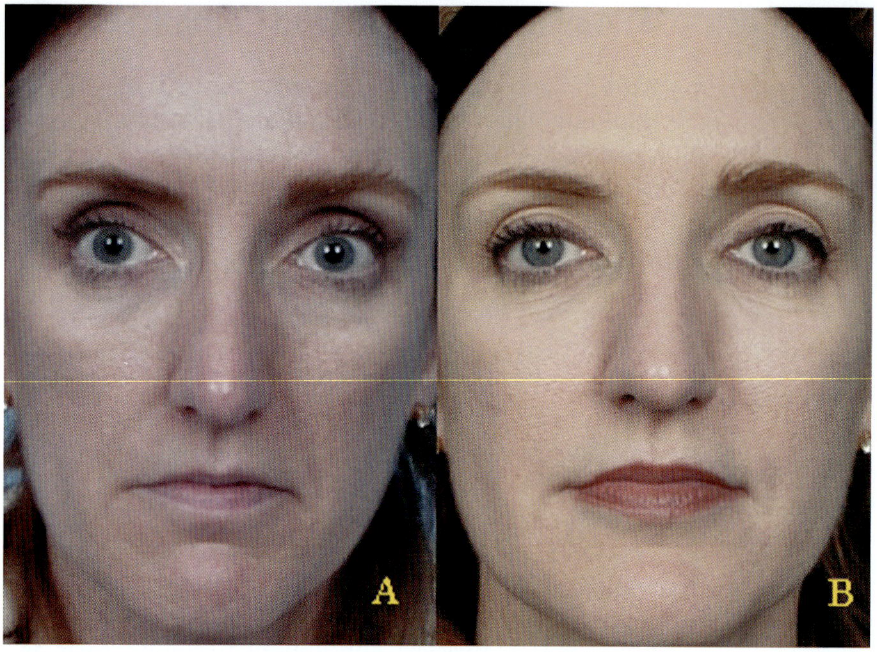

Figure 7–5 (**A**) A middle-aged woman before facial lipoinjection. (**B**) Five months after last injection.

technique enhances the patient's natural features (Fig. **7–5A,B**).

◆ Controversies

Most of the controversy regarding lipotransfer surrounds the viability of the grafted adipocytes. Different authors have varying theories as to how much fat survives and how this is accomplished. Thus many different techniques have developed. Due to the proliferation of techniques, many of the fundamental questions regarding lipotransfer have remained unanswered. The estimates of fat graft survivability are reported, in part, through results with two-dimensional photography, which are difficult to compare with an actual three-dimensional change with augmentation. The patients themselves may also pursue other techniques of rejuvenation simultaneously. This may confound the results of one technique versus combined techniques. As we all do, the patient continues to intrinsically age, and thus the evidence-based criteria, when applied 6 months, 1 year, and 2 years out from the procedure, are difficult to assess. Controversy remains concerning adipocyte cell viability and its relation to the harvesting technique, storage, and freezing of fat, and recipient site characteristics.

Some degree of debate exists as to the preferred site for harvesting fat. Some prefer areas with high lipogenic activity, including the outer thighs, buttocks, and abdominal regions.[32] Others prefer areas that are resistant to weight change: abdominal fat in men and outer thigh fat in women.[16,22,33]

One of the controversies regarding the harvesting technique centers around the concern whether adipocyte trauma affects ultimate adipocyte cell viability. Different authors feel that the use of machine-assisted or syringe liposuction results in different degrees of trauma to the cells. Those supporting machine-assisted liposuction advocate blunt-tipped microcannulas with diameters of 1.5 to 3 mm because the multihole cannulas allow for constant low suction pressure with minimal trauma and fibrous tissue.[34] Others caution against using high negative-pressure suction systems because they may cause excess fat traumatization.[24] When using machine-assisted suction for harvesting, however, one needs a special trap to catch the fat and to maintain a sterile environment. Thus many support the use of a closed syringe system to minimize possible contamination. However, even among syringe harvesters, there is still considerable debate as to the size of the syringe and whether to use an attached cannula or needle. Dr. Fournier advocates obtaining fat with a 14-gauge, 2 mm needle to get "cores of adipose tissue."[35] Various authors use either 30 or 60 mL syringes to harvest, although proponents of 10 mL syringes feel that the smaller syringes minimize pressure-induced fat trauma.[24] Fat that has been harvested with 60 mL syringes and washed in saline has been maintained in cell cultures for up to 2 months.[36] In spite of varying opinions, similar fat survival rates have been demonstrated with both techniques as evaluated by glycerol-3-phosphate dehydrogenase enzyme assay.[37]

The presence or absence of lidocaine in the tumescent and/or storage material has also been debated. Some feel that lidocaine is helpful for fat viability. Studies support that it inhibits glucose transport and fat lipolysis[38] and provides a supportive environment for wound healing.[39,40] Others note that high levels of lidocaine are toxic to adipocytes and recommend minimal lidocaine concentrations.[38] One group supports the use of prilocaine instead of lidocaine because it is eliminated by the lungs and kidneys as well as the liver with minimal cytochrome P450 3A4 enzyme interactions.[34] However, safety studies with large doses of prilocaine have not been conducted and lidocaine has a well-established safety record in tumescent anesthesia.

Another area of disagreement is whether to wash the harvested fat samples once they are obtained. There is overall agreement that the presence of blood in transplanted fat samples leads to fat degradation.[41] The premise is that washing leads to decreased blood in the fat and decreased free lipids with improved healing and less of an inflammatory response with macrophages.[2] Decreased specimen manipulation without washing may have the advantage of increased fat survival.

How and what to wash the fat with sparks other debates. Some wash with normal saline; some prefer Ringer's lactate solution due to decreased stimulation of glucose metabolism in fat.[16] Centrifugation may also be used to remove residual lidocaine or heme from the adipose specimen. Many centrifuge the fat for 2 minutes to separate the supernatant from the infranatant and to define the triglyceride layer.[42,43] In addition to removing heme, lidocaine, and triglycerides, centrifugation will also compact the fat cells. Proponents of this technique support more consistent results with a more concentrated fat sample injection. Varying amounts of residual tumescent liquid make it more difficult for the surgeon to accurately judge the true volume of adipocytes injected. In a study of 14 patients, a greater degree of long-term correction was obtained with the injection of centrifuged fat as compared with noncentrifuged fat during dorsal hand fat augmentation.[44] Comparison of the degree of fat trauma demonstrated no difference between washing, centrifugation, or no washing.[41]

The controversy over the use of frozen adipose tissue is at the center of most debates on this technique of facial rejuvenation. If fat can be stored in a frozen state, the ideal storage time and method of freezing are also controversial. Coleman reports no bacterial contamination of frozen fat at 6 months.[42] Other groups have used stored frozen fat for successful augmentation without complications at 1, 2, and even 7 years after the original harvest.[45,46] We have stored fat for 2 years and also have found no bacterial contamination. When examining the reabsorption rates of both freshly injected and frozen fat, both result in reabsorption rates of 30 to 70% within the first 6 weeks of injection.[46] Some groups believe that using frozen fat is better than fresh fat because thawing leads to increased fat density with less swelling and bruising.[47]

Whether fat cells remain viable after freezing has come to the forefront in this controversy. Many clinicians have injected frozen fat with good clinical outcomes.[5,24,30] However, others believe that only fresh fat will graft and retain long-term correction with live adipocytes. At least two groups show that fat cells survive freezing to −20°C followed by thawing because the majority of cells did not take up trypan blue dye.[48,49] Sommer and Sattler demonstrate significant cell viability after 3 years at −20°C with the trypan blue dye method.[41] Despite these demonstrations of cell viability with staining methods, however, it was not possible to culture viable adipocytes or stem cells from fat that had been frozen to −20°C without using cryoprotectant.[50] To store the harvested fat, most slow freeze to −20°C[41] because flash freezing may destroy adipocytes.[43]

How the adipocytes are transferred into the tissue may also affect graft viability. Coleman advocates the "lipostructure" approach where the face is structurally augmented through layers of fat, which are bluntly injected at multiple levels upward from the periosteum level.[29] Tiny amounts of tissue are injected with each pass, resulting in numerous criss-crossing thin tunnels of fat because, in order for cells to graft, they need to be in contact with viable tissue to provide nutrients via diffusion. Angiogenesis also needs to occur to allow true cell graft survival. Although there is documented success with this approach, there is a relatively long recovery time from this procedure.[29,42] Donofrio uses a "panfacial" technique to restore the face to its youthful natural rotundity by injecting small amounts of fat into multiple layers from just above the bone level upward to the subcutaneous area and upward to create a three-dimensional, pleasing augmentation.[30,51] The fat autograft muscle injection (FAMI) technique developed by Amar promotes the injection of fat into seven muscle groups of the face with cannulas.[52] The "liporecycling" technique of Sattler and Sommer describes machine-assisted liposuction and then injection through a 24-gauge needle to dermal and subdermal areas.[34]

Other authors support the use of single-layered subdermal injections. Many authors have combined or blended these two techniques to optimize the potential theoretical benefits of each one. All of these approaches try to place the fat in close proximity to vascular supportive environments to encourage the graft to take and provide longer-term correction. Carpaneta's key study in this area emphasizes success with fat placement within 1.5 mm of viable vascularized tissue.[18] Relative recipient site vascularity has also been reported to support the grafting of cells.[47,52,53] At the same time, fat transfer tissue survives in relatively less vascular tissue such as facial hemiatrophy and scars.[48] In our practice, we use a gently layered, multiinjection technique, which allows for an even layering of facial fat. There is concern that the volume of injected fat may alter potential tissue vascularization. It may be helpful to transfer less than 0.5 mL to the same site to ensure vascularization,[19,54] although we have routinely injected larger volumes than this without adverse affect.

Much of the controversy regarding lipotransfer surrounds the viability of the grafted adipocytes. Different authors have varying theories as to how much fat survives and how this survival is obtained. Numerous factors go into the final result obtained. Because there are numerous fat injection techniques, long-term studies are difficult to compare. Some feel that correction is due to true adipocyte graft and survival, others to fibrosis, and others to a blend of the above. Several histological studies addressing the fate of injected fat have been conducted. The mechanism of augmentation involves both adipocyte augmentation through the fat cells' continued survival via neovascularization and a mass effect of fibroblastic proliferation.[19,43] Most agree that the bulk of fat survival is attributed to the cell survival theory. After fat transfer, some cells die and some original adipocytes survive. Some other adipocytes dedifferentiate into preadipocyte cells. These preadipocytes over time accumulate fat and mature into adipocytes. The fat graft establishes its own blood supply. The cells that have not survived are replaced eventually by fibrosis.[21,55,56]

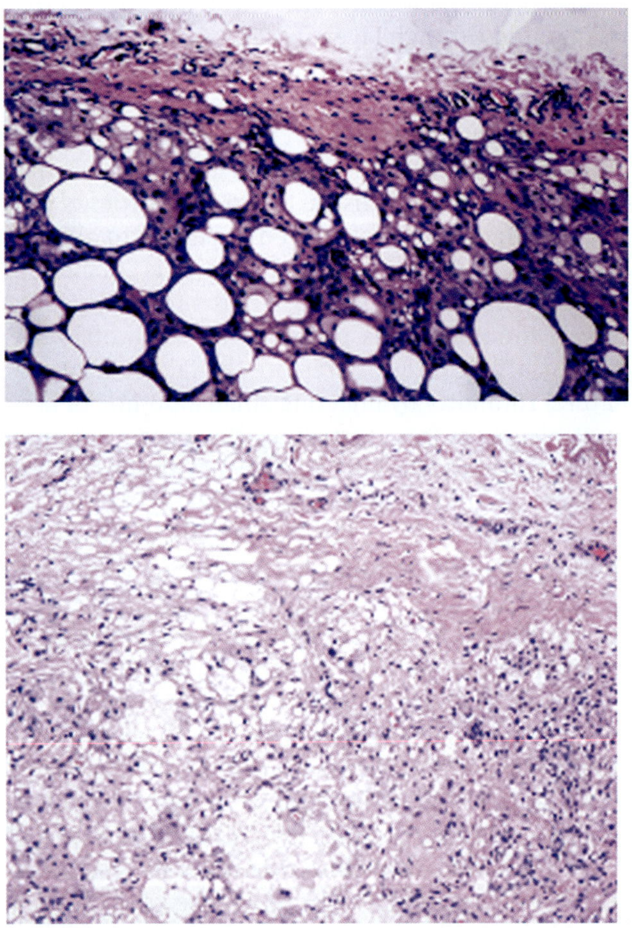

A

B

Figure 7–6 (**A,B**) Biopsies from two patients, 2 months after frozen fat injection. Both biopsies demonstrate adipocytes with surrounding fibrohistiocytic hyperplasia.

◆ Techniques and Outcomes

For the technique described by the authors, two histological samples have been taken. Both specimens were obtained from small fat nodules that occurred after the injection of frozen fat. These bumps were excised more than 2 months after the original injection. Both slides (Fig. **7–6A,B**) were read out as normal adipocytes with surrounding fibrohistiocytic hyperplasia. Our two patients have long-lasting correction, apparently due to a combination of individual adipocyte grafting and survival, in addition to the mass effect of the fibrohistiocytic fibroplasia. Depending upon different techniques, there are probably variable histological patterns that are responsible for the long-term results. Whether the clinical results seen are from the grafting of viable cells or from the space occupying fibrohistiocytic hyperplasia may be an intellectual exercise because both of these patterns are capable of providing long-lasting and sustainable results for the patients.

Overall, objective measurements of the mechanism of augmentation and persistence of augmentation are difficult to obtain. Patients will continue to age, and many patients also have multiple procedures over years. Also, cosmetic patients are typically reticent to have any biopsies. Two-dimensional photos carefully selected by each person who performs the technique add inherent bias to a result that is experienced three-dimensionally. Older literature describes 50% of the maintained volume of autologous fat transplants at 1 year.[9] Both animal models[57,58] and human studies[20,59] provide good evidence of fat survival. A small but interesting study demonstrates that fatty acid composition from the outer thighs, which is different from the recipient site at the nasolabial fold, persists after 4 months when sampled from the recipient site.[60] Magnetic resonance imaging (MRI) studies following 10 patients out over 1 year show maximum substance loss by 6 months (~55%), and then volume maintenance out to 12 months.[61] Ultrasound studies also show fat maintenance in transplanted sites for up to 1 year in congenital and acquired lipodystrophies.[62,63] The best sites for fat retention are the buccal fat pad, chin, and cheekbones. Lips and nasolabial folds show decreased retention, possibly secondary to increased mobility in these areas.[3] Eremia and Newman performed a retrospective review of 116 patients, who had at least two treatment sessions, and at least 12 months of follow-up after their last fat injections.[64] They report rapid loss of correction with the glabellar area, relatively rapid loss with the lips within 3 to 6 months, and, even, with initial correction early on, 97% loss of correction of nasolabial fold areas within 12 months. These results are in direct contrast to average reports of 50% survivability or correction in the literature, and, although they can be tempered with the fact that the study was evaluated retrospectively and with photographs, it clearly highlights the need for additional longer-term studies on fat injection.

◆ Conclusions

A general consensus on autologous fat transfer for facial rejuvenation maintains the following principles for success: harvest sites with lower vasculature and recipient sites with higher vasculature, syringe-aspirated fat after lidocaine tumescence, gravity to separate the fat supernatant, larger-bore needle/cannula for injection to prevent fat trauma, subdermal deposition of fat, and slight overcorrection for best graft survival.

There is increasing interest in using fat to rejuvenate the face. Patients are looking for injectable fillers that are safe and provide long-term correction. Although there are numerous techniques to inject fat and numerous controversies as to the best and most predictable technique, fat provides a long-lasting option to create both a filling and a lifting effect in the skin.

References

1. Neuber F. Fettransplantation. Chir Kongr Verhandl Dsch Gesellsch Chir. 1893;22:66
2. Skouge JW. Autologous fat transplantation in facial surgery. In Coleman WP, Hanks CW, Alt TH, Asken S, eds. Cosmetic Surgery of the Skin: Principles and Techniques. Philadelphia: BC Decker Publishers; 1991:239–249
3. Fulton JE, Suarez M, Silverton K. Small volume fat transfer. Dermatol Surg 1998;24:857–865
4. Newman J, Ftaiha Z. The biographical history of fat transplant surgery. Am J Cosmet Surg 1987;4:85
5. Perez MI. Update on autologous fat transplantation. Cosmetic Dermatology 2002;15:36–40
6. Billings EJ, May JJ. Historical review and present status of free fat graft autotransplantation in plastic and reconstructive surgery. Plast Reconstr Surg 1989;83:368–381
7. Klein AW, Elson ML. The history of substances for soft tissue augmentation. Dermatol Surg 2000;26:1096–2005
8. Brunning P. Contribution e l'etude des greffes adipeuses. Bull Acad R Med Belg 1914;28:440
9. Peer LA. The neglected free fat graft. Plast Reconstr Surg 1956; 18:233
10. Fischer A, Fischer G. First surgical treatment for molding body's cellulite with three 5 mm incisions. Bull Int Acad Cosmetic Surg. 1976;3:35
11. Illouz YG. De l'utilization de la graisse aspiree pour combler les defauts cutanes. Rev Chir Esth Langue Fr 1985;10:19–22
12. Illouz YG. The fat cell "graft": a new technique to fill depressions. Plast Reconstr Surg 1986;78:122–123
13. Fournier PF. Microlipoextraction et microlipoinjection. Rev Chir Esthet Lang Franc 1985;10:36–40
14. Klein JA. The tumescent technique for liposuction surgery. Am J Cosm Surg 1987;4:236–237
15. Ellenbogen R. Free autogenous pearl fat grafts in the face: a preliminary report of a rediscovered technique. Ann Plast Surg 1986;16:179–194
16. Asken S. Autologous fat transplantation: micro and macro techniques. Am J Cosmet Surg 1987;4:111–121
17. Campbell GL, Laudenslager N, Newman J. The effect of mechanical stress on adipocyte morphology and metabolism. Am J Cosmet Surg 1987;4:89–93
18. Carpaneta C. Percentage of graft viability versus injection volume in adipose auto transplant. Adv Plast Surg 1994;18:16–19
19. Niechajev I, Sevcuk O. Long-term results of fat transplantation: clinical and histologic studies. Plast Reconstr Surg 1994; 5:87–90
20. Chajchir A, Benzaquen I. Liposuction fat grafts in face wrinkles and hemifacial atrophy. Aesthetic Plast Surg 1986;10:115–117
21. Pinski JB, Roenigk HH Jr. Autologous fat transplantation: long-term follow-up. J Dermatol Surg Oncol 1992;18:179–184
22. Chairman EL. Restoration of the plantar fat pad with autopilotransplantation. J Foot Ankle Surg 1994;33:373–379
23. Brandenburg JH, Unger JM, Koschkee D. Vocal cord injection with autogenous fat: a long-term magnetic resonance imaging evaluation. Laryngoscope 1996;106:174–180
24. Markey AC, Glogau RG. Autologous fat grafting: comparison of techniques. Dermatol Surg 2000;26:1135–1139
25. Vita VT. Lipoinjection and aging hands. Am J Cosmetic Surg 1989;6:27–32
26. Teimourian B. Blindness following fat injections [letter to the editor]. Plast Reconstr Surg 1988;82:361
27. Lee DH, Yang HN, Kim JC, Shyn KH. Sudden unilateral visual loss and brain infarction after autologous fat injection into nasolabial groove. Br J Ophthalmol 1996;80:1026–1027
28. Feinendegen DL, Baumgartner RW, Vuadens P, et al. Autologous fat injection for soft tissue augmentation in the face: a safe procedure? Aesthetic Plast Surg 1998;22:163–167
29. Coleman SR. Facial recontouring with lipostructure. Clin Plast Surg 1997;24:347–367
30. Donofrio LM. Structural autologous lipoaugmentation: a panfacial technique. Dermatol Surg 2000;26:1129–1134
31. Berman M. Rejuvenation of the upper eyelid complex with autologous fat transplantation. Dermatol Surg 2000;26:1113–1116
32. Lilleth H, Boberg J. The lipoprotein-lipase activity of adipose tissue from different sites in obese women and relationship to cell size. Int J Obes 1978;2:47–52
33. Hudson DA, Lambert EV, Bloch CE. Site selection for rat autotransplantation: some observations. Aesthetic Plast Surg 1990;14:195–197
34. Sattler G, Sommer B. Liporecycling: a technique for facial rejuvenation and body contouring. Dermatol Surg 2000;26: 1140–1144

35. Fournier PF. Fat grafting: my technique. Dermatol Surg 2000;26:1117–1128
36. Jones JU, Lyles ME. The viability of human adipocytes after closed syringe liposuction harvest. Am J Cosmet Surg 1997;14:275–280
37. Lalikos JF, Li YQ, Roth TP, Doyle JW, Matory WE, Lawrence WT. Biochemical assessment of cellular damage after adipocyte harvest. J Surg Res 1997;70:95–100
38. Moore JH, Kolacynski JW, Morales LM, et al. Viability of fat obtained with syringe suction lipectomy: effects of local anesthesia with lidocaine. Aesthetic Plast Surg 1995;19:335–339
39. Skidmore RA, Patterson JD, Tomsick RS. Local anesthetics. Dermatol Surg 1996;22:511–522
40. Eriksson AS, Sinclair R, Cassuto J, Thomsen P. Influence of lidocaine on leukocyte function in the surgical wound. Anesthesiology 1992;77:74–78
41. Sommer B, Sattler G. Current concepts of fat graft survival: histology of aspirated adipose tissue and review of the literature. Dermatol Surg 2000;26:1159–1166
42. Coleman SR. Long-term survival of fat transplants: controlled demonstrations. Aesthetic Plast Surg 1995;19:421–425
43. Coleman WP, Lawrence N, Sherman RN, et al. Autologous collagen? Lipocytic dermal augmentation: a histopathological study. J Dermatol Surg Oncol 1993;19:1032–1040
44. Butterwick KJ. Lipoaugmentation for aging hands: a comparison of the longevity and aesthetic results of centrifuged versus noncentrifuged fat. Dermatol Surg 2002;28:987–991
45. Sattler G, Sommer B. Liporecycling: immediate and delayed. Am J Cosmet Surg 1997;14:311–316
46. Takasu K, Takasu S. Long-term frozen fat transplantation. Int J Cosmet Surg 1999;7:33–38
47. Saylan Z. Frozen fat: better than fresh fat. Int J Cosm Surg 1999;7:39–42
48. Schuller-Petrovic S. Improving the aesthetic aspect of soft tissue defects on the face using autologous fat transplantation. Facial Plast Surg 1997;13:119–124
49. Jackson RF. Frozen fat-does it work? Am J Cosmet Surg 1997;14:339–343
50. Moscatello DK, Dougherty M, Lawrence N, Narins R. Cryopreservation of human fat for soft tissue augmentation: viability requires use of cryoprotectant and controlled freezing and storage. J Dermatolog Surg. In press
51. Donofrio LM. Fat distribution: a morphologic study of the aging face. Dermatol Surg 2000;26:1107–1112
52. Amar RE. Microinfiltration adipocytaire (MIA) au niveau de la face ou restructuration tissulaire par graffe de tissue adipeux. Ann Ch Plast Esthet 199;44:593–608
53. Guerrerosantos J, Gonzalez-Mendoza A, Masmela Y, Gonzalez MA, Deos M, Diaz P. Long-term survival of free fat grafts in muscle: an experimental study in rats. Aesthetic Plast Surg 1996;20:403–408
54. Fournier PF. Facial recontouring with fat grafting. Dermatol Clin 1990;8:523–537
55. Van RL, Bayliss CE, Roncari DA. Cytological and enzymological characterization of adult human adipocyte precursors in culture. J Clin Invest 1976;58:699–704
56. Nguyen A, Pasyk KA, Bouvier TN, Hassett CA, Argenta LC. Comparative study of survival of autologous adipose tissue taken and transplanted by different techniques. Plast Reconstr Surg 1990;85:378–386
57. Kononas TC, Bucky LP, Hurley C, May JW Jr. The fate of suctioned and surgically removed fat after reimplantation for soft-tissue augmentation: a volumetric and histologic study in the rabbit. Plast Reconstr Surg 1993;91:763–768
58. Eppley BL, Sidner RA, Platis JM, Sadove AM. Bioactivation of free-fat transfers: a potential new approach to improving graft survival. Plast Reconstr Surg 1992;90:1022–1030
59. Ersek RA, Chang P, Salisbury MA. Lipo layering of autologous fat: an improved technique with promising results. Plast Reconstr Surg 1998;101:820–826
60. Sadick NS, Hudgins LC. Fatty acid analysis of transplanted adipose tissue. Arch Dermatol 2001;137:723–727
61. Horl HW, Feller AM, Biemer E. Technique for liposuction fat reimplantaion and long-term volume evaluation by magnetic resonance imaging. Ann Plast Surg 1991;26:248–258
62. Goldman R, Carmargo CP, Goldman B. Fat transplantation and facial contour. Am J Cosmet Surg 1998;15:41–44
63. Glogau RG. Microlipoinjection: autologous fat grafting. Arch Dermatol 1988;124:1340–1343
64. Eremia S, Newman N. Long-term follow-up after autologous fat grafting: analysis of results from 116 patients followed at least 12 months after receiving the last of a minimum of two treatments. Dermatol Surg 2000;26:1150–1158

8

Noninvasive Neck Rejuvenation

Ioannis P. Glavas and Stephen Bosniak

The neck plays an important role in patients' self-perception. Neck characteristics and qualities are idealized in the perception of feminine beauty and youth in different cultures. It is widely accepted that a long, thin, slender, "swan's" neck is a pleasant and graceful characteristic in a woman's appearance. It is not by chance that jewelry and clothing are created by fashion designers with ambition to attract the eye to the beautiful lines of the female neck. A different set of characteristics is assigned to the male neck. The ideal man's neck is more often described as a strong, muscular, thick "bull's" neck, giving an aggressive, dominant quality.

Neck rejuvenation has a balancing and complementary role in the whole approach to a youthful appearance of an individual. The chin and jawline frame the facial characteristics. The elements that influence the appearance of the neck are: the quality and texture of the skin; the amount and firmness of the subcutaneous fat; the platysma muscle strength, thickness, and form; subplatysmal fat; anatomy and prominence of submaxillary glands, thyroid cartilage, and the surrounding bones. The bony structures of the face, neck, and upper chest provide the framework for the attachment of the soft tissues.

It is apparent that the inevitable changes of time upon the tissues can affect the neck to different degrees. The skin loses its turgor and becomes wrinkled and saggy. The platysma muscle may atrophy while hypertrophic medial bands become noticeable, running from the chin down to the clavicles. Submental subcutaneous fat may increase in volume and result in a "double" chin. Jowls may become prominent and sag, further altering the midfacial contours by dragging the facial tissues inferiorly.[1–4] The above multifactorial changes cannot be corrected with any single noninvasive treatment.

Available choices for neck rejuvenation to this point have been largely surgical. Among the surgical techniques are: facialplasty, cervicofacial rhytidectomy, platysmaplasty, corset platysma repair, digastric muscle recontouring, submandibular gland resection, deep plane facelift, and suture suspension. Their goal is to restore youthful facial anatomy by removing redundant tissue or repositioning lax tissue or both.

We have developed a noninvasive, nonsurgical, three-staged approach to neck rejuvenation.[5] The skin texture and resilience are corrected with superficial chemical peels, privately compounded home care products, nonablative lasers (1320 and 1064 nm), intense pulsed light (IPL), and Thermage (radiofrequency-mediated collagen tightening) therapies (Thermage, Hayward, California). Phosphatidylcholine (Lipostabil, Aventis, France) injections reduce submental fat accumulation. Botox injections relax platysmal banding. The goal of these therapies is to globally rejuvenate the neck by promoting collagen remodeling and regeneration rather than by resection or plication.

◆ Principles of Treatment

Minimally invasive neck rejuvenation can be achieved with a combination of multiple modalities and techniques with different mechanisms of action. The ultimate goal is to combine these actions to get the maximum neck rejuvenating effect with minimum healing and recovery downtime.[6] Surgical techniques of neck rejuvenation may target specific types of tissues (skin, fat, muscle) depending on their contribution to the aging effect on the neck. But unlike the noninvasive approach, the healing time and recovery period after surgical procedures ranges from weeks to months. The ecchymosis and edema following surgical procedures may restrict the social and professional activities of the patient. For this reason many patients prefer the less invasive rejuvenation modalities even if it means that they will need repeat treatments to obtain the desirable effect and to maintain it.

◆ Pretreatment Evaluation

Establishing Patient Priorities

Sitting directly in front of the patient allows the physician to examine the patient at rest and in animation while building rapport and hearing exactly what the patient's concerns are. While looking in a mirror, the patient can point to the areas of concern, which will give the patient and the physician an opportunity to establish priorities, discuss the options, and confirm realistic expectations.[7,8]

Evaluating the Patient

The patient is examined at rest and while speaking, from the front and from each side. The patient is asked to raise the chin and to depress the chin to the chest. The quality, texture, pigmentation, and resilience of the skin are noted. The amount and location of submental fat deposits are noted. The prominence of the submandibular glands is noted. The extent and location of anterior and posterior platysmal bands are also noted. These notations are correlated to the patient's list of complaints and priorities. In this manner a treatment plan can be suggested and augmented.

Discussing Posttreatment Follow-up and Complications

Even though nonsurgical techniques are much less invasive than surgical techniques are, they are not devoid of possible complications. The risks, possible adverse effects, and alternative treatments should be discussed with the patient. Each of the different therapeutic modalities will have its own set of limitations and possible adverse effects. It is important to explain the usual course following each treatment and when the patient will begin to notice improvement following each treatment. It is also important to emphasize the need for effective maintenance.

Photographic Documentation

Photographic documentation before and after each procedure is essential for patient discussion. It facilitates implementation of future procedures and confirms the results of the recently performed procedure. Patients are photographed before each treatment, immediately after each treatment, 1 to 2 weeks following each treatment, and again after the final result has been achieved. It is most convenient to perform digital flash photographs. These can be downloaded directly into a computer for patient comparison. Although angled soft lighting is better than straight, hard light, it requires special equipment and a more complex setup in the exam/treatment room. The physician or technician taking the photographs should establish a protocol so as to obtain patient poses with the same subject angle, facial expression, magnification, and luminosity. This will make before and after comparisons more accurate and meaningful.

◆ The Setting

Minimally invasive procedures are performed in the office with the patients dressed comfortably in their own clothes while seated in an examination or treatment room. To put the patient further at ease, this should be made a relaxing and nonthreatening environment. Although there is no need for extensive preoperative evaluation and patient preparation, the physician must take all the precautions for infection control and bloodborne pathogens when performing injections or minor procedures. In addition, the room should be adequately equipped with the proper medications and equipment to efficiently address any allergic reactions, syncope episodes, or other emergency conditions related to the performed treatments.

◆ Treatment Options

There is no preset combination of treatments. Each patient is carefully examined and an individualized treatment plan is recommended. Changes in the appearance of the neck may look similar to the patient, but may result from different causes. One example is the "double chin" deformity. The patient sees a double chin regardless of its etiology. From the physician's standpoint the cause may be excess fat, lax and redundant skin, or a hypertrophic anterior platysmal muscle insertion.

The principle of rejuvenating the neck using noninvasive techniques lies on a simple concept: to rejuvenate each tissue type of the neck independently using tissue specific treatments and to combine the effects of those treatments to achieve a better result. The rationale behind this concept is that the effect of each tissue on the appearance of the neck has a different underlying mechanism. For example, skin gets wrinkled because of degenerating tissue changes, the platysma muscle degenerates and forms hypertrophic bands, and submental fat accumulates. Noninvasive neck treatments fall into one of the following groups based on their ability to:

1. Improve the texture, tone, and resilience of the skin (i.e., rejuvenate the skin)
2. Relax the neck musculature
3. Reduce the amount of unwanted fat
4. Tighten the skin

Treatments can be offered in any order and at any time independently. Our personal experience has proved that performing some treatments first helps improve the effectiveness of other subsequent treatments. We recommend addressing issues of skin quality and texture before performing skin-tightening treatments. Also, relaxing the neck musculature and reducing unwanted fat from the submental area can provide an improved anatomical foundation for the subsequent aesthetic improvement of the overlying skin and yield the desired neck contour.

Rejuvenating the Skin

Actinic damage plays a significant role in the degeneration of neck skin. Years of ultraviolet (UV) exposure contribute to the development of rhytidosis, poikiloderma, and actinic keratoses. The treatment of postmenopausal hair growth on the chin and submental areas must also be considered. The goal is to improve the texture, tone, and resilience of the skin. This can be accomplished with several treatment modalities.

Alpha hydroxy acid (AHA) peels can be used as an initial treatment. These superficial peels are the least invasive of all skin treatments. They have no downtime. They essentially exfoliate the top layers of the epidermis. The result is a soft and silky texture on the skin. Skin pigmentation can be treated with a series of weekly AHA peels.[9] A series of at least five peels, one per week, should be recommended to the patient initially to accelerate early improvement. Patients who can see some result early in the treatment regimen will be encouraged to continue and to complete the program. Although the initial concentration of AHA to be used may depend on the skin quality, it is practical to start with a 70% buffered solution, observe the patient's response, and advance to higher concentrations during subsequent treatments. After washing the face with a mild cleanser, the skin is degreased with 5% acetone to remove any residual makeup or secretions. Using cotton swab applicators the AHA is applied to the skin of the neck. A timer is set to 10 minutes. After that time (or sooner if the skin becomes erythematous) the AHA is washed from the face with water. Application of a moisturizing serum and sunblock concludes the treatment. The effects of these treatments can be maintained and prolonged by having the patient use home care products daily. The daily use of topical sunscreen and oral antioxidants is essential to prevent further actinic exposure and degeneration. If the patient will not use sunscreen on a daily basis, continued skin care is pointless.

Photorejuvenation of the skin with nonablative light-emitting devices offers impressive results with minimal downtime and minimal patient discomfort (see Chapter 2). These devices emit intense polychromatic noncoherent light in a broad wavelength spectrum of 515 to 1,200 nm.[10] IPL can be used to treat diffuse and discrete pigmented and vascular lesions of the neck skin, including poikiloderma and telangiectasias. This instrumentation can also be used to soften the demarcation between a laser-resurfaced face and an actinically damaged neck.

Specific tissue chromophores can be targeted by using the appropriate wavelength filter for the emitting light. Hemoglobin is targeted mainly at a wavelength of 580 nm. Melanin is targeted within the visible range (400–750 nm). For specifically treating pigmented lesions, a 560 nm filter is used. With a 590 nm filter both pigmented and vascular lesions can be treated[11–13] (see Chapter 2).

We prefer to pretest darker-skinned patients (Fitzpatrick type IV–VI) by treating the skin behind the ear, where any skin changes will not be visible, with two pulses of lower energy (18–20 J/cm^2), utilizing the 640 nm filter and a longer interval between pulses (40 msec). We observe the area for 30 minutes and then reexamine the area again in 1 week. We look for initial and prolonged erythema or late hyperpigmentation. If there is no evidence of transient or persistant hyperpigmentation, we proceed with the treatment. We do not treat patients with a recently acquired tan.

Clear cool gel is applied to the skin of the neck. In addition, gel applied directly to the crystal is allowed to freeze before treatment is begun. Protective goggles or dark protective glasses are worn by the patient and all other persons in the treatment room. The power is adjusted to a sufficient level so that slight erythema is observed after the treatment. When using the 590 filter, treatments typically begin with a power setting of 25 J/cm^2. Blistering and/or erythema lasting longer than several days and hyperpigmentation are rare sequelae. These usually occur when higher power settings are used or when treating patients with darker skin types. They are transient and subside with time. A series of weekly AHA peels (beginning with 70% buffered and gradually increased to 50% unbuffered) and the use of topical retinoids (0.05%), hydroquinone

(4–6%), and kojic acid can improve any residual hyperpigmentation.

Most patients report a tingling or warm sensation and only minimal discomfort while the IPL procedure is being performed. Rarely, when higher power settings are being used, topical anesthetic is applied for 15 minutes before the treatment. At the conclusion of the treatment the gel is wiped off. Residual hyperpigmentation can be treated with one or two coats of 25 or 30% trichloroacetic acid (TCA), although this will require 4 to 5 days of downtime.

The CoolTouch II (Cutera, Brisbane, California), a dynamically cooled, long-pulse 1320 nm neodymium:yttrium-aluminum-garnet (Nd:YAG) is a nonablative laser that can be added to the menu of treatments for aging and photodamaged skin. It can improve the appearance of rhytids, reduce the size of skin pores, and improve skin texture. Four to six monthly treatments are recommended. The results are initially subtle but improve over 3 to 6 months. It can be used in all skin types because its target chromophore is not melanin. Its main action is stimulation of fibroblasts to form new collagen in the skin. The epidermal layer of the skin is cooled with a cryogen spray device while the beam heats the dermal tissue beneath the surface. The cooling effect allows the laser to penetrate to depths of 200 to 400 μm in the dermal layer. The temperature of the surface of the skin is monitored before, during, and after each laser application. The maximum temperature (T_{max}) at the skin surface during the pre-cooled treatment application is 40 to 43°C. The applications should be spaced 10 to 15 mm apart because the laser light at this wavelength has the property of horizontal scattering and heat spread. At the conclusion of the treatment, mild erythematous spots are visible on the skin surface; typically they disappear within 20 to 30 minutes. Natragel cool masks (Gel Concepts, Whippany, New Jersey) can reduce this period of erythema very effectively.[14–24]

Cosmetically undesirable hypertrichosis can be treated with laser hair removal. The mechanism of action is thought to be selective thermal damage to cutaneous microvessels and melanosomes. The mechanism for hair reduction is not completely understood. Although collagen regeneration and rhytid ablation are not the primary functions of this modality, there is definite improvement in skin texture and rhytidosis following this course of treatment. Four to six treatment sessions may be necessary to achieve the desired affect. The Coolglide (Cutera, Brisbane, California) long-pulsed Nd:YAG laser devices are available for hair removal using the 1064 nm wavelength. For the hair follicle to effectively absorb the maximum laser energy and to avoid singeing of long hairs, the area to be treated is shaved before treatment and topical anesthetic cream (Photocaine, University Pharmacy, Salt Lake City, Utah) can be applied to the sensitive patient. The anesthetic cream is removed after 20 minutes and chilled clear aloe gel is applied to the area. This serves as coupling gel to minimize the scattering of light and as a cooling and soothing medium to maximize patient comfort. The brass cooling tip then cools the skin immediately before treatment. A 10 mm spot and 30 to 50 mJ/cm^2 are used. Mild erythema of the skin subsides ~30 minutes after the treatment. Because not all hairs are in the anagen growth phase at the time of treatment (a requirement for the laser application to be effective), destruction of hair follicles usually takes 4 to 6 treatment sessions, 3 to 4 weeks apart.[25]

Small benign superficial skin lesions such as papillomas, nevi, and seborrheic keratoses can be individually removed, with topical anesthetic, using high radiofrequency technology, such as the Surgitron (Ellman International Inc., Hewlett, New York). Ablation of small telangiectatic vascular lesions using this technology is also impressively successful. This technology achieves excellent hemostasis with minimal cicatrix formation.

Relaxing the Muscles

Relaxing the muscles of the neck using chemodenervation agents can improve the appearance of the neck and at the same time prepare the overlying tissues to be maximally rejuvenated with complementary treatments.[26,27] The relaxation effect is not only confined to the injected muscles but also extends indirectly to all the soft tissues (skin, fat) to which these muscles are attached. The theoretical advantage of this secondary effect is that skin rejuvenation, by means of collagen regeneration, can be maximized after the muscles have been treated. For this reason it is important to perform chemodenervation before skin tightening procedures. The relaxing of the muscles reduces platysmal bands and the overlying skin wrinkles of the neck. A smoother scaffold is provided for the regenerating skin that has been treated with nonablative lasers, IPL, or ThermaLifting (Thermage) (Fig. **8–1A–B**).

Botulinum toxin type A (Botox Cosmetic, Allergan, Irvine, California) is the most commonly used agent in the United States. Even though its current U.S. Food and Drug Administration (FDA) cosmetic approval is for the treatment of glabellar furrows, many physicians have been utilizing it off-label to treat other areas of the face and neck with dramatic results[28] (see Chapter 5). Botox Cosmetic is not recommended for use in patients with albumin allergy, for those taking aminoglycoside antibiotics, or for pregnant women.[29]

The platysma muscle is a pair of skeletal muscles originating from the deep fascia and skin of the lower

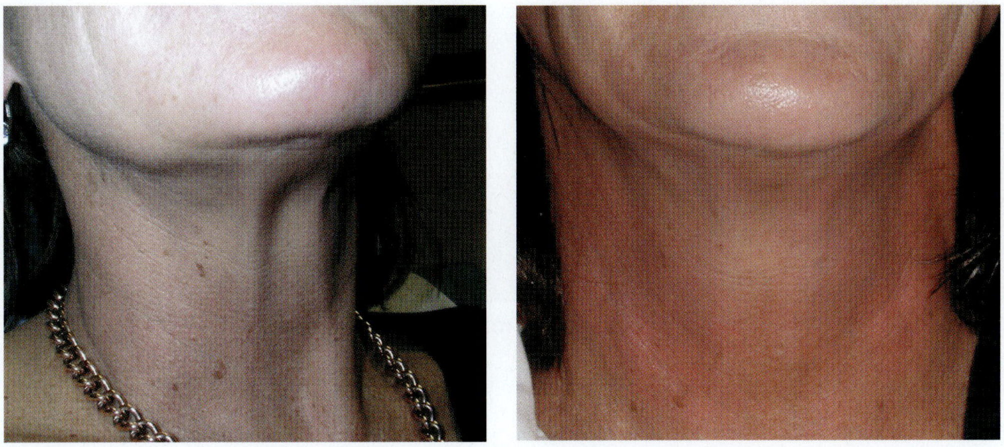

A B

Figure 8–1 (**A**) Prominent platysmal bands, mild submental fat accumulation, and moderate skin laxity were this patient's complaints. (**B**) Thermage following Botox pretreatment of this patient's platysmal bands resulted in a significant improvement of her neck contour and skin texture.

neck and upper chest, extending laterally to the anterior surface of the deltoid muscles and inserting at the inferior border of the mandible and the skin inferior to the mouth. Its main functions are drawing the corners of the mouth inferiorly and assisting in opening the mouth by depressing the mandible. Hyperkinetic activity and loss of tone of the platysma muscle due to senescence of the neck may result in vertical muscle bands and horizontal neck rhytid formation.[30]

Fifteen to 20 minutes of topical anesthesia (Photocaine) can be augmented by applying a Natragel mask (Gel Concepts) over the areas to be injected. This cools the skin and provides additional vasoconstriction. After the anesthetic cream is removed iced compresses are applied to the injection sites. While grasping the platysmal band, 0.1 mL injections (2.5 units of Botox Cosmetic) are given directly into the band, spaced 1 cm apart along its entire vertical length. This is usually enough to relax and soften the appearance of platysmal bands. If the total dose is less than 50 units, it is unlikely that there will be enough diffusion to affect the deeper muscles. Swallowing difficulty and weakness of the strap muscles are remote but possible complications. After the injection, squeezing the band and applying iced compresses reduces the possibility of bruising. We advise patients not to rub the injected areas for at least 4 hours after the injection to avoid diffusion. We prefer to perform touch-up injections 1 week later rather than risking overdosing the patient during the initial treatment session.

The relaxing effect of Botox Cosmetic starts appearing in 3 to 5 days after the injection. It may take up to 10 days for the full effect to take place. It is important to clearly communicate this information with the patients before they leave the office. A follow-up visit is scheduled for 1 to 2 weeks later. The result may last 3 to 6 months. Besides relaxing platysmal bands, Botox may also be used to reduce horizontal neck wrinkles. One or two units are given along each horizontal wrinkle, spaced 1 cm apart. Botox Cosmetic may also be used to improve the appearance of jowls and elevate the corners of the mouth with injections to the depressor angulii oris and the platysma. Maintenance with neuromodulation is very important especially for patients who have had other procedures such as nonablative laser skin rejuvenation and Thermage (see Chapter 5).

Contouring the Fat

Subcutaneous submental fat may blunt the cervicomental angle and cause sagging of the neck skin. Fat in this location is responsive to noninvasive techniques. The subplatysmal fat lies deeper and is not accessible without surgical intervention.

Lipostabil (Aventis, France) is phosphatidylcholine. This enzyme dissolves the fatty acids and also protects the liver from alcohol-induced oxidative stress.[31] It has been used for many years in Brazil, Germany, Italy, and South America as a systemic lipid-lowering drug. It has also been used off label as an injectable fat-dissolving agent. It is supplied in 5 mL vials containing 250 mg. It is not approved by the FDA in the United States. Injections of Lipostabil have been reportedly successful in treating prominent periorbital fat with no recurrences and no significant short-term adverse effects.[32] However, we have found that significant facial edema that persists for 1 to 2 weeks follows facial injections and we prefer not to use it in these areas. Phosphatidylcholine injections to the submental fat, on the other hand, improve the neck and jaw contours, and the subsequent

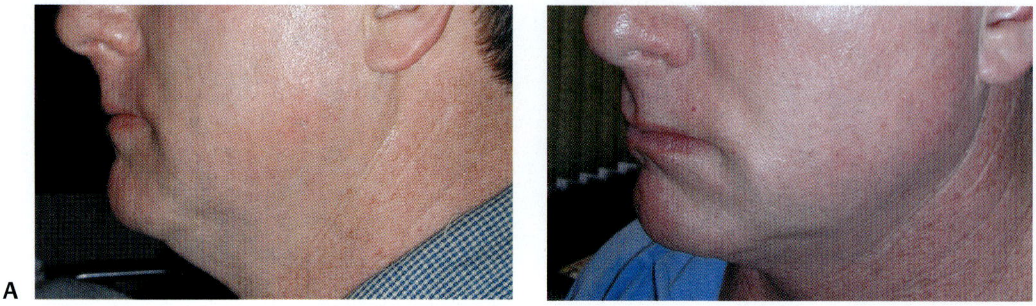

Figure 8–2 (A,B) Three sessions of Lipostabil injections followed by a Thermage treatment improved this patient's jawline and neck contour.

edema is not as obvious.[33,34] More than one injection session is necessary; usually two to five treatments spaced about 3 to 4 weeks apart are effective. Transient mild swelling and itching, lasting 30 to 90 minutes, are common immediately following the treatment. For maximum effect, 0.5 mL of the undiluted solution is injected subcutaneously at 1 cm intervals. Often no response is noted for 10 to 14 days.

Thermage (to de discussed more fully under skin tightening) can also be used to reduce the amount and improve the contour of submental fat (Fig. **8–2A,B**).

Any residual submental fat can be removed with minimal incision submental tumescent liposuction performed under local anesthesia with or without intravenous sedation. The margins of the submental fat are first marked with the patient sitting in the upright position. This will identify the margins of the fatty tissue during the procedure after the infiltration has tumesced the area. A 3 mm submental crease incision is sufficient to accommodate blunt infiltration and dissection cannulas and a 2 mm Mercedes liposuction cannula. 1000 mL of Klein solution (1 mL of adrenaline, 50 mL of xylocaine in 1000 mL of normal saline), using a three-way stopcock and a blunt infiltrating cannula, is instilled 20 minutes before the procedure is begun. The tumescent technique minimizes bleeding by providing adequate vasoconstriction and hydrodissection.[35–37]

Recovery is very rapid. After the procedure, the patient wears an elastic band that provides pressure to the submental area, encouraging subcutaneous adhesions and reducing edema.

Tightening the Skin

After improving the appearance of the skin, reducing the horizontal skin wrinkles and the vertical platysmal bands, and sculpting the submental fat, the final step in noninvasive neck rejuvenation is to tighten the skin. Success of the previous steps will augment the final result. Until recently, surgical techniques such as neck lift and platysmaplasty were the primary choices. Laser resurfacing of the neck skin has been unpredictable and its use is limited today.

ThermaCool TC (Thermage, Hayward, California) was approved by the FDA in November 2002 for periorbital applications. It is a noninvasive, nonablative system that uses radiofrequency technology to deliver heat energy to the deep levels of the skin while protecting the epidermis by monitoring surface temperature and using a cryogen cooling apparatus. Radiofrequency energy causes movement of charged particles within the tissue, and the resultant molecular motion generates heat. The heat in turn causes collagen shrinkage and new collagen deposition.[38] Immediate collagen contraction is followed by long-term collagen remodeling. Off-label uses include treatment of the forehead, midface, and neck.[39–41] Forty minutes before the procedure is begun, the patient is given Percocet (10 mg p.o. $\times$ 1) and Atavan (1 mg p.o. $\times$ 1). The patient's neuromodulation pretreatment administered at least 1 to 2 weeks before to the platysmal bands and submental platysma will facilitate the lifting and tightening of the Thermage treatment by reducing downward pulling. Posttreatment soothing Natragel masks (Gel Concepts LLC, Whippany, New Jersey) are applied following the procedure.

A temporary stencil grid is applied to the skin in the areas to be treated. This delineates the areas to be treated and avoids overlapping. These include the submental areas and the lateral aspects of the neck as far posterior as the strap muscles and avoiding the midline. For the neck treatment the patient should be in the supine position facing away from the side being treated and with the chin elevated. In this manner, the tip can be more easily applied in a perpendicular fashion to the skin being treated. Sufficient conducting fluid must be applied. And exact, complete apposition of the tip to the surface of skin is necessary for treatment.

Using the grid of 1.5 cm squares as a guide, two complete passes using a setting of 62.5 (92 J) with the new fast, large tips the area of the neck is treated while retracting the skin laterally. Two fingerbreadths above and below the angle of the mandible are treated with two or three or three passes of 62.5 (92 J). Two or three additional passes over the complete neck area (excluding the midline) using 61.5 (75 J) are performed. After the procedure the residual coupling fluid and the stencil grid are removed using alcohol sponges. Minimal erythema and swelling may be observed. With sufficient treatment, discrete subcutaneous nodules and surface irregularity may be evident at the conclusion of the procedure. They will typically subside in 1 to 2 days but may persist longer.

Results appear gradually over 3 to 6 months. Besides the tightening effect there may also be some improvement in the overall skin quality. This could be explained by the formation and deposition of new collagen. The longevity of the effect may be several years. Repeat treatments may be necessary to maintain or augment the result.

◆ Conclusion

We have recommended a series of minimally invasive treatments for the rejuvenation of the neck. These treatments have minimal downtime and offer impressive results. Not all the treatments are appropriate for every patient. Patients should receive a customized recommendation based on their individual needs and desires. The combination of treatments has an additive effect on the rejuvenating effort. We recommend performing procedures in a specific order. For example relaxing the muscles with Botox and treating the skin with chemical peels is recommended before the Thermage procedure. The use of home care products, UV protection, and cessation of smoking are important actions patients can take to participate in their skin care. Their role is important in the maintenance of the rejuvenating effect. Regular follow-up visits and photographic documentation may establish treatment goals and facilitate the maintenance of the overall rejuvenating effect.

References

1. Beaty MM. Treatment of neck laxity with a Gore-Tex cervical sling for patients with heavy neck tissues. Facial Plast Surg 2001;17:117–122
2. Wall SJ, Adamson PA. Surgical options for aesthetic enhancement of the neck. Facial Plast Surg 2001;17:109–115
3. Sykes JM. Rejuvenation of the aging neck. Facial Plast Surg 2001;17:99–107
4. Ramirez OM, Robertson KM. Comprehensive approach to rejuvenation of the neck. Facial Plast Surg 2001;17:129–140
5. Bosniak S, Cantisano-Zilkha M, Glavas IP. Noninvasive neck rejuvenation: a multi-disciplinary approach. Presented at the 34th Annual Meeting of the American Society of Ophthalmic Plastic and Reconstructive Surgeons, Anaheim, California, Nov. 13–14, 2003
6. Jasin ME. Submentoplasty as an isolated rejuvenative procedure for the neck. Arch Facial Plast Surg 2003;5:180–183
7. Castle DJ, Honigman RJ, Phillips KA. Does cosmetic surgery improve psychosocial wellbeing? Med J Aust 2002;176:601–604
8. Rohrich RJ. Mirror, mirror on the wall: when the postoperative reflection does not meet patients' expectations. Plast Reconstr Surg 2001;108:507–509
9. Perez-Bernal A, Munoz-Perez MA, Camacho F. Management of facial hyperpigmentation. Am J Clin Dermatol 2000;1:261–268
10. Raulin C, Greve B, Grema H. IPL technology: a review. Lasers Surg Med 2003;32:78–87
11. Weiss RA, Weiss MA, Beasley KL. Rejuvenation of photoaged skin: 5 years results with intense pulsed light of the face, neck, and chest. Dermatol Surg 2002;28:1115–1119
12. Anderson RR, Parrish JA. Selective photothermolysis: precise microsurgery by selective absorption of pulsed radiation. Science 1983;220:524–527
13. Sadick NS, Weiss R, Kilmer S, Bitter P. Photorejuvenation with intense pulsed light: results of a multi-center study. J Drugs Dermatol 2004;3:41–49
14. Tanzi EL, Alster TS. Comparison of a 1450-nm diode laser and a 1320-nm Nd:YAG laser in the treatment of atrophic facial scars: a prospective clinical and histologic study. Dermatol Surg 2004;30:152–157
15. Cassuto D, Emanuelli G. Nonablative scar revision using a long pulsed frequency doubled Nd:YAG laser. J Cosmet Laser Ther 2003;5:135–139
16. Tanzi EL, Alster TS. Long-pulsed 1064-nm Nd:YAG laser-assisted hair removal in all skin types. Dermatol Surg 2004;30:13–17
17. Trelles MA, Allones I. The CoolTouch laser: too much of a good thing? Lasers Med Sci 2001;16:304–305
18. Pham RT. Nonablative laser resurfacing. Facial Plast Surg Clin North Am 2001;9:303–310; ix
19. Rogachefsky AS, Hussain M, Goldberg DJ. Atrophic and a mixed pattern of acne scars improved with a 1320-nm Nd:YAG laser. Dermatol Surg 2003;29:904–908
20. Lee MW. Combination visible and infrared lasers for skin rejuvenation. Semin Cutan Med Surg 2002;21:288–300
21. Romero P, Alster TS. Skin rejuvenation with Cool Touch 1320 nm Nd:YAG laser: the nurse's role. Dermatol Nurs 2001;13:122,125–127
22. Fatemi A, Weiss MA, Weiss RA. Short-term histologic effects of nonablative resurfacing: results with a dynamically cooled millisecond-domain 1320 nm Nd:YAG laser. Dermatol Surg 2002;28:172–176
23. Goldberg DJ. Nonablative subsurface remodeling: clinical and histologic evaluation of a 1320-nm Nd:YAG laser. J Cutan Laser Ther 1999;1:153–157
24. Goldberg DJ. Full-face nonablative dermal remodeling with a 1320 nm Nd:YAG laser. Dermatol Surg 2000;26:915–918
25. Kelly KM, Nelson JS, Lask GP, Geronemus RG, Bernstein LJ. Cryogen spray cooling in combination with nonablative laser treatment of facial rhytides. Arch Dermatol 1999;135:691–694

26. Carruthers J, Carruthers A. Botox use in the mid and lower face and neck. Semin Cutan Med Surg 2001;20:85–92

27. Brandt FS, Bellman B. Cosmetic use of botulinum A exotoxin for the aging neck. Dermatol Surg 1998;24:1232–1234

28. Brandt FS, Boker A. Botulinum toxin for rejuvenation of the neck. Clin Dermatol 2003;21:513–520

29. Molgo J, Lemeignan M, Thesleff S. Aminoglycosides and 3,4-diaminopyridine on neuromuscular block caused by botulinum type A toxin. Muscle Nerve 1987;10:464–470

30. Matarasso A, Matarasso SL. Botulinum A exotoxin for the management of platysma bands. Plast Reconstr Surg 2003;112(5 suppl):138S–140S

31. Aleynik SI, Lieber CS. Polyenylphosphatidylcholine corrects the alcohol-induced hepatic oxidative stress by restoring s-adenosylmethionine. Alcohol Alcohol 2003;38:208–212

32. Rittes PG. The use of phosphatidylcholine for correction of lower lid bulging due to prominent fat pads. Dermatol Surg 2001;27:391–392

33. Hexsel D, Serra M, Mazzuco R, Dal Forno T, Zechmeister D. Phosphatidylcholine in the treatment of localized fat. J Drugs Dermatol 2003;2:511–518

34. Hexsel D, Serra M, Dal Forno A, Zechmeister D. Cosmetic uses of injectable phosphatidylcholine in the face. Operative Techniques in Oculoplastic, Orbital, and Reconstructive Surgery 2004. In press

35. Gryskiewicz JM. Submental suction-assisted lipectomy without platysmaplasty: pushing the (skin) envelope to avoid a face lift for unsuitable candidates. Plast Reconstr Surg 2003; 112:1393–1405

36. Jacob CI, Berkes BJ, Kaminer MS. Liposuction and surgical recontouring of the neck: a retrospective analysis. Dermatol Surg 2000;26:625–632

37. Jones BM, Grover R. Reducing complications in cervicofacial rhytidectomy by tumescent infiltration: a comparative trial evaluating 678 consecutive face lifts. Plast Reconstr Surg 2004;113:398–403

38. Hsu TS, Kaminer MS. The use of nonablative radiofrequency technology to tighten the lower face and neck. Semin Cutan Med Surg 2003;22:115–123

39. Fitzpatrick R, Geronemus R, Goldberg D, Kaminer M, Kilmer S, Ruiz-Esparza J. Multicenter study of noninvasive radiofrequency for periorbital tissue tightening. Lasers Surg Med 2003;33:232–242

40. Narins DJ, Narins RS. Nonsurgical radiofrequency facelift. J Drugs Dermatol 2003;2:495–500

41. Iyer S, Suthamjariya K, Fitzpatrick RE. Using a radiofrequency energy device to treat the lower face: a treatment paradigm for a nonsurgical facelift. Cosmetic Dermatology 2003; 18:37–40

Section II

Less Invasive Surgical Options

9

Minimally Invasive Eyelid Rejuvenation

Stephen Bosniak

Neuromodulation, filling agents, nonablative lasers, and therma-lifting can noninvasively rejuvenate the periorbital tissues. These techniques can be dramatic nonsurgical surgical alternatives for many patients. For other patients these techniques are an essential step to prepare them for laser-assisted surgical procedures. Eyelid skin redundancy and marked loss of elasticity, fatty prolapse, levator aponeurotic disinsertion, lacrimal gland prolapse, and lateral canthal tendon and lower lid margin laxity need to be addressed surgically. Carbon dioxide (CO_2) laser techniques allow us to perform skin and skin–muscle resections, levator aponeurotic repairs, lacrimal gland suspensions, lateral canthal plications, lipovaporization, fat transposition, and eyelid skin resurfacing efficiently, with great accuracy and minimal downtime, in a virtually bloodless field.

◆ Patient Evaluation

The best way to start with these patients is to sit down with them, listen to their comments, look in the mirror with them, and review their old photographs. At the same time you will be observing their face at rest and in animation. Obviously, individual patients have their own anatomic variations. But patients also have their own insights into what they do not like about their faces. We are directed by what the patients see. We listen. We examine them and analyze their faces. And then we make our recommendations, discussing each patient's options and realistic expectations.

Gender and ethnic variations in blepharoplasty are essential considerations. Male upper eyelids are typically full and their eyebrows are low and flat (Fig. **9–1A,B**) whereas female upper lids may have a more defined superior sulcus and a more accentuated brow arch. Oversculpting a male superior sulcus or creating an overly arched brow will feminize the man's appearance

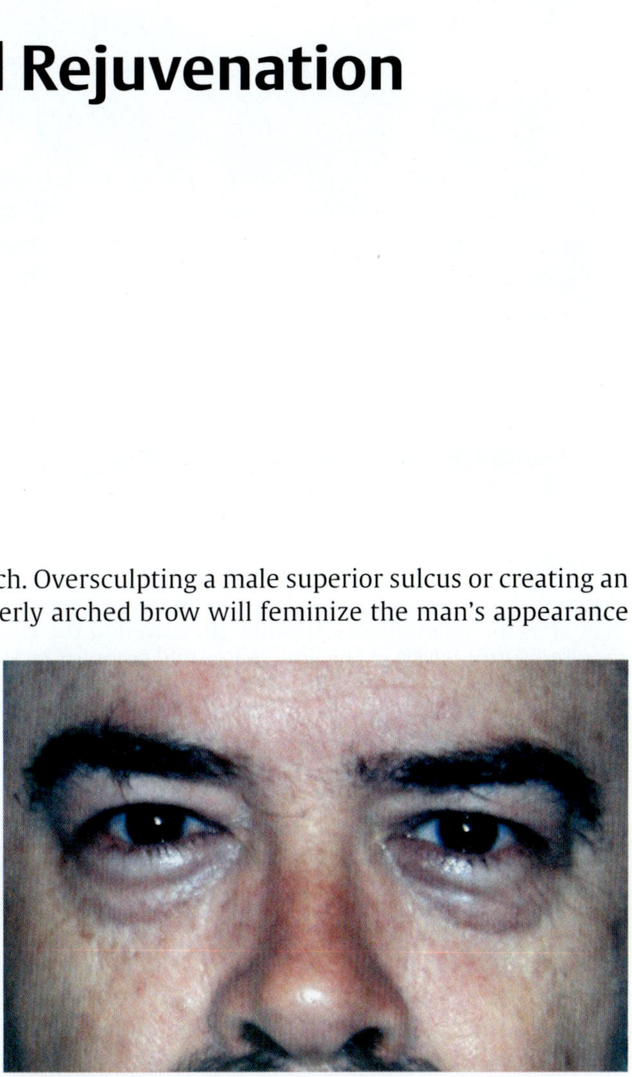

A

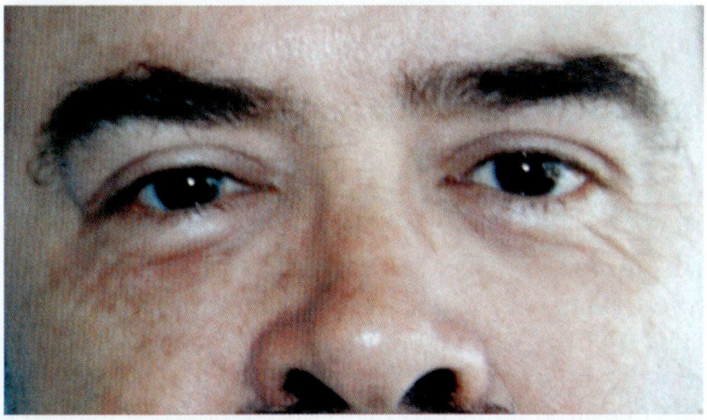

B

Figure 9–1 (**A**) A low flat brow and heavy upper lid folds are male eyelid characteristics. Heavy lower facial musculature and lateral canthal laxity may predispose them to lower lid retraction following a transcutaneous approach. (**B**) Internal brow stabilization followed by cautious trimming of a male patient's upper lid without oversculpting the preaponeurotic fat can give a more youthful appearance without feminizing. Transconjunctival carbon dioxide laser–assisted lipovaporization will improve the lower lid contours without risk of lower lid margin displacement.

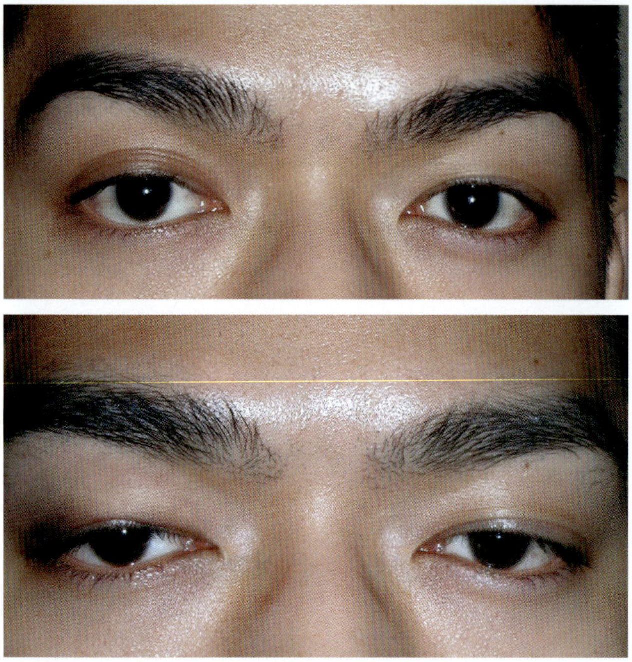

A

B

Figure 9–2 (**A**) An elevated right upper lid crease became evident after an inflammatory episode. (**B**) Lowering the crease required surgical lysis of the lid–crease–fold complex internal cutaneous adhesions and interpositioning of a layer of Restylane between the skin and orbicularis muscle.

and should be avoided. We discourage Asian patients from occidentalizing their eyelids. Redundant upper eyelid folds can be trimmed and reduced via a very low supraciliary incision, thus avoiding the creation of a double eyelid or elevating a low lid–crease–fold complex. Multiple eyelid creases can be eliminated and asymmetric lid–crease–fold complexes can be corrected (Fig. **9–2A,B**).

◆ Anatomical Structure and Position

Facial structures cannot be examined in a vacuum (Fig. **9–3**). The upper lids are intimately related to the level and contour of the eyebrows (Fig. **9–4A,B**), just as the lower lids are related to the lateral and medial canthi and the midface. The vertical height of the palpebral aperture may be diminished because of upper lid ptosis (Fig. **9–5A,B**) or may be increased because of upper or lower eyelid retraction (Fig. **9–6A,B**). Some surgeons use the marginal reflex distance (MRD) measurement to further qualify absolute measurements of the vertical palpebral aperture. In any case the relationship of the upper lid margin to the pupil and the lower lid margin to the inferior limbus must be noted.

Lower lid margin and/or lateral canthal laxity may be significant even in the absence of overt lower lid margin retraction and inferior scleral show (Fig. **9–7A,B**). The

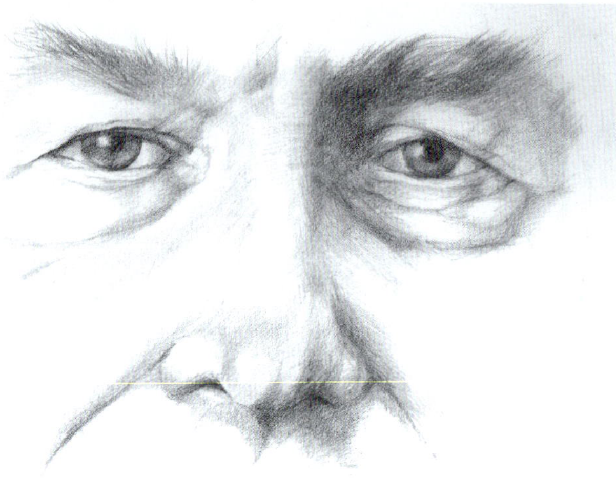

Figure 9–3 Male upper lid blepharoplasties may need internal brow fixation to stabilize the brow before upper lid fold resection. Male lower lid blepharoplasties may need lateral canthal suspension to stabilize the lower lid margin before cutaneous resurfacing.

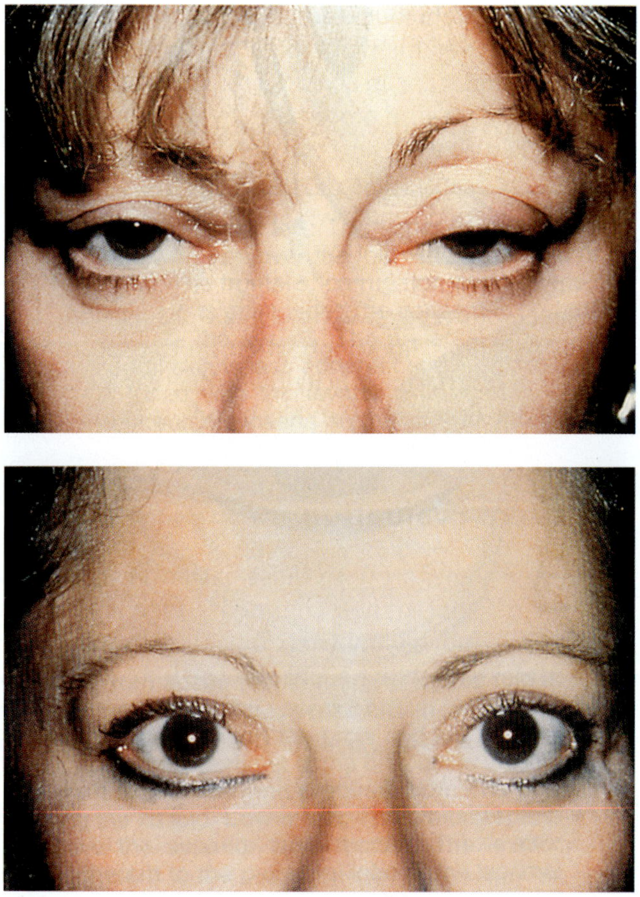

A

B

Figure 9–4 (**A**) This patient exhibited the hallmarks of blepharoptosis—narrowed palpebral apertures, elevated lid crease-fold complexes, and secondary compensatory brow elevation. (**B**) Marked bilateral upper lid blepharoptosis and lower lid retraction were improved with laser-assisted upper lid blepharoplasty, levator aponeurotic repair, recession of lower lid retractors, and lateral canthal plication.

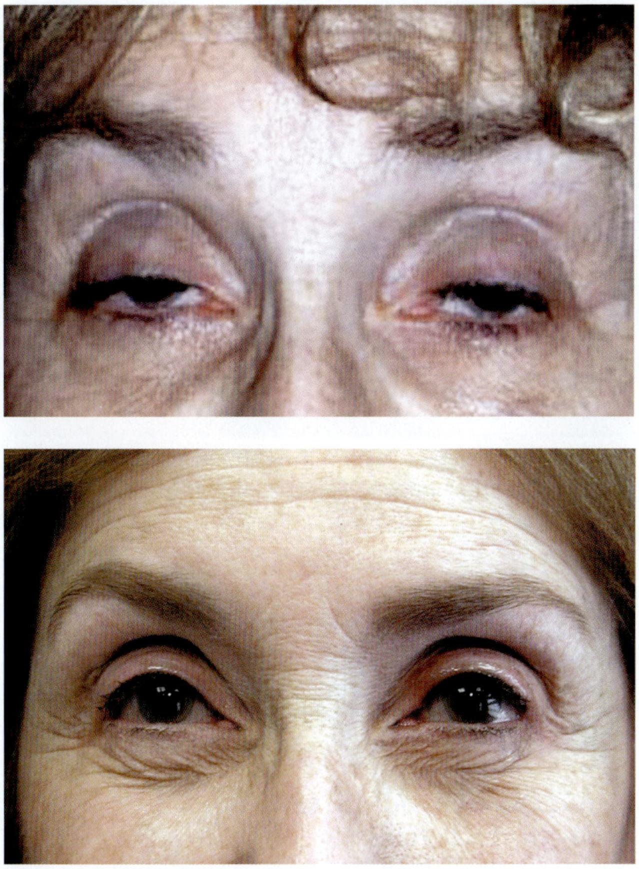

A

B

Figure 9–5 (**A**) When repairing prominent levator aponeurotic disinsertions that create marked blepharoptosis and deep superior sulci, old photographs may be helpful to determine placement of the lid crease incision and the depth of the reconstructed superior sulcus. (**B**) This patient's final result after levator aponeurotic repair was enhanced with micropigmentation of her superior eyelid margin.

snap test and the distraction test alone are not the only relevant factors in predicting lower lid margin displacement after a procedure. Granted, the amount of lid margin laxity (distraction test) that can be demonstrated by pulling the eyelid away from the globe (greater than 8 mm is deemed lax) and the rapidity of the lid margin returning to its normal anatomic position against the globe (snap test) will demonstrate the stability of the lower lid margin. But the amount of inferior scleral show, lower lid margin retraction, and prominence of the globe (whether secondary to high myopia and a large globe or shallow bony orbits) have a significant impact on the potential for postoperative lower lid margin displacement (Fig. **9–8A,B**).

◆ Surgical Plan

We use carbon dioxide laser assisted techniques for all of our procedures. We use the 0.2 mm handpiece as a cutting tool and the Lumenis Ultra Pulse C5000 computer

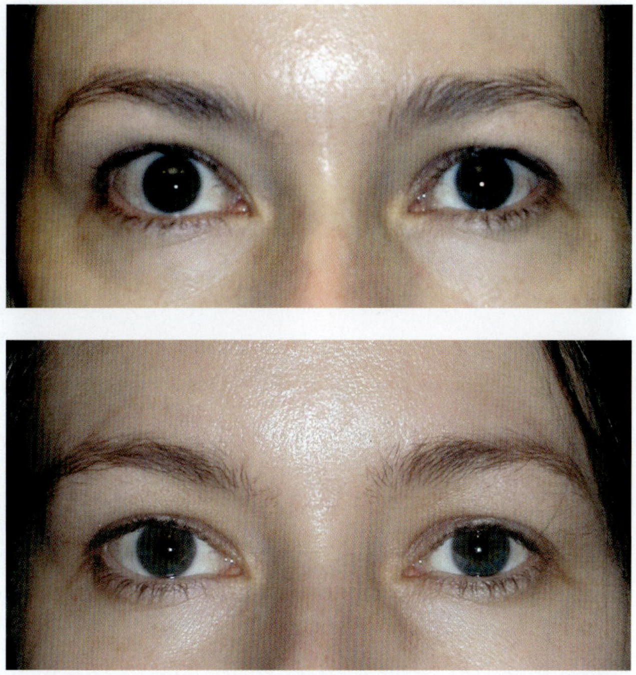

A

B

Figure 9–6 (**A**) Idiopathic retraction of this patient's right upper lid (normal thryroid workup) exposes the superior limbus and enlarges the palpebral aperture. (**B**) Her apertures are symmetric following recession of her right upper lid retractors.

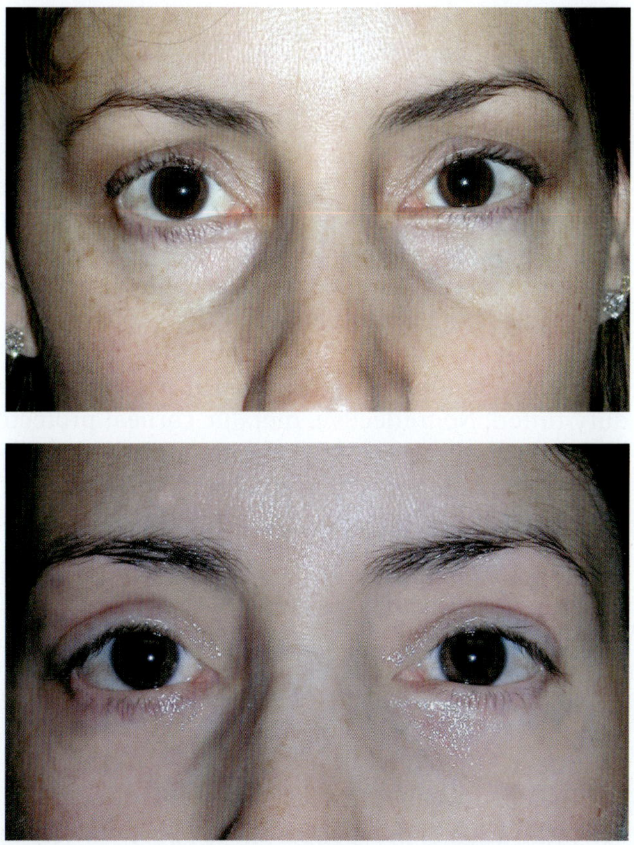

A

B

Figure 9–7 (**A**) A right lower lid retraction and a tear trough deformity following a transcutaneous lower lid blepharoplasty. (**B**) It was corrected with a right lateral canthal plication, bilateral transconjunctival fat transposition, and lower lid CO_2 laser resurfacing (150 mJ, one pass, pattern 3, size 4, density 6).

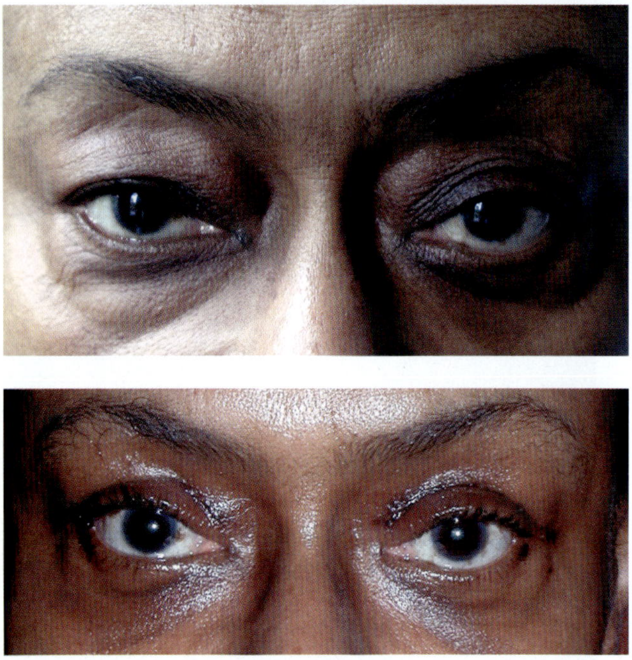

A

B

Figure 9–8 (**A**) Shallow orbits create inferior scleral show. (**B**) Lateral canthal support is essential to stabilize the lower lid margins when performing a transconjunctival lower lid blepharoplasty.

pattern generator (CPG) (Lumenis, Santa Clara, California) as a resurfacing tool. We also use the Lumenis Ultra Fine (Lumenis) erbium: yttrium-aluminum-garnet (Er:YAG) CPG as a resurfacing tool in selected patients.

For the comfort and safety of the patient and operating room staff, a high-power plume evacuator is utilized to remove the vapor plume from the surgical field. All personnel in the operating room suite wear protective goggles and filtration masks.

Topical tetracaine drops are applied to each eye. The patient is prepped and then draped in sterile heavy-duty tinfoil. Nonreflective, metallic corneal protectors are applied to each eye. After the preoperative decisions have been made for the surgical plan, the following is our customary order of surgical procedures:

1. Demarcation of upper lid crease incision and cutaneous or myocutaneous resection
2. Xylocaine infiltration of upper lid cutaneous incision, resection, and resurfacing sites (<1 mL per side is injected if levator aponeurotic adjustment is to be performed)
3. Upper lid crease incision (Fig. **9–9**)
4. Levator aponeurotic repair (Fig. **9–10**)
5. Infiltration of preaponeurotic fat, brow, lateral canthus, lower lid
6. Suspension of prolapsed lacrimal gland (Fig. **9–11**)
7. Vaporization of upper lid preaponeurotic fat
8. Internal brow stabilization (Fig. **9–12**)

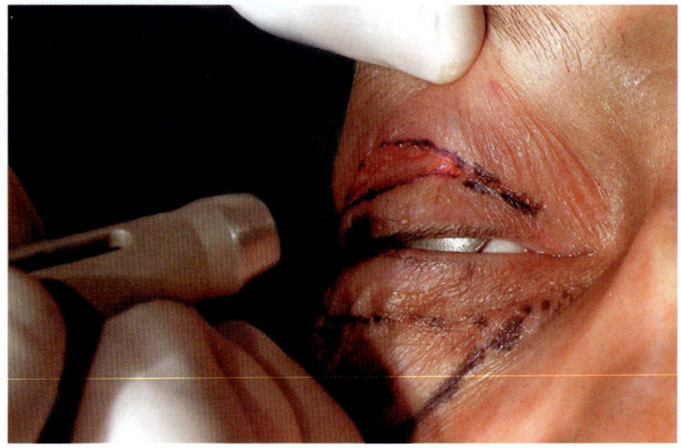

Figure 9–9 The CO_2 laser (ultrapulse mode, 400 Hz, 5 mJ) is used to incise the upper lid skin.

9. Lower lid transconjunctival lipovaporization and fat transposition (Fig. **9–7A,B**)
10. Lateral canthal plication
11. Eyelid laser resurfacing (Fig. **9–13A,B**)
12. Wound closure

Skin Texture Rhytidosis, Lesions, and Periorbital Veins

Patients often perceive eyelid wrinkling as excess skin. And indeed in the past our proposed surgical remedy encouraged this manner of thinking: skin resection. True skin excess may exist, but a loss of skin elasticity or a deterioration of skin texture can give the appearance of rhytidosis. When evaluating the upper eyelid, the patient and physician have to decide if they wish to

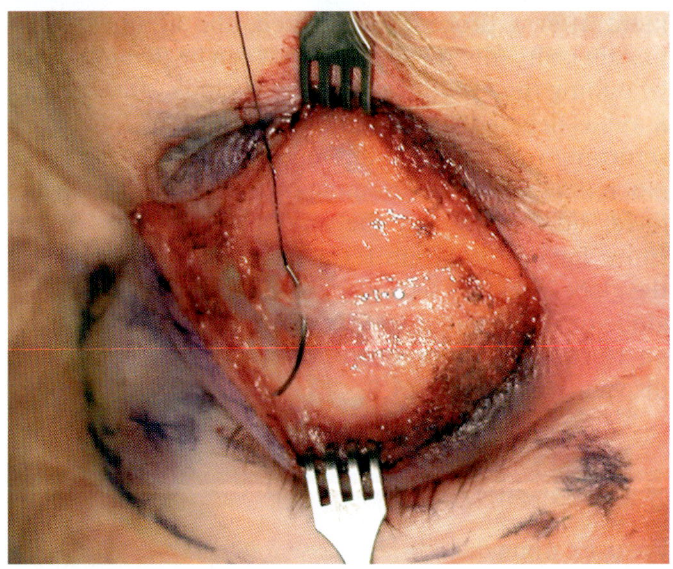

Figure 9–10 A 6–0 black silk suture is used to reapproximate a disinserted levator aponeurosis to the anterior tarsal surface.

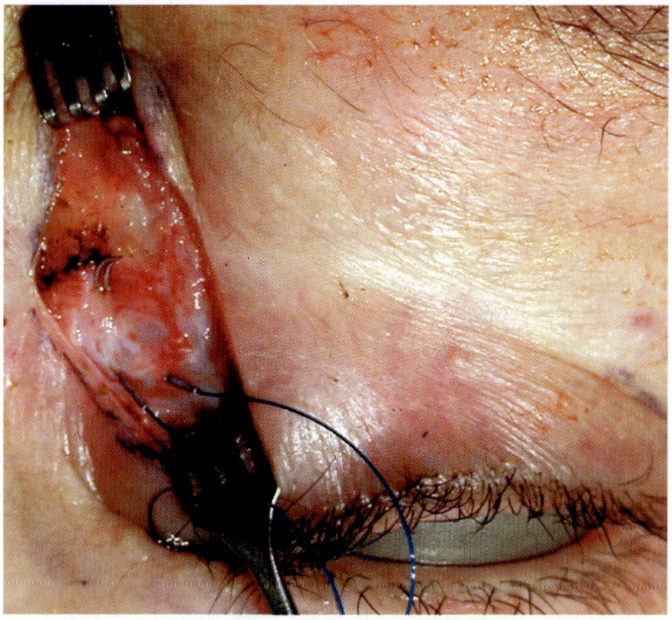

Figure 9–11 A double-armed 4–0 Prolene suture is used to suspend the orbital lobe of the lacrimal gland to the periosteum of the lacrimal fossa.

reduce the size of the fold, to improve the texture of the skin, or both. Upper lid skin management requires a blending of resection and laser resurfacing. Lower lid skin management requires either or both chemical peeling or laser resurfacing with lateral canthal support when necessary (Fig. **9–14A,B**). Resurfacing the pretarsal lower lid skin is avoided when possible, particularly medially anterior to the inferior punctum. Laser resurfacing in this area may predispose the lower lid to inferior retraction and punctal eversion.

Intradermal nevi, adenomas, and keratoses are shaved with a radiosurgical loop (Ellman International, Hewlett,

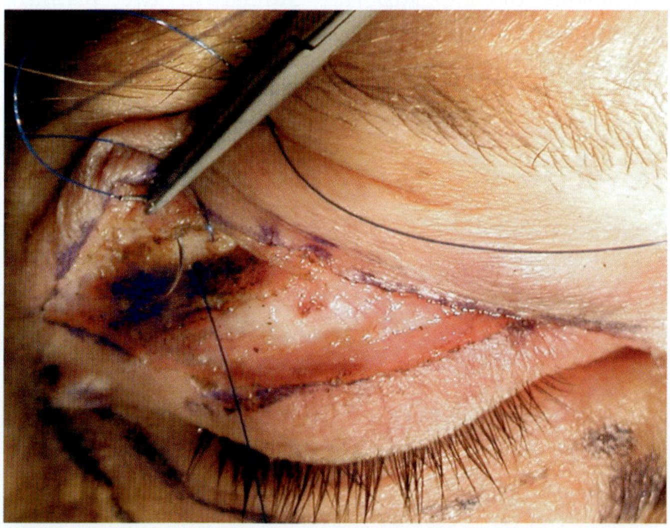

Figure 9–12 Internal brow suspension. The Prolene suture is passed through the brow subcutaneous tissue and anchored to the periosteum 5 mm superior to the superior orbital rim.

A

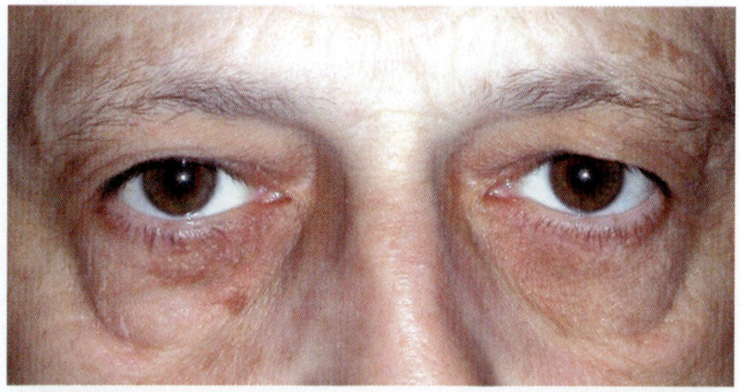

B

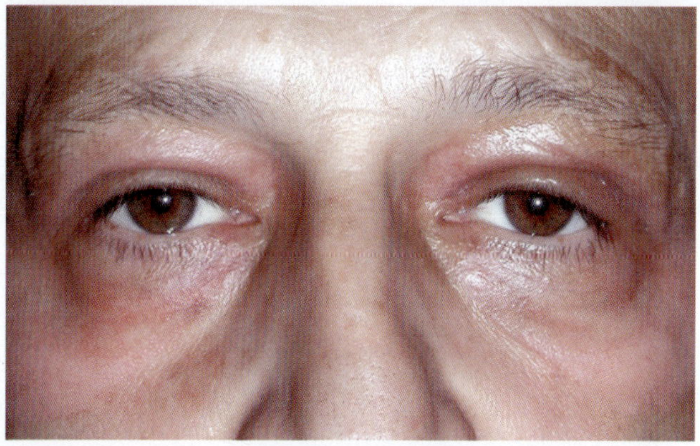

Figure 9–13 (**A**) Low, flat, masculine brows must be stabilized before upper lid skin redundancy can be addressed. (**B**) Pretreated with a "Botox browlift," internal brow stabilization facilitated creation of a natural-appearing masculine upper lid following myocutaneous resection and laser resurfacing. Transconjunctival lipovaporization, lateral canthal plication, and carbon dioxide laser resurfacing were used to improve this patient's lower lid and malar contours.

A

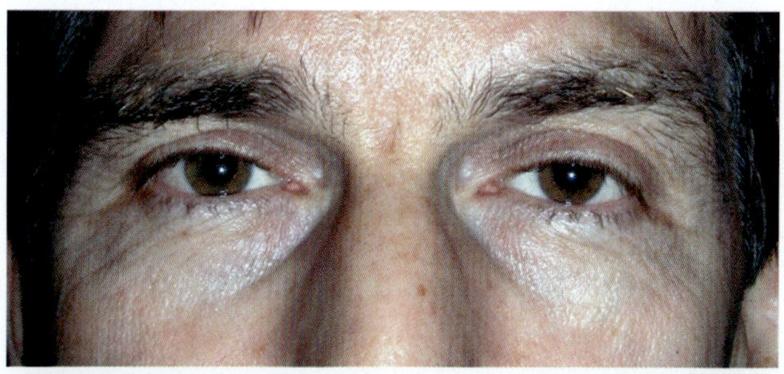

B

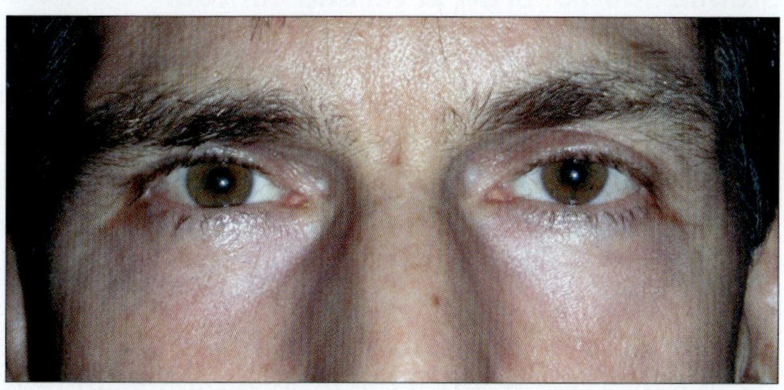

Figure 9–14 (**A**) Mild fatty prolapse and moderate lower lid skin rhytidosis were this patient's complaints. (**B**) Transconjunctival lipovaporization and laser resurfacing provided a smoother lower eyelid contour for this patient.

A

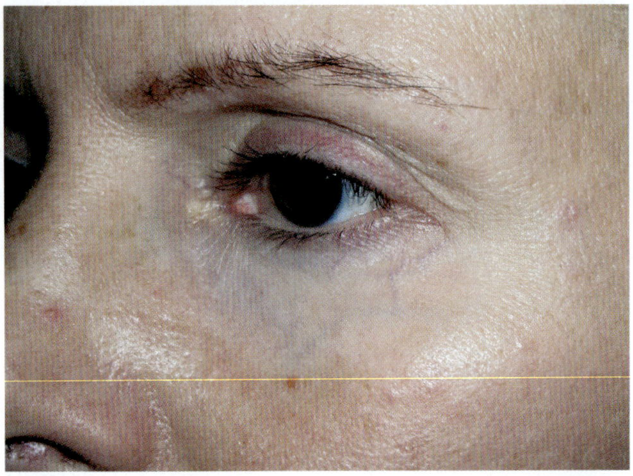

B

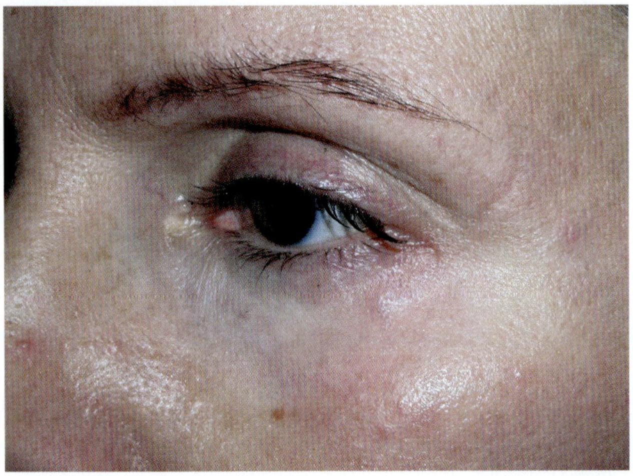

Figure 9–15 (**A**) Lower eyelid veins may be visible through translucent skin. (**B**) Lower lid and periorbital varices were effectively treated with a 1064 nm laser (Cutera Cool Glide; 140 J/cm; 3 mm spot).

New York) to make them flush with the eyelid surface before laser resurfacing. Perioperatively periorbital veins that are apparent through translucent skin can be ablated with a 1064 nm laser utilizing 120 to 140 J/cm^2 with a 3 mm spot (Cutera Cool Glide, Bristane, CA) (Fig. **9–15A,B**).

Stabilization of Brow Level and Contour

With the patient seated in an upright position, facing the surgeon, the brow arch and relation to the superior orbital rim are determined. Old photos are reviewed with the patient to determine if there has been any change in brow level and contour.

In males, a flat contour and a position at the level of the superior orbital are acceptable. A level inferior to the rim will cause excessive hooding and upper lid fold redundancy (Fig. **9–16**). If the brow is mobile and easily elevated, the amount of elevation laterally (at the tail of the brow), and centrally (in line with the lateral limbus) is noted. If there is medial brow ptosis, it is noted.

Female patients who have always had a flat brow contour and want to maintain it are managed in the same fashion as male patients. In female patients who have lost their brow contour and want to re-create it, the amount of elevation laterally, centrally, and medially is noted.

Patients are pretreated with neuromodulation of the brow depressors to modify brow level and contour (see Chapter 5). This will give the patient a partial preview of the final result as well as enhancing the surgical result by relaxing the brow depressors during the postoperative period.

For brow stabilization and minimal elevation, in cases where only 1 or 2 mm of elevation are necessary, we prefer the transblepharoplasty approach, utilizing the CO_2 laser 0.2 mm handpiece as an incisional tool. Through an upper lid crease incision, a myocutaneous flap is elevated superiorly 5 mm above the superior orbital rim. Defocusing the laser handpiece, the brow fat pocket is vaporized, exposing the periosteum overlying the superior orbital rim. Two vertical mattress sutures of 4–0 Prolene are used to fixate the brow. One is placed laterally from the periosteum 3 mm above the lateral superior orbital rim to the undersurface of the orbicularis muscle at the tail of the brow (Fig. **9–12**). The second is placed more medially from the periosteum 4 to 5 mm above the superior orbital rim, and in a line with the lateral limbus, to the undersurface of the orbicularis in the central portion of the brow. The contour of the brow arch can be changed to suit the patient by modifying the placement of the central internal suspension suture. Superficial placement of the suborbicularis suture can give dimpling of the brow. Aggressive resection of the brow fat pocket and postseptal fat in the superior sulcus can result in segmental retraction of the superior sulcus in the primary position and in downgaze. Defocused CO_2 laser vaporization of the brow suborbicularis fat and eyelid

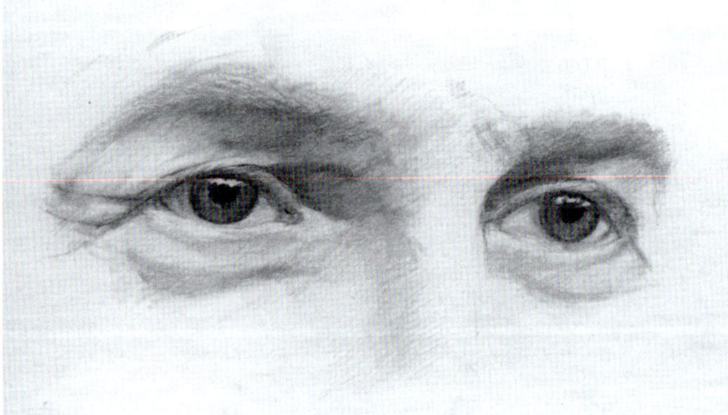

Figure 9–16 A ptotic brow creates a secondary upper lid fold redundancy and upper lid hooding.

preaponeurotic fat minimizes the occurrence of this potential complication.

After the brow has been stabilized, the lid crease incision is closed or the upper blepharoplasty is completed. More prominent lateral and central brow ptosis and marked medial brow ptosis are treated with endoscopic techniques (see Chapter 10).

Upper Lid Rejuvenation

Once the eyebrow level and contour are appropriately positioned and adjusted, when necessary, the upper eyelids can be addressed. During the preoperative examination, a ptotic brow is manually elevated and an overactive brow manually depressed so the extent and contour of the upper lid crease, height of the palpebral aperture, and levator excursions can be determined accurately. Patients with structural integrity of their eyebrows and eyelids can be managed with an artful blend of upper lid resection and laser resurfacing, using old photographs as a guide.

Although the level of the upper lid crease is generally 8 to 10 mm above the lid margin, the level of the lid crease incision is determined after examining the patient's old photos and determining the action and position of the levator aponeurosis. Classically, a disinserted levator aponeurosis presents as an elevated upper lid crease with a retracted upper lid fold, a narrowed vertical palpebral aperture, an elevated brow, and normal levator excursions (Fig. **9–5A,B**). The vertical palpebral aperture may even appear normal if the brow elevation has completely compensated for the ptosis.

The proposed depth of the superior sulcus is determined by reviewing the patient's old photographs and discussing the proposed outcome with the patient. We use an old photo as a guide to how we would like to shape the upper lid fold. Remembering the dictum: "We want to make patients look well-rested and rejuvenated, but still retain their own characteristics" is of paramount importance. Patients are rarely pleased when a technically perfect procedure has been performed, yet they don't recognize themselves. Patients who have always had a full superior sulcus should maintain a full superior sulcus and may not feel comfortable with a deep, oversculpted superior sulcus. Giving a male patient a deep superior sulcus may feminize the appearance of his eyelids. Often patients with full upper lids do not require skin resection but, rather, cutaneous laser resurfacing to restore smoothness and resilience to the upper lid fold contour (Figs. **9–7A,B; 9–17A,B**). Patients with large aponeurotic disinsertions and retracted upper lid folds will appear to have a deep superior sulcus. Once the levator aponeurosis is repositioned, their upper lid fold will also be advanced. The advanced

A

B

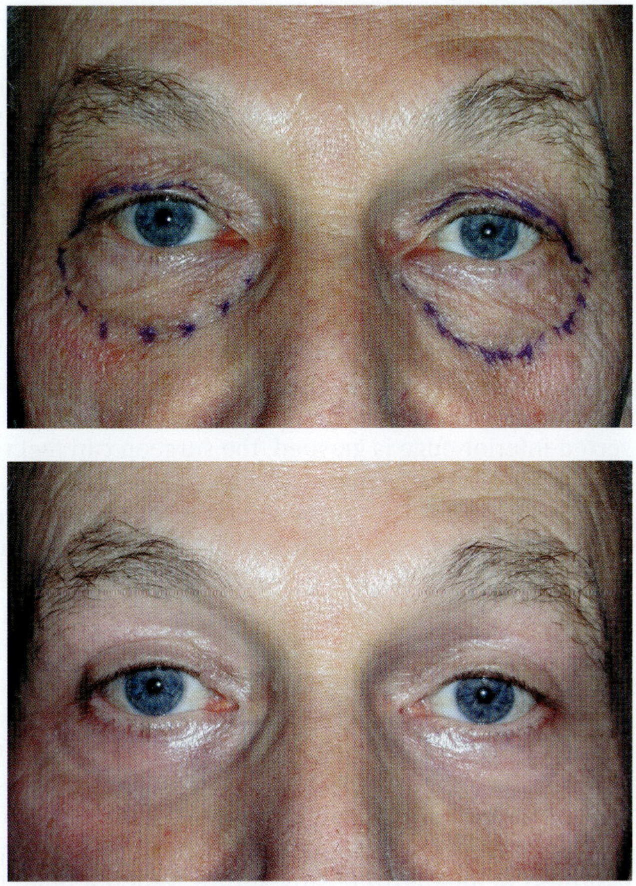

Figure 9–17 (**A**) This patient exhibited marked actinic changes and rhytidosis of his eyelids. (**B**) Eyelid resurfacing (CO_2, two passes, 200 and 150 mJ, pattern 3, size 4) improved this patient's eyelid contours and texture.

upper lid fold will often require trimming. Patients accustomed to their deep superior sulci have to be informed that after their ptosis has been corrected, their levator apponeurosis has been reattached, and their lid–crease–fold complex has been restored, their eyelids will have the more "normal" appearance of an upper eyelid fold. Patients may not understand this at first and may be surprised postoperatively unless they have been made aware of this beforehand.

Bulging of the upper outer segment of the upper lid should not be confused with a fat pocket. Although the nasal upper lid fat pocket is often quite prominent, and the central pocket can create a full superior sulcus, a lateral fat pocket does not exist in the upper lid. Temporal bulging is most commonly secondary to a prolapsed orbital lobe of the lacrimal gland. This may occur in patients with shallow bony orbits (i.e., most commonly with patients of African or Asian descent) or an enlarged lacrimal gland (i.e., sarcoidosis).

An upper lid crease incision is made with a 0.2 mm CO_2 laser handpiece, utilizing the ultrapulse mode, 5 mJ 1000 Hz, and a focused beam. The superior edge of the cultaneous resection is made in a similar fashion. If the levator aponeurosis is being repaired, an inferior skin flap is developed, exposing the pretarsal orbicularis muscle but avoiding damage to the upper lid lashes. A 4 mm strip of the superior portion of the pretarsal orbicularis muscle is resected, exposing the underlying anterior surface of the tarsus and providing a platform for reinserting the advanced aponeurosis. Superiorly a myocutaneous flap is developed, exposing the orbital septum. The septum is opened exposing the preaponeurotic fat and the disinserted levator aponeurosis. The surgeon can confirm the location of the disinserted aponeurosis by asking the patient to look up and look down and watching the diaphanous white structure move. When the disinserted inferior edge is grasped, the surgeon can feel the pull. While feeling the pull of the aponeurosis, and palpating the superior sulcus, there should be no transmission of movement or tautness palpated in the superior sulcus.

If the inferior cut edge of the orbital septum is grasped, a tautness can be palpated in the superior sulcus where it attaches to the arcus marginalis. Three mattress sutures of 6–0 black silk are used to reapproximate the disinserted aponeurosis to the anterior surface of the tarsus (Fig. **9–10**). The patient is asked to open and close the eyes and to look up and down to confirm the appropriate lid margin elevation, contour, and lack of lid lag on downgaze: a sign that the orbital septum is captured in an anastomosing suture. When a bilateral procedure is performed, both lid margins are adjusted before the lid crease incisions are closed.

If the grayish, lobular, orbital portion of the lacrimal gland is visible and prolapsed, it can be repositioned into the lacrimal fossa with a 4–0 Prolene mattress suture (Fig. **9–11**). Two superficial bites are placed in the anterior surface of the gland and are then anchored to the periosteum within the bony lacrimal fossa. When the suture is tightened, the gland retracts into the fossa.

The preaponeurotic fat is then vaporized with a defocused beam (CW mode 5 mJ), and sculpted in a bloodless field. The wound is closed with interrupted 6–0 black silk sutures, which are left in place for 5 to 7 days.

Lower Eyelid Rejuvenation

Lower eyelid rejuvenation can, in most cases, be accomplished without skin resection. A combination of transconjunctival lipovaporization, lateral canthal tendon plication, and cutaneous laser resurfacing techniques are effective in correcting fatty prolapse, lid margin laxity, and cutaneous rhytidosis. If there is no lid margin or lateral canthal tendon laxity and no significant cutaneous rhytidosis, lipovaporization alone via a transconjunctival approach will be effective.

With the patient sitting upright, in primary gaze, abducting, adducting, and supraducting, the location and extent of each prolapsed fatty pocket is noted preoperatively. On some occasions the three inferior fat pockets are distinctly visible. On other occasions they may appear confluent. Of particular note is the lateral pocket, which may not be visible until the patient abducts each eye. A concave contour just lateral to a prominent anterior lacrimal crest may create a tear trough deformity. These are best addressed with a technique of combined lipovaporization, fat transposition, and laser resurfacing (Fig. **9–7A,B**).

The lower lid level, contour, and acuteness of the lateral canthal angle are noted. The degree of horizontal lower lid margin laxity is noted. The amount, location, and extent—in relation to the inferior orbital rim—of lower lid rhytidosis are noted. Malar festoons, their cutaneous, orbicularis muscle, and fatty components, are noted (Fig. **9–13A,B**).

Lipovaporization, bloodless sculpting, of the prolapsed inferior fat pockets is performed via the transconjunctival approach. Using a 0.2 mm handpiece, 5 mJ ultrapulse, 1000 Hz, and a focused beam, the globe is gently compressed and the conjunctiva is opened over the bulge of orbital fat, ~4 mm inferior to the inferior tarsal margin (Fig. **9–18**). The conjunctival edges are retracted with small rakes, a defocused beam [0.2 mm handpiece 5 W continuous wave (CW)] vaporizes the fat and sculpts its anterior contour (Fig. **9–19A,B**). Cotton-tipped applicators keep the field dry (they must be lightly moistened to avoid being singed by the laser beam). Intermittent gentle pressure on the globe exposes residual fat in each of the three compartments for additional sculpting. The inferior oblique muscle is prominently visible during the transconjunctival approach to lower lid blepharoplasty. It courses between the medial and central fat pockets. The surgeon must be aware of its location during vaporization of the medial

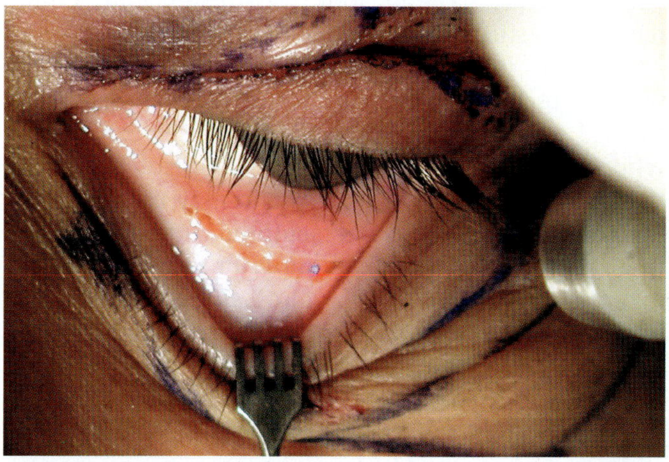

Figure 9–18 The conjunctival incision is made 3–4 mm inferior to the inferior tarsal margin using a 0.2 mm CO_2 laser incisional handpiece.

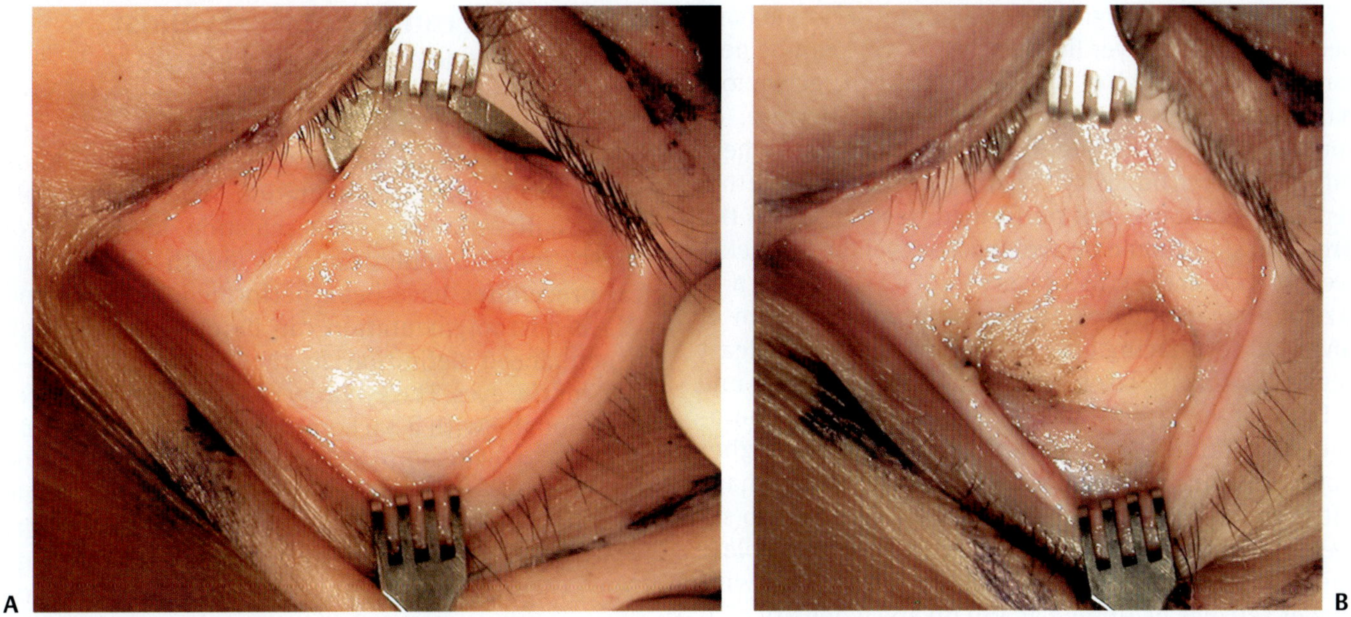

Figure 9–19 (**A,B**) The three inferior fat pockets are exposed and vaporized one pocket at a time with a defocused CO_2 laser (0.2 mm handpiece, 5 W continuous wave).

fat pocket to avoid inadvertent vaporization or charring of the muscle. Wide exposure, diligence, and repeated pressure on the globe facilitate localizing and effectively sculpting the lateral fat pocket.

Fat transposition is performed medially after the central pocket has been recontoured. The base of the medial pocket is mobilized with a defocused beam, using 5 mJ CW, sealing any visible vessels. A mattress suture of 6–0 plain gut is placed through the anterior portion of the medial pocket and then brought through the skin overlying the anterior lacrimal crest.

If lateral canthal tendon laxity is evident or has been demonstrated preoperatively, it is plicated with a 4–0 Prolene suture via a 2 mm lateral subciliary incision and an upper lid crease incision extended to the lateral orbital rim. Each arm of the suture is passed from the lateral inferior palebral conjunctiva, through the cutaneous incision (Fig. **9–20**). They are then replaced into the small lateral subciliary incision, passed deeply, laterally, and superiorly to engage the deep expansions of the lateral canthal tendon 4 mm posterior to the lateral orbital rim, and exiting in the lateral lid crease incision. The sutures are then anchored to the periosteum of the superior aspect of the lateral orbital rim. The incisions are closed.

If there is excessive lower lid margin laxity, and the lid margin is pleated after a lateral canthal plication, then lid margin resection and a lateral tarsal strip procedure are necessary for proper lid margin apposition to the globe and lateral canthal angle rejuvenation. A lateral canthotomy and cantholysis are performed. The lateral severed edge of lid margin and tarsus are pulled over the lateral orbital rim. The lid margin is notched where it overlaps the orbital rim. The lid margin, lash line, orbicularis muscle, and skin lateral to the notch are resected. The tarsus is preserved. A double-armed 4–0 Prolene suture anchors the lateral tarsal strip to the periosteum posterior to the lateral orbital rim and to the superior crus of the lateral canthal tendon. The lateral canthal angle is re-created with interrupted 6–0 silk sutures anastomosing the inferior and superior gray lines, lash lines, and meibomian orifices. The suture ends are left long and folded over the skin to avoid corneal irritation.

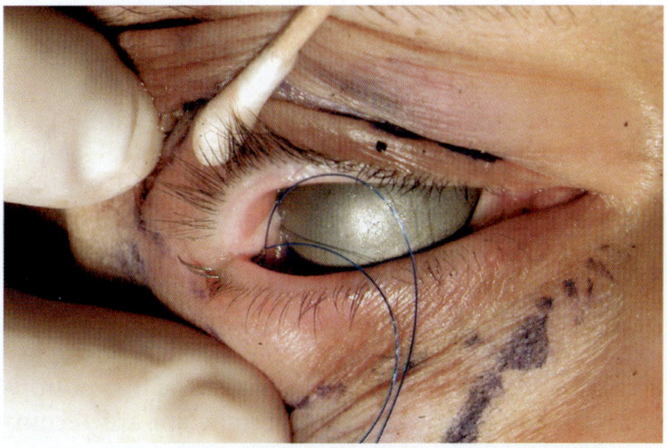

Figure 9–20 Lateral canthal plication. A mattress suture of 4–0 Prolene is passed from the lateral palpebral conjunctiva through a lateral subciliary incision.

Once the lid margin and lateral canthal angle have been stabilized, lower lid laser resurfacing can be performed without risk of lower lid retraction, ectropion, narrowing of the horizontal palpebral aperture, or rounding of the lateral canthal angle. In patients where minimal lower lid laxity is evident but lateral canthal tendon plication is not performed, resurfacing of the pretarsal skin should be avoided. For eyelid resurfacing we use CO_2 and Er:YAG lasers with CPGs (pattern 3, size 4, a small square). There is a broad spectrum of lower lid resurfacing options. Beginning with the least severe rhytidosis, laser resurfacing can begin with one 2-J pass of the Er:YAG, anesthetized with topical Photocaine. As more passes, more potent lasers, and higher power settings are used, local infiltration and perhaps intravenous sedation will be necessary. If three to six passes with an Er:YAG laser do not adequately ablate the rhytids, we proceed to CO_2 laser resurfacing, with power settings beginning at 150 mJ and a density of 5. Our highest eyelid settings are typically 250 mJ, density 6. For moderately severe rhytids, we will treat with a second pass of 200 to 250 mJ, avoiding the prepunctal, pretarsal area on the second pass. For malar festoons that are primarily cutaneous and muscular, we use settings as high as 300 mJ for two to three passes.

Resurfaced lower eyelids and malar festoons are covered with Flexan (Bentek/Hickman Research Triangle Park, North Carolina) dressings for 5 to 7 days. Upper lid crease incisions and resurfaced eyelid skin are treated with erythromycin ophthalmic ointment three times daily until the sutures are removed on the seventh postoperative day. Immediately following the procedure Natragel Eye Ovals (Gel Concepts, Whipanny, New Jersey) are applied to the eyes for 20 minutes, refrigerated, then reapplied. This is continued for the first 36 postoperative hours.

◆ Perioperative Care

Beginning at least 2 weeks preoperatively 1000 mg of oral vitamin C is recommended after each meal, and all antiinflammatory medications and vitamin E are discontinued. To reduce ecchymosis and edema all patients begin taking sublingual *Arnica montana* C_{12} pellets 3 days preoperatively and continue for 7 to 10 days postoperatively. Lymphatic drainage massage is recommended pre- and postoperatively on the day of surgery and, when possible, continued daily for the first postoperative week. Oral papain and bromelain are recommended three times daily during the first postoperative week.

◆ The Final Framing of the Eyelids: Micropigmentation and Single Follicular Unit Hair Transplantation

Although all of the procedures described in this book are art forms, micropigmentation requires multiple artistic skills—drawing, color selection, knowledge of cosmetic makeup application. One month after the surgical procedures have been performed, eyebrow and eyelash micropigmentation can be applied. This will give enhanced definition to the periorbital area—a frame for the eyes. The eyebrow can be enhanced three-dimensionally with a background color (Fig. **9–21A,B**). Later hair strokes with a slightly darker color can be applied. This can be further augmented with single follicular unit hair transplantation (Fig. **9–22A,B**). The eyelashes can also be enhanced by applying a fine line of micropigmentation between the eyelashes or just anterior to them. Care is taken not to create a thick line or to make a fashion statement. This technique is used as a basic lash enhancement technique. Makeup can be applied in addition for special occasions. Following micropigmentation, areas of lash alopecia can be remedied with single-follicle grafts.

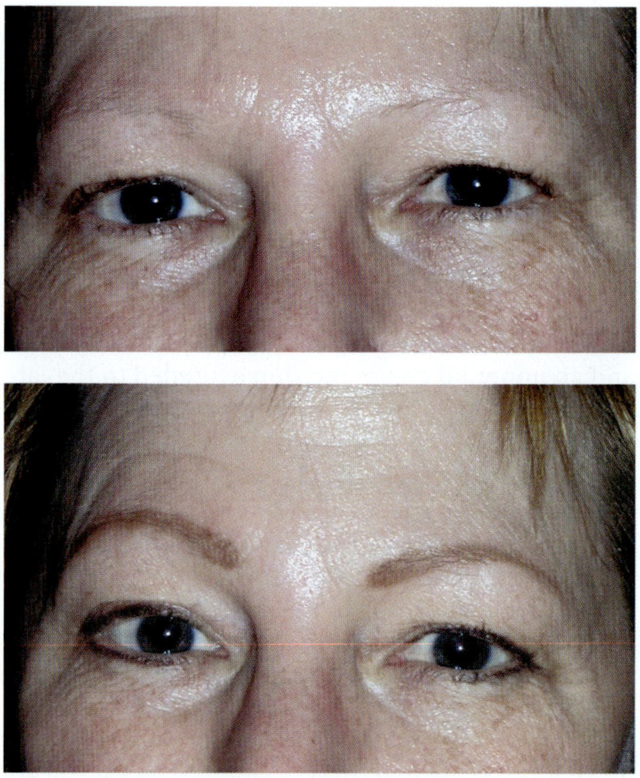

A

B

Figure 9–21 (**A**) This patient has few eyebrow hairs. Her eyes disappear in a monochromatic field. (**B**) Background micropigmentation of the eyebrows creates periorbital definition and enhances the appearance of the eyes.

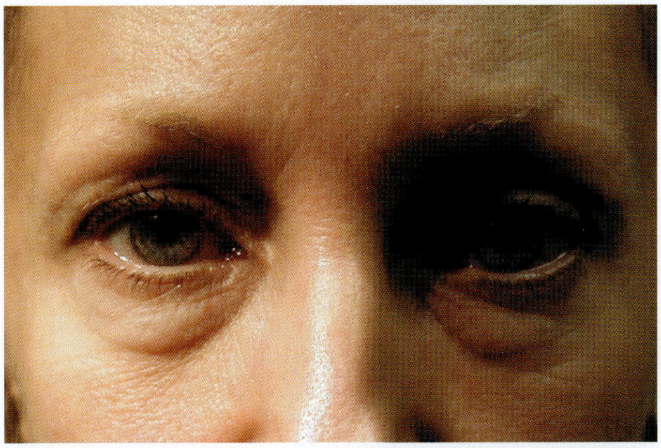

A

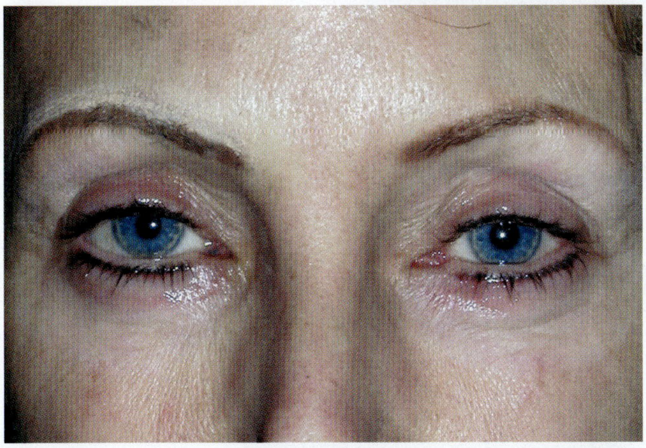

B

Figure 9–22 (**A**) The preoperative image is side-lit to emphasize the patient's eyelid skin texture and contour irregularities as well as redundant upper lid folds, prolapsing orbital fat, and eyebrow alopecia. (**B**) Upper and lower blepharoplasty and eyelid resurfacing are further enhanced with single hair follicular unit transplantation and micropigmentation of the eyebrows and lid margins.

Basic Principles of Micropigmentation

Pigment Selection

For eyebrows the color that is selected should match the patient's hair color; it may be slightly darker but should never be black or overly bright (extreme reds are also to be avoided). The patient's underlying skin tone must also be taken into consideration. The color in the bottle will not appear the same once it has been applied to the skin. Remembering the color wheel (Fig. **9–23**) is essential: green balances red and violet balances yellow. That is why implanted black pigment may appear blue in certain patients. Ruddy-complexioned Irish patients, Native Americans, and "peaches and cream golden girls" are warm. If a cool pigment is applied to them without first balancing their underlying skin tones, the effect will be muddy. Conversely, cool-complexioned Scandinavian, Mediterranean, and Asian patients will need their underlying skin tone balanced before warm pigments can be applied to them.

All colors fade with time and some colors oxidize faster than others. Shades of brown and gray are more discrete, appear more natural when implanted, and fade more uniformly. Buying pigment from a reputable source is also exceptionally important. Contaminated, commercial grade, and not cosmetic grade pigment may cause localized granulomatous reactions. Organic pigments (brighter colors) may be more prone to granulomatous reactions. For eyeliner micropigmentation, the darkest brown should always be used and black should be avoided.

Brow Shaping and Eyelash Enhancement

Eyebrow level and contour and their relationship to the bony superior orbital rim, upper lid superior sulcus, and lid–crease–fold complex must all be considered. Judicious plucking may be the first step. Although subject to personal variations and desires, the traditional female brow arch is highest at the level of the outer corneal limbus. The medial aspect customarily extends to the vertical line draw from the outer aspect of the nostril to where it intersects the brow (Fig. **9–24**). And the lateral aspect customarily extends to the line drawn from the external aspect of the nostril, through the lateral canthal angle where it intersects the brow (Fig. **9–25**). Past and future procedures and their effect on brow level and contour must also be considered. Brow shaping with Botox neuromodulation is a frequently performed procedure in our office. If the patient maintains a satifactory result with this procedure, micropigmentation of the brow can be performed. If further elevation is desired, surgical browlifting procedures can be performed before the micropigmentation is applied. Patients not desiring further surgical brow elevation can be treated with complete removal of eyebrow follicles and micropigmentation and follicle transplantation at the desired level.

Eyelash enhancement with micropigmentation is applied discretely either between the lashes or just anterior to the lash line in the lower lid or just superior to the lash line in the upper lid. The line should not be extended further medially than the punctum, not further laterally than the lateral canthal angle. Thick, wide applications of pigment are discouraged. Applications of pigment into the palpebral conjunctiva and peripunctal areas are also avoided.

Technique

The areas to be treated are painted with topical Photocaine. During the procedure, the areas can be painted with topical anesthetic gel and epinephrine. Rarely local

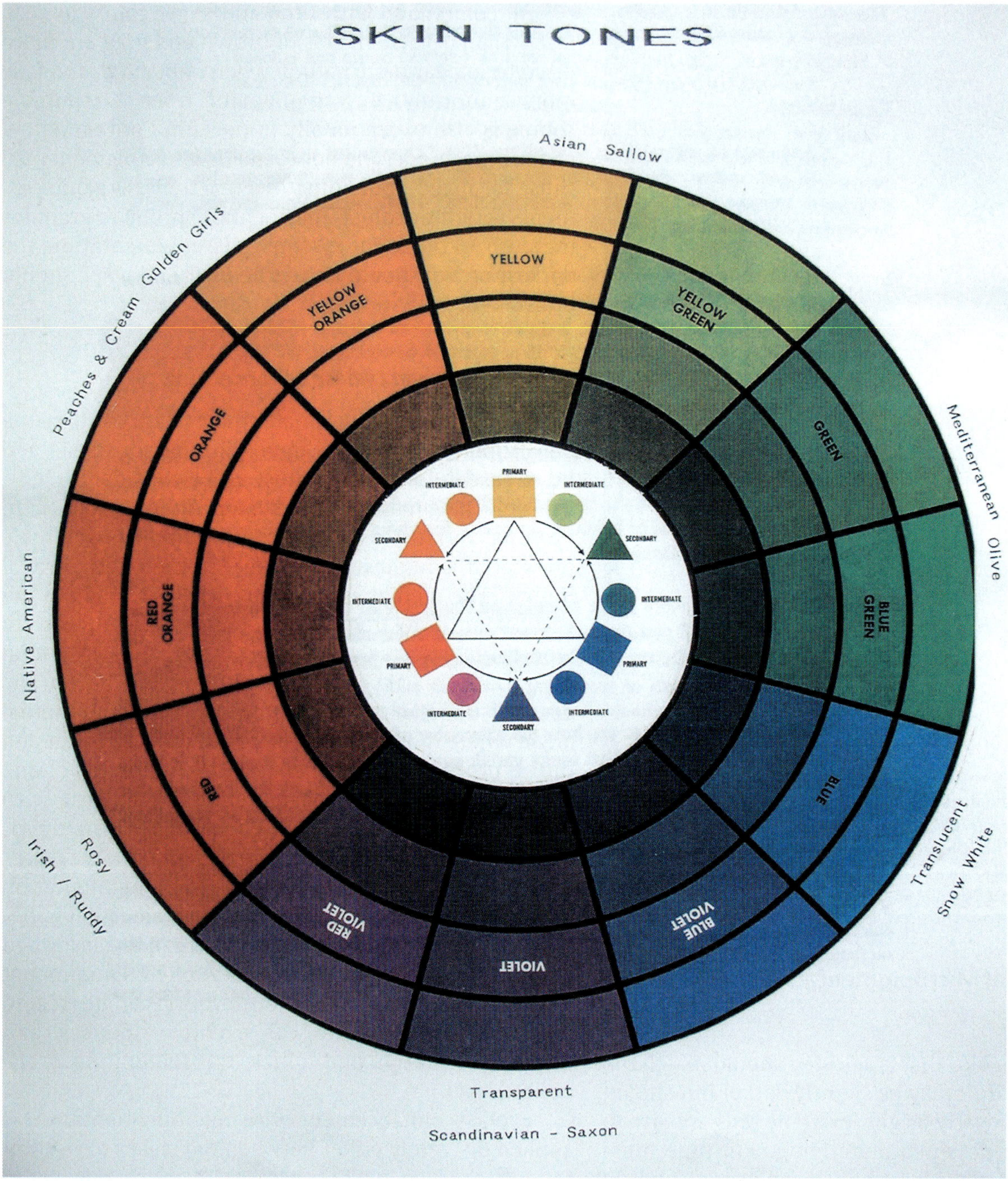

Figure 9–23 The color wheel depicts color balance and ethnic skin undertones. (*Courtesy of the Society of Permanent Cosmetic Professionals.*)

infiltration with xylocaine and epinephrine is required. For greater accuracy, this procedure should be performed while wearing surgical loupes.

A sturdy, easy to hold, powerful device, with controlled speed and depth penetration, operated with a foot pedal (Harmonix, Boca Raton, Florida) makes the procedure more efficient, effective, and reliable while avoiding complications. The Harmonix device has a digital display of the needle speed (most often used between 90 and 130) for a controlled depth of penetration (between 1.25 and 1.57 mm). Although held like a pen device, it has the power of a coil machine, but is easier to use. This instrumentation minimizes tissue trauma, bleeding, and edema and facilitates exact pigment implantation. This is especially important, not only regarding making the experience more pleasant for the patient, but because if there is bleeding, crusting or marked edema, the pigment will not stay in place and overly deep implantation of pigment will lead to pigment migration.

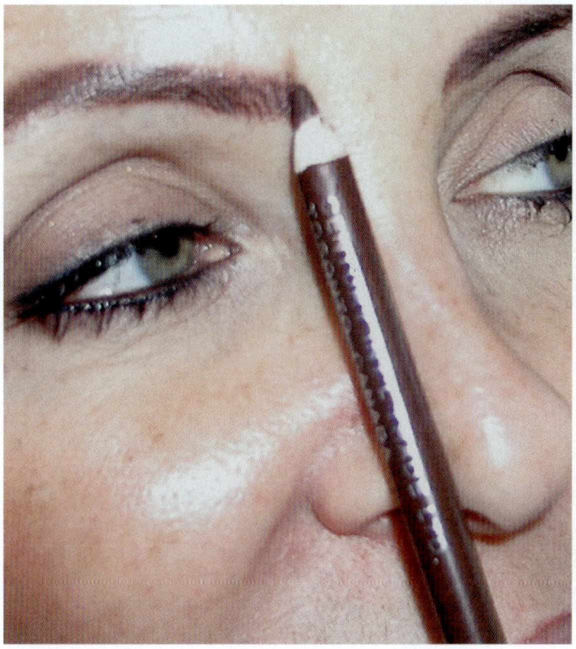

Figure 9–24 The medial extent of the brow is determined by extending a straight line from the side of the nose to the orbital rim.

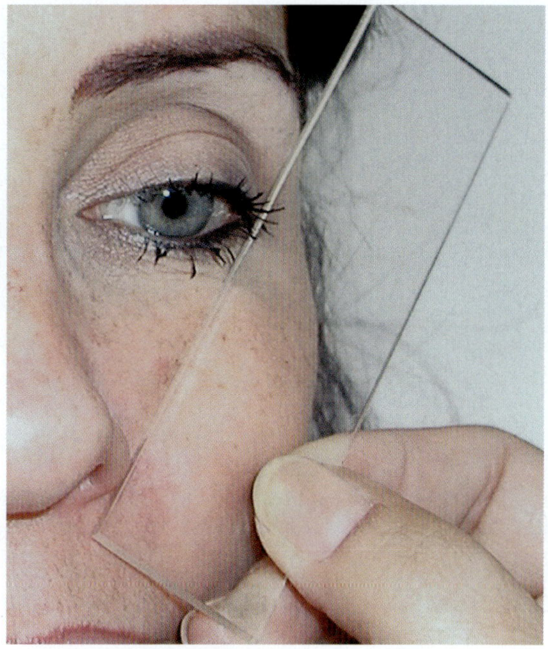

Figure 9–25 The lateral extent of the brow is determined by extending a straight line from the side of the nose through the lateral canthal angle.

For background brow shading, a #3 needle is used with a circular pattern of application. Hair strokes are created with a #3 outline needle or a #1 needle. Hair strokes must be applied deliberately to avoid tissue masceration. Bland ointment is applied to the micropigmented areas four times daily for 1 week to avoid crusting. The micropigmented areas are also kept dry during that first week. For eyelash enhancement a #3 outline or #1 needle is used.

Single Follicular Unit Hair Transplantation

For use as a procedure for correcting complete eyebrow or eyelash alopecia, for correcting segmental hair loss, or to enhance the results of micropigmentation, single follicular unit hair transplantation is an effective technique. An elliptical resection of occipital scalp in the area of highest hair density provides the graft material. Under magnification and retroillumination single follicular units are dissected free (Fig. **9–26**). In the eyebrow,

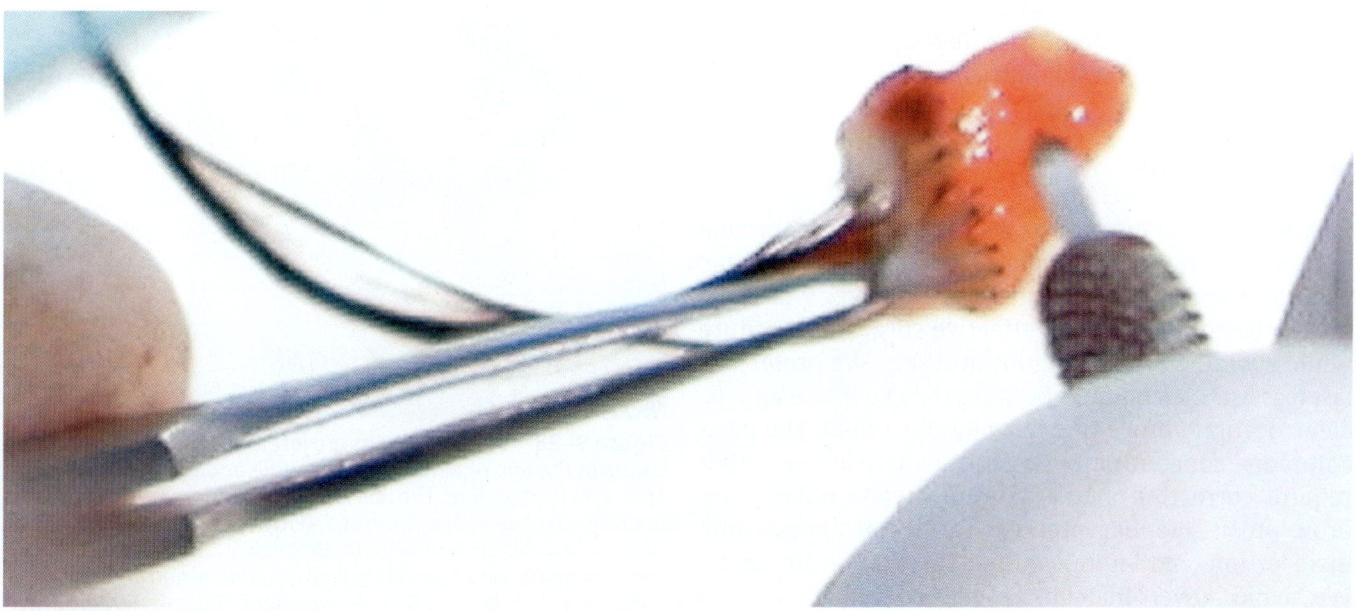

Figure 9–26 Single follicular units are dissected with magnification and retroillumination.

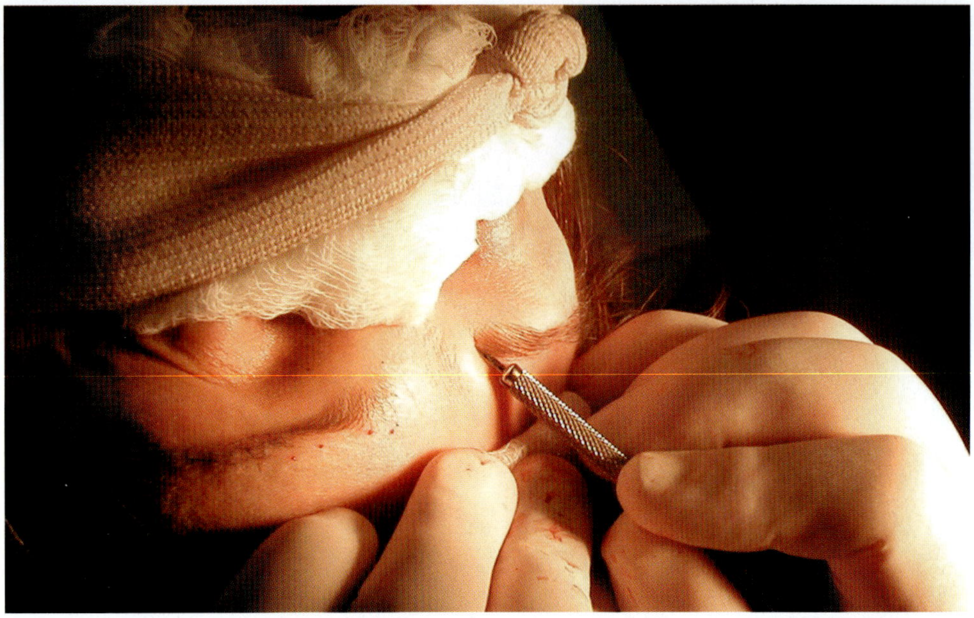

Figure 9–27 Brow implantation sites are created with a solid-core 27-gauge needle in the direction of the proposed hair grafts, which will follow the direction of the normal brow hairs, more vertically oriented nasally and more horizontally directed laterally.

a solid-core 27-gauge needle is used to create the recipient sites, angling them in the appropriate direction of normal brow hair growth (more vertical nasally and more horizontal laterally) (Fig. **9–27**). The individual follicular units are placed into the holes with a jeweler's forceps. For complete brow restoration 50 to 100 units may be necessary per brow. Hair growth may not be evident for several months after implantation and in most cases will require trimming.

For eyelash restoration, the hair is left long and threaded into the eye of a #16 free French needle. The needle enters the lid pretarsally and exits in the lash line (Fig. **9–28**). The hair is advanced until the follicle remains in place. Then the hair is trimmed. This procedure is only performed on the upper lid where the lashes are more evident. Also lower lid margin hair transplantation may result in trichiasis.

◆ Conclusion

Enhancing eyelid function as well as cosmesis is the goal of reconstructive blepharoplasty. Recognizing anatomic variations and age-related structural changes will allow for the performance of an effective surgical procedure while avoiding potential complications. We prefer CO_2 laser-assisted techniques because they facilitate an efficient, accurate procedure in a bloodless field. The most common concomitant structural deficiencies that require correction at the time of blepharoplasty are brow ptosis, blepharoptosis with levator aponeurotic disinsertion, and lateral canthal and lid margin laxity. We avoid lower lid skin resection and advocate a transconjunctival approach with lateral canthal plication and cutaneous laser resurfacing. Adjunctive procedures that enhance the final result include periorbital rejuvenation with Botox (Allergan), Restylane (Medicis, Scottsdale, Arizona), Perlane (Q-Med, Uppsala, Sweden), and micropigmentation, with or without single follicular unit hair transplantation of the brows and lid margins.

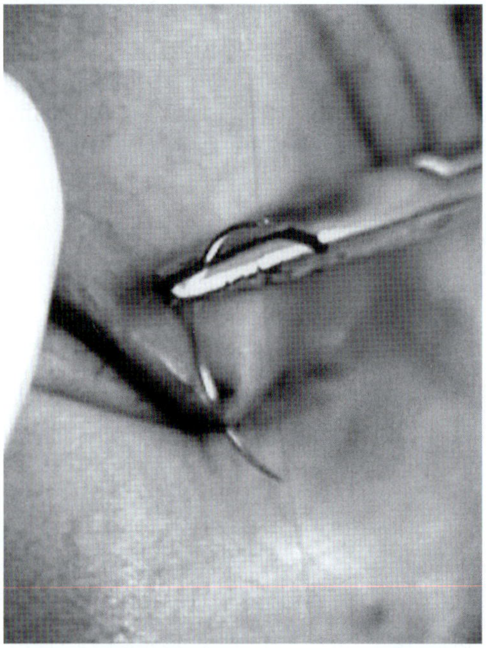

Figure 9–28 Lash graft hairs are left long. The hair is threaded through the eye of a free French needle and passed pretarsally, exiting in the lash line. The hair is pulled anterior until the follicle is in place. The hair is then trimmed. (From Gandelman M. Eyebrow and eyelash reconstruction. In: Bosniak S, Cantisano-Zilkha M, eds. *Operative Techniques in Oculoplastic Orbital and Reconstructive Surgery, Vol. 4, No. 2, 2003*. Amsterdam: Swets and Zeitlinger. With permission.)

Suggested Readings

1. Bosniak S. Cosmetic Blepharoplasty. New York: Raven; 1990
2. Bosniak S, ed. Principles and Practice of Ophthalmic Plastic and Reconstructive Surgery. Philadelphia: Saunders; 1996
3. Bosniak S, Cantisano-Zilkha M. Lymphatic drainage massage: a double blind study of effectiveness. Operative Techniques in Oculoplastic, Orbital, and Reconstructive Surgery. 1999;2: 214–217
4. Bosniak S, Cantisano-Zilkha M. Total eyelid rejuvenation. Operative Techniques in Oculoplastic, Orbital, and Reconstructive Surgery. 1999;2:198–203
5. Bosniak S, Cantisano-Zilkha M. Cosmetic Blepharoplasty and Facial Rejuvenation. New York: Lippincott-Raven; 1999
6. Bosniak S, Cantisano-Zilkha M, Nestor M. Therma-lifting of the face, neck, and brows. Operative Techniques in Oculoplastic, Orbital, and Reconstructive Surgery 2001;4:113–119
7. Bosniak S, Cantisano-Zilkha M, Ziering C, et al. Eyebrow rejuvenation: a multidisciplinary approach. Operative Techniques in Oculoplastic, Orbital, and Reconstructive Surgery 2001;4: 100–103
8. Bosniak S, McDebitt T, Wojno TH. Alternative techniques of fat removal. In Bosniak S, ed. Principles and Practice of Ophthalmic Plastic and Reconstructive Surgery, Vol. 1. Philadelphia: Saunders; 1996:632–638
9. Custer PL. Lower eyelid blepharoplasty. In Bosniak S, ed. Principles and Practice of Ophthalmic Plastic and Reconstructive Surgery. Philadelphia: Saunders; 1996:617–626
10. Gandelman M. Eyebrow and eyelash reconstruction. Operative Techniques in Oculoplastic, Orbital, and Reconstructive Surgery 2001;4:94–99
11. Goldberg RA, Baylis HI, Golden SH. Transconjunctival lower blepharoplasty. In Bosniak S, ed. Principles and Practice of Ophthalmic Plastic and Reconstructive Surgery. Philadelphia: Saunders; 1996:626–632
12. Maries HM, Patrinely JR. Male blepharoplasty. In Bosniak S, ed. Principles and Practice of Ophthalmic Plastic and Reconstructive Surgery. Philadelphia: Saunders; 1996:632–638
13. Mazza JF, Roger C. Blepharopigmentation: techniques, indications and comparison of modalities. In Bosniak S, ed. Principles and Practice of Ophthalmic Plastic and Reconstructive Surgery. Philadelphia: Saunders; 1996:682–688
14. Meneuzes. The principles of permanent facial makeup. Operative Techniques in Oculoplastic, Orbital, and Reconstructive Surgery 1999;2:182–187
15. Ploof H. Electropigmentation and the cosmetic surgery patient. In Bosniak S, ed. Principles and Practice of Ophthalmic Plastic and Reconstructive Surgery. Philadelphia: Saunders; 1996:676–681
16. Reifler DM. Upper eyelid blepharoplasty. In Bosniak S, ed. Principles and Practice of Ophthalmic Plastic and Reconstructive Surgery. Philadelphia: Saunders; 1996:596–617
17. Weiss RA. Brow ptosis. In Bosniak S, ed. Principles and Practice of Ophthalmic Plastic and Reconstructive Surgery. Philadephia: Saunders; 1996:578–589
18. Wojno TH, Bosniak S. Cosmetic surgery. In Bosniak S, ed. Principles and Practice of Ophthalmic Plastic and Reconstructive Surgery. Philadelphia: Saunders; 1996:543–545

10

Endoscopic Forehead Rejuvenation

Thomas Romo III, Haresh Yalamanchili, and Kyle Seung Choe

The symmetry and balance of the face, which are essential components of an aesthetically pleasing visage, are gradually altered as a result of various aging factors. The resulting dissonance of various facial features poses a challenge to the facial plastic surgeon. The dissonance from aging is often most dramatically reflected in the upper third of the face: development of forehead rhytids, sagging of the eyebrows, and hooding of the upper eyelids.

The aesthetic importance of the upper third of the face is well established, and efforts at facial rejuvenation typically focus on this region. For nearly a century, aesthetic rejuvenation of the aging face has involved the surgical elevation of the brow. Several different techniques have been widely utilized to reverse the forehead aging process and to restore a youthful appearance. Three classic approaches to forehead rejuvenation include the coronal forehead lift, the high forehead lift, and the midforehead lift. Despite their popularity, these approaches have carried significant disadvantages such as visible scars, hypoesthesia, alopecia, and the unnecessary removal of healthy hair-bearing skin.

The advent of endoscopic facial plastic surgery has allowed present-day aesthetic surgeons to avoid many of these morbidities without compromising the result. First introduced by Keller in 1991, the endoscopic forehead lift is a minimally invasive technique for forehead rejuvenation. Under endoscopic visualization the surgeon may perform myotomies of the muscles contributing to brow ptosis and forehead rhytids, as well as temple lifts. When compared with the classic approaches, several advantages are evident with the endoscopic technique: preservation of the scalp sensory nerves, better control of brow position, accurate resection of brow depressor muscles, decreased postsurgical numbness and edema with a shorter recovery period, and preservation of hair-bearing skin.

Since its introduction many authors have reported their personal experiences and have offered various modifications of the endoscopic technique. There has been great success with the technique, with long-lasting results equivalent to those of the traditional open approaches, yet without the associated morbidity of the traditional procedures. Accordingly, many surgeons are now choosing the endoscopic technique in preference to coronal brow lift procedures.

◆ The Aging Process

Aging is a gradual process in which the smooth, wrinkle-free skin of youth is altered. This process begins to manifest itself in the forehead region as early as the fourth decade, at which point horizontal lines begin to appear. These lines begin to deepen and vertical lines form in the glabella during the fifth decade. Concurrently, the eyebrows begin to descend and flatten with prolapse of the infrabrow tissue over the thin eyelid skin, leading to medial and lateral hooding of the upper eyelid. These various changes combine to alter the aesthetically appealing Y-shaped sweep between the eyebrow, medial orbit, and lateral nose to a T-shaped impression. The result is a countenance seemingly conveying anger, sadness, or fatigue (Fig. **10–1A–D**).

The aging effects on forehead skin are pronounced because of the uniquely intimate relationship between the skin and muscle of the upper third of the face. With minimal subcutaneous tissue present to separate skin

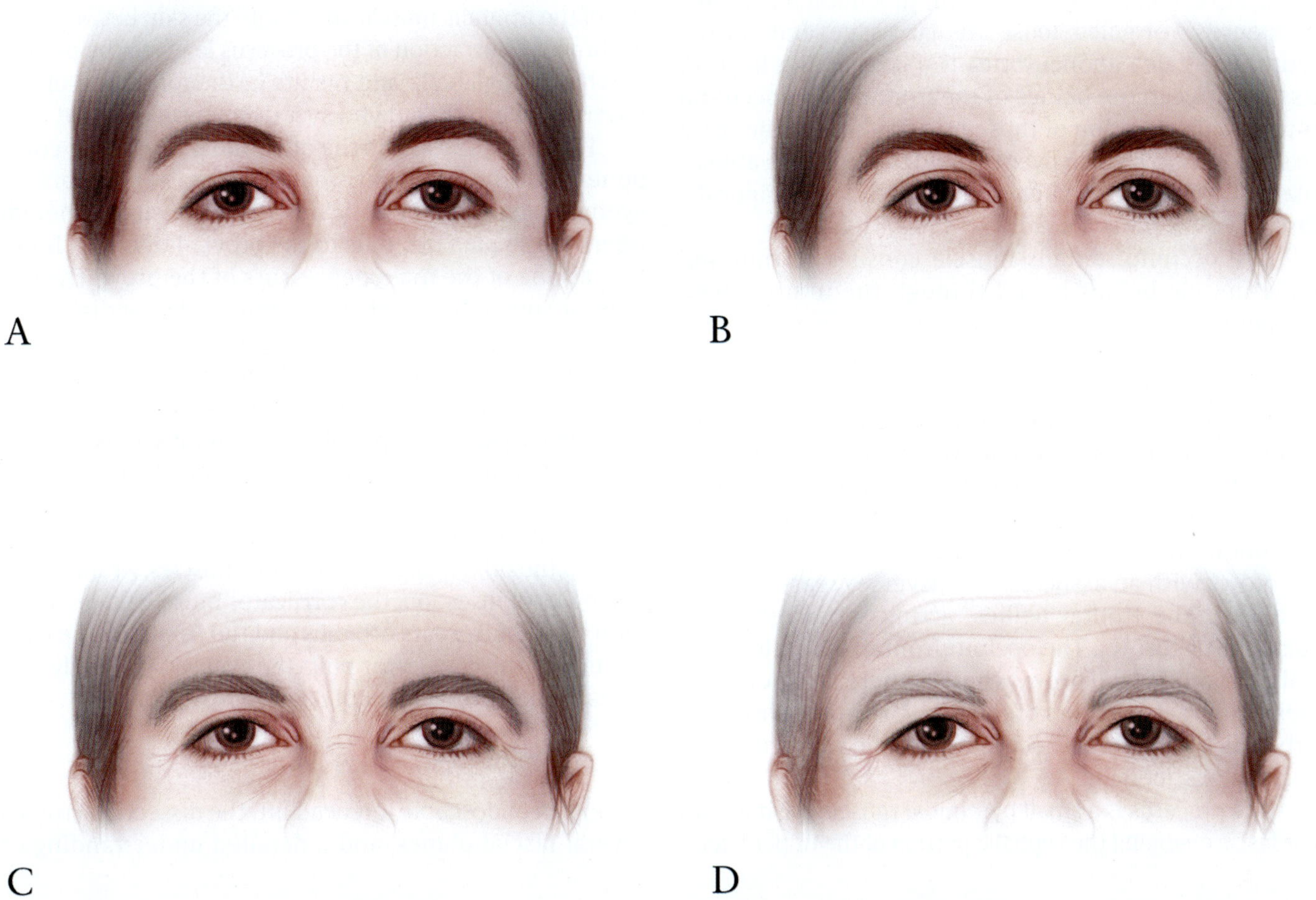

Figure 10–1 Aging process in the forehead region. (A) A young wrinkle-free forehead develops (B) horizontal rhytids by the fourth decade. (C) Vertical glabellar furrows begin to develop subsequently. (D) Ultimately, an appearance seemingly conveying anger, sadness, or fatigue results. (Courtesy of Karl Storz Endoscopy-America, Inc., Culver City, California.)

from muscle, the repetitive actions of facial muscles are directly transmitted to the overlying skin, predisposing this region to develop deep wrinkles and furrows. Ellis and Masai[1] have previously discussed three basic patterns of facial animation that lead to the development of rhytids and brow ptosis: eyebrow raising, frowning, and squinting. Eyebrow raising, which involves the contraction of the frontalis muscles, gradually but permanently establishes horizontal wrinkles on the forehead. The most inferior horizontal rhytid, over the radix of the nose, is due to the action of the procerus muscle. Frowning reflects the action of the corrugator supercilli muscles to bring the medial club heads of the eyebrows together, resulting in deep vertical glabellar rhytids. Lastly, repeated squinting—contraction of the orbicularis oculi—causes "crow's feet" at the lateral canthus.

Aesthetic balance requires that the vertical proportion of the middle third of the face be equivalent to that of the lower third. With forehead aging and the resultant brow ptosis, the middle third of the face becomes increasingly compressed and narrowed in comparison to the lower third. Rejuvenation of the upper third of the face serves to restore balance and symmetry to the lower two thirds of the face.

◆ Forehead Anatomy

A comprehensive understanding of surgical anatomy is a prerequisite for any successful cosmetic surgical procedure. This is particularly true with the use of the endoscope, which necessitates a different perspective on the forehead anatomy. Appreciation of the various features of forehead musculature, fascia, and neurovascular structures will afford the surgeon superior results while avoiding potential complications.

Scalp and Forehead Musculature

The scalp is composed of the skin, subcutaneous tissue, aponeurosis or galea, loose areolar tissue, and periosteum. The galea aponeurotica is a connecting band of tissue between the bellies of the frontalis and occipital muscles. Contraction of these muscles causes the scalp to slide back and forth over the underlying loose areolar plane. Laterally, the galea merges with the temporalis fascia.

The occipitofrontalis muscle consists of thin and wide muscle bellies joined through the intermediate aponeurosis. At the coronal suture, the galea gives rise to the insertion of the frontal bellies, which frequently appear in a quadrilateral shape. The frontalis is contiguous with the procerus muscle (via medial fibers), corrugator supercilii muscle (via intermediate fibers), and the pars orbitalis of the orbicularis oculi muscle (via lateral fibers) (Fig. **10–2**). The perceived action of the occipitofrontalis muscle, functioning as a unit, is to raise the eyebrows with an associated transverse creasing of the forehead. The frontal bellies, acting separately, only raise the eyebrows. The occipitofrontalis muscle is the only elevator of the brow, whereas there are four muscles that are depressors of the brow: the procerus, pars orbitalis of orbicularis oculi, depressor supercilii, and corrugator supercilii.

The procerus is a small pyramidal muscle arising from the fascia overlying the cephalic portion of the upper lateral nasal cartilages and the inferior aspect of the nasal bones. The muscle fibers, which interdigitate with the medial border of the frontalis muscle, insert into the skin between the eyebrows. Contraction of the procerus leads to the pulling down of the glabella and results in the formation of the lowermost horizontal rhytid over the radix of the nose.

The pars orbitalis is the only one of the three components of the orbicularis oculi that has an impact on eyebrow motion. The attachment of the superomedial fibers of the pars orbitalis to the brow allows it to function as one of the main depressors of the brow. The depressor supercilii muscle is located on the medial arc of the orbicularis oculi and is considered by some to be a part of the larger muscle. This muscle acts in concert with the corrugators to depress the medial brow.

The corrugator supercilii is a complex muscle consisting of both transverse and oblique heads. The muscle originates from the medial portion of the supraorbital rim and inserts into the dermis of the medial eyebrow, deep to the orbicularis and frontalis muscles. At their medial point of insertion, the corrugator muscle fibers blend with those of the pars orbitalis and the frontalis. The contraction of the corrugator pulls the eyebrow medially and leads to the development of deep vertical furrows.

Fascia

During an endoscopic forehead lift, the dissection crosses several fascial planes, and a detailed understanding of

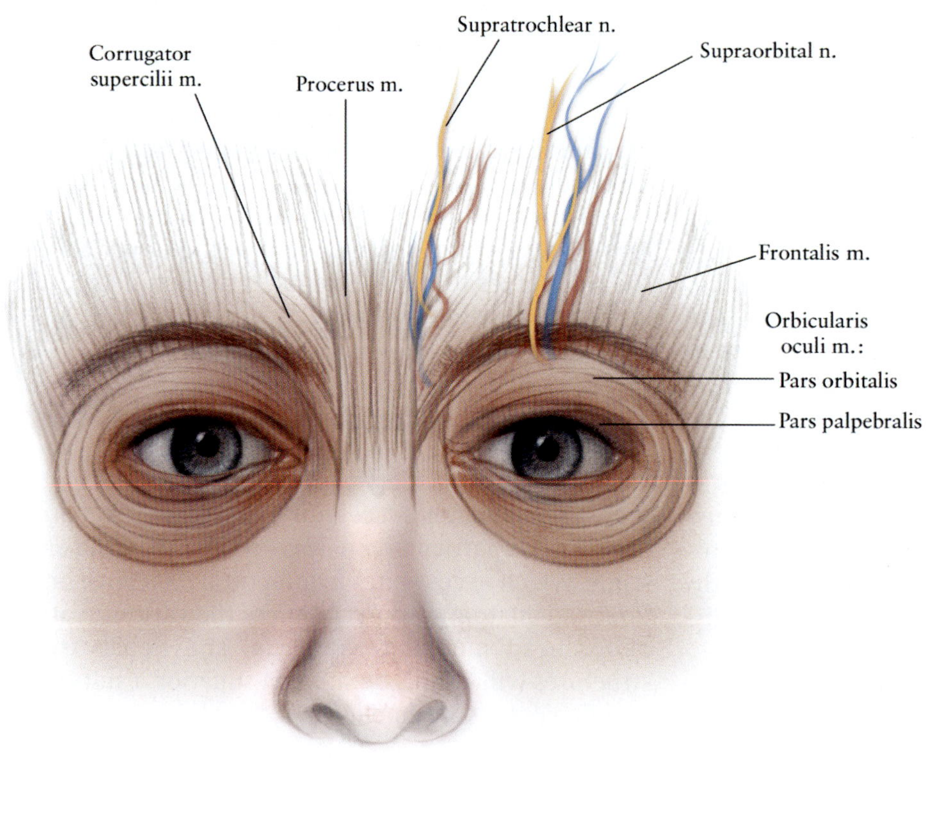

Figure 10–2 Musculature and neurovascular structures of the forehead. The frontalis is the sole elevator of the brow, the remaining forehead muscles function as brow depressors. The supraorbital and supratrochlear nerves provide sensation to the forehead. (Courtesy of Karl Storz Endoscopy-America, Inc., Culver City, California.)

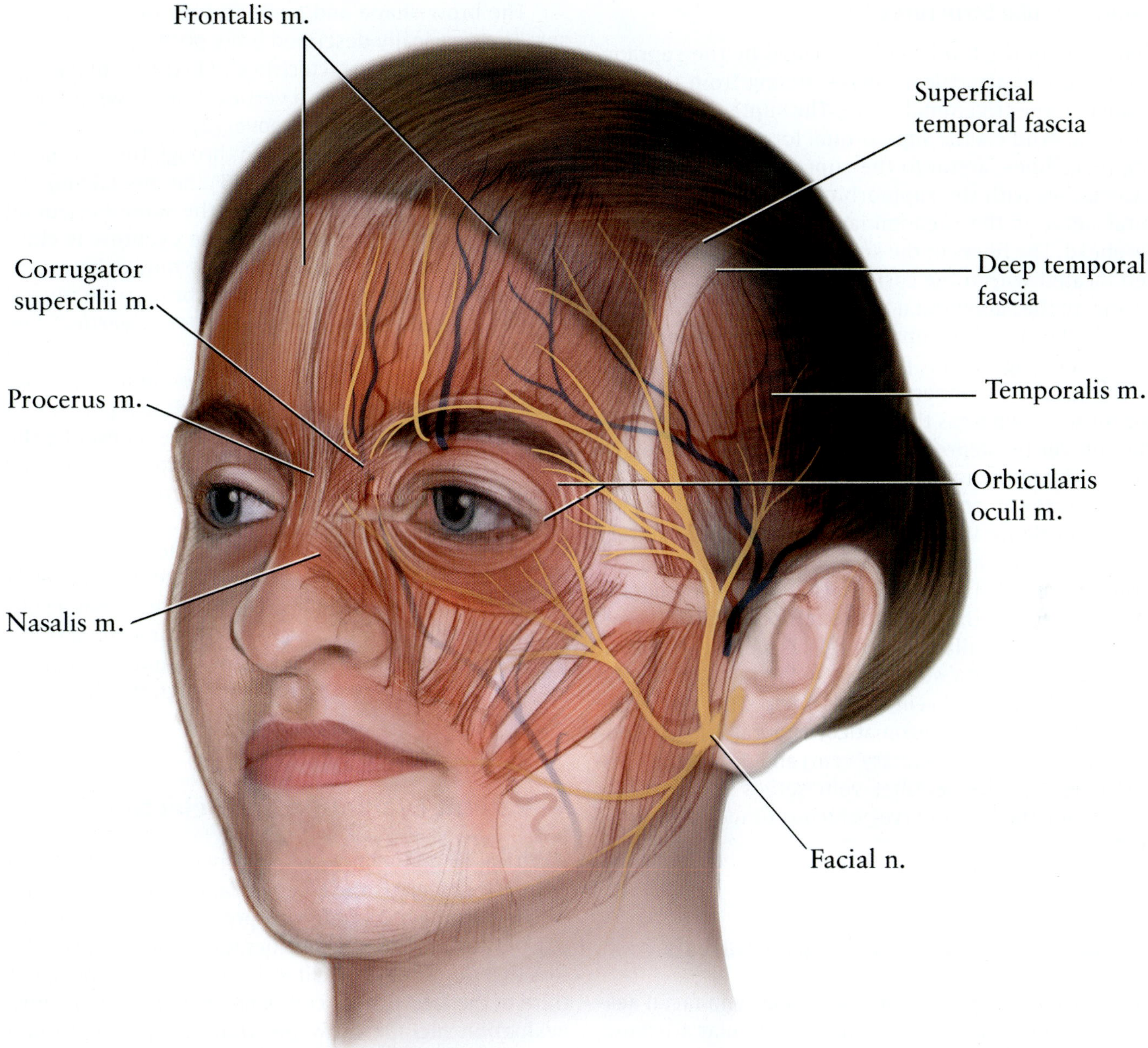

Figure 10–3 Relevant surgical anatomy of the forehead and midforehead. The surgeon should appreciate the various fascial planes and their relationship to relevant neurovascular structures. (Courtesy of Karl Storz Endoscopy-America, Inc., Culver City, California.)

these planes allows the surgeon to safely approach the brow. The superficial temporal fascia (i.e., temporoparietal fascia) is the first fascial plane encountered just underneath the skin and subcutaneous fat of the temporal area. Within this plane the temporal artery and vein may be found superiorly. The superficial temporal fascia merges inferiorly with the extensive superficial musculoaponeurotic system (SMAS) of the lower face and is in continuity with the galea superiorly, the frontalis anteriorly, and the occipitalis posteriorly.[2] This fascial layer lies superficial to the zygomatic arch and encompasses the temporal branch of the facial nerve (Fig. **10–3**).[3] Beneath the superficial temporal fascia lies the subaponeurotic plane, which is a loose areolar plane separating the superficial temporal fascia from the layer of deep temporal fascia.[4] Dissection in the temporal region should proceed within this plane, just on the deep temporal fascia. This allows the surgeon to avoid the temporal branch adherent to the undersurface of the superficial temporal fascia. Violation of the deep temporalis fascia exposes the underlying deep temporal fat pad, which may then atrophy and result in temporal wasting.

Neurovascular Structures

Sensation of the forehead is provided by the supraorbital and supratrochlear nerves arising from the first branch of the trigeminal nerve. The supraorbital nerve exits the skull via the supraorbital foramen in the midpupillary line—lateral to the supratrochlear nerve—in association with the supraorbital artery. The supraorbital nerve is the predominant sensory nerve of the forehead. The fibers of the supratrochlear nerve are often located within the corrugator muscle, 8 to 12 mm medial to the supraorbital nerve (Fig. **10–2**).

The facial nerve supplies all the muscles of facial expression (Fig. **10–3**). Specifically, the temporal branch of the facial nerve innervates the frontalis and corrugator muscles, whereas the zygomatic branch innervates the procerus, depressor supercilii, and orbicularis oculi.[5] The temporal branch of the facial nerve may be found during an endoscopic approach by locating a series of bridging vessels between the superficial and deep temporal fascial layers. The point at which the bridging vessels insert into the superficial temporalis fascia identifies the site of the temporal branch as it courses superficially through the fascia. At the level of the frontozygomatic suture, 1.5 cm lateral to the lateral canthus, the sentinel vein can be found. This vein is the medial branch of the zygomaticotemporal vein (a tributary of the internal maxillary vein) and drains the temporal region. The sentinel vein serves as a reliable marker for the facial nerve, which is found just lateral to it.[6]

◆ Forehead and Brow Facial Analysis

The concept of attractiveness and beauty in facial aesthetics is not defined by any single particular attribute, but rather by the combination of facial features and aesthetic balance. It is the facial plastic surgeon's objective to identify and improve upon any distinct qualities or proportions of the face that are perceived to be undesirable by the patient and society. With this in mind, authors have proposed numerous methodologies for facial analysis. The concept of the ideal forehead and brow has been extensively explored, and several common principles have emerged.

Facial height in Caucasians can be evaluated by dividing the face into equal thirds. The upper third of the face contains the forehead and extends from the trichion to the glabella and superior aspects of the eyebrows laterally. In men there is a greater prominence of the supraorbital ridge with more supraorbital bossing as compared with women, who have a more gradual curvature of the forehead.

The brow shape and position vary on the basis of sex. The classically described brow position in a female has the following characteristics[7]: (1) the medial origin of the brow is defined by a vertical line drawn perpendicular to the alar–facial groove, (2) the lateral aspect extends to an oblique line drawn through the alar–facial groove and the lateral canthus, (3) the medial and lateral ends of the eyebrow rest on the same horizontal level, and (4) the medial end of the eyebrow is club-shaped and tapers laterally. There is some debate as to the ideal position of the apex of the brow, with several authors agreeing that it should lie on a vertical line drawn tangential to the lateral limbus of the eye. Many authors believe, however, that the apex should be more lateral, coinciding with a vertical line drawn perpendicularly through the lateral canthus. Others describe the ideal apex as being found at the junction between the medial two thirds and lateral one third of the brow (Fig. **10–4A,B**).

Many of these criteria apply to the male brow as well, such as the medial and lateral extent of the brow and the position of the apex. The male brow has a subdued arch situated directly over the supraorbital ridge, however, whereas the female brow should have a high, graceful arch and be positioned slightly above the supraorbital ridge.

◆ Patient Evaluation and Selection

A critical component of preoperative planning for facial cosmetic surgery is the careful evaluation and selection of the patient. A decision to proceed with foreheadplasty warrants careful consideration of a variety of factors that determine the clinical appearance of the upper third of the face. Crucial components of the preoperative evaluation include brow position and ptosis, frontal hairline height and general hair density, the presence of forehead and glabellar rhytids, and the patient's skin quality. The need for ancillary procedures such as a blepharoplasty should also be recognized.

The accurate assessment of brow ptosis and brow position is critical to the evaluation of the upper third of the face. As discussed earlier, the dynamic forces imparted by various upper facial muscles eventually lead to the development of a ptotic brow, which manifests as a tired, sad, or stern look. McKinney et al[8] found that the normal distance from the midpupil to the center of the upper edge of the brow is 2.5 cm. Brow ptosis is present when this distance is less than 2.5 cm, in which case the patient will likely benefit from a forehead lift. Another valuable preoperative assessment of brow ptosis requires the examiner to manually lift the brow and record the maximal excursion of the medial,

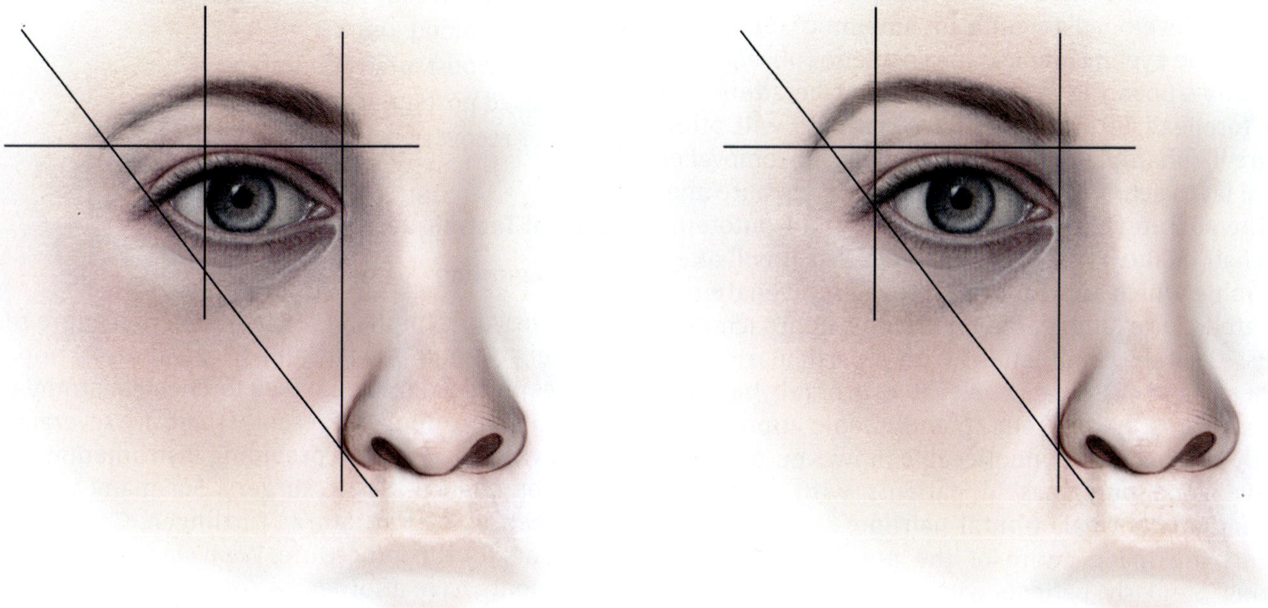

A B

Figure 10–4 Ideal brow shape and position in the female. Debate persists regarding the ideal position of the brow apex: intersecting the line tangential to (**A**) the lateral limbus, or (**B**) the lateral canthus. (Courtesy of Karl Storz Endoscopy-America, Inc., Culver City, California.)

central, and lateral portions of the brow from resting position. The typical measurement lies between 1 and 2 cm; however, certain ethnic groups (Asian; African American; Mediterranean) often display reduced excursion.[6] As one might surmise, a patient with a greater amount of brow excursion preoperatively may not enjoy the same results from an endoscopic forehead lift as a patient with a lower degree of excursion. Patients with mild to moderate brow ptosis—those requiring less than 1.5 cm elevation of the midbrow—are considered the best candidates for endoscopic foreheadplasty. Those requiring greater elevation may be better served by an open procedure incorporating skin resection into the forehead/brow lift.[9]

Many patients will subconsciously elevate their brow with eye opening to alleviate visual field obstruction caused by hooding or ptosis.[1] This repetitive frontalis action leads to the formation of horizontal forehead rhytids, which are often amenable to surgery. Postoperative results for this group of patients may be unimpressive if the surgeon does not take into account the artificial elevation of the brow associated with opening of the eyes. This pitfall can be avoided with preoperative assessment of the patient for this behavior, consisting of evaluation of the patient's brow position with the eyes closed. Patients in this subgroup should also be evaluated for eyelid ptosis because brow elevation serves as a compensatory mechanism for this problem. Indeed, forehead rejuvenation in a patient with unaddressed eyelid ptosis may result in an unfavorable cosmetic result with increased apparent ptosis.

The presence of glabellar furrows at rest should be appreciated. Chronic frowning or hyperdynamic action of the brow depressors will often lead to vertical rhytids at an early age. Upon endoscopic evaluation, these patients will likely demonstrate hypertrophy of the procerus, corrugator, and depressor supercilii muscles, requiring meticulous attention and appropriate debulking maneuvers.[10]

The patient's skin quality is another important determinant of success for any facial cosmetic procedure and should be included in the preoperative assessment for forehead rejuvenation. If the potential for visible scarring is present, then patients with thin, nonsebaceous, less pigmented skin are preferred candidates for the endoscopic approach. Patients with a history of hypertrophic scarring and skin pigmentation changes in response to previous surgery should be recognized and the surgical approach should be tailored appropriately. The mobility of the skin must also be considered. Ramirez[11] proposed that people of certain ethnic groups, such as Asians and American Indians, have tight or thick forehead skin with significant bony attachments of the frontal/periorbital soft tissues. It was believed that these patient groups were not as amenable to an endoscopic approach unless an extended periorbital release was made in conjunction with a more reliable fixation of the advanced soft tissue. More recent experiences, however, have shown excellent results using endoscopic techniques for face lifts in Asian patients.[12] In aging patients who have developed a significant amount of redundant tissue in the eyelid complex, the cosmetic consequence is a puffy-appearing eyelid that cannot be addressed with forehead lifting alone. Such patients will often require blepharoplasty with repositioning or removal of orbital fat to achieve an aesthetically pleasing outcome.

The position of the frontal hairline and frontotemporal hair quality must be assessed because it will often determine which approach to forehead rejuvenation is indicated. For example, the endoscopic approach may be less desirable in a patient with a particularly high forehead and associated elevated frontal hairline. Because the scarring from an endoscopic approach is usually minimal and unnoticeable, however, one may achieve good outcomes in patients with a slightly higher than "normal" frontal hairline, as long as the patients are made aware of the possibility of slight scarring. Similarly, patients with male pattern baldness may also benefit from the endoscopic approach, after having been counseled of the potential risk of visible scarring.

◆ Endoscopic Forehead Rejuvenation

Over the past decade, the application of the endoscope has revolutionized how aesthetic surgeons approach mild to moderate ptotic brows and forehead rhytids. As one of the pioneers in endoscopic forehead rejuvenation, Keller described using endoscopic visualization to incise the procerus, corrugator, and depressor musculature and to perform a temple lift. Isse and Ramirez further advanced the endoscopic technique by modifying it on the basis of the configuration of the skull, bony architecture, and soft tissue characteristics.[11]

Numerous authors have since reported their own experiences with modifications to the original technique that they have found to be useful. Nevertheless, the basic concept of endoscopic forehead rejuvenation remains unchanged: (1) a sub- or supraperiosteal dissection of the scalp to the level of the superior and lateral orbital rims and zygomatic arch, (2) incision and release of orbital periosteum, and (3) selective myotomies of the brow depressors.

The endoscopic approach to forehead rejuvenation offers many advantages when compared with the traditional, open procedures:

- Accurate resection or manipulation of the brow depressor muscles
- Less recurrent brow ptosis
- Preservation of the sensory nerves to the scalp
- Minimal rate of alopecia
- Minimal elevation of the hairline
- Can be used in thin-haired or bald patients
- Decreased blood loss
- Decreased postsurgical numbness
- Decreased postsurgical edema
- Shorter recovery period

Surgical Technique

Instrumentation

The endoscopic forehead rejuvenation procedure relies on extensive and precise subperiosteal dissection and endoscopic visualization of key forehead anatomy with subsequent myotomies. Presently there are several companies who specialize in providing instrumentation for endoscopic facial plastic surgery. For many years, we have been using Karl Storz (Tuttlingen, Germany) instruments for this procedure. We have found that their instruments have afforded us consistent precision and accuracy, which is essential in obtaining superior results.

The basic setup consists of a 7-inch long, 5 mm diameter endoscope with a 30-degree down-angled lens connected to a single-chip digital video camera. A xenon light source provides the most natural-appearing surgical field, which allows for better appreciation of the anatomy. The video output may be optimally viewed on a 19- or 20-inch high-resolution monitor.

Other required instruments include a complete selection of angled dissectors, spreaders, and periosteal elevators. Specialized instruments such as nerve protectors, angled punches, scissors, and needle holders will also prove invaluable as advanced endoscopic skills are developed.

Marking

All patients are marked preoperatively in an upright position in the presurgical waiting area, marking the anticipated course of the temporal branch of the facial nerve, placement of the temporal and parietal incisions, and desired brow elevation (5–8 mm medially and 8–10 mm laterally).

The desired amount of brow elevation is marked in the following way. The position of the ptotic brow is marked using a fine-tip marker pen at its medial head, above the lateral limbus and the lateral canthus. Next, using accepted aesthetic norms,[13] the brow is elevated manually to the desired position. The brow is then released, and the corresponding area of the frontal skin is marked. The distances between the pairs of marks are measured. Palpation and marking of the supraorbital notch create a useful landmark when later aggressive

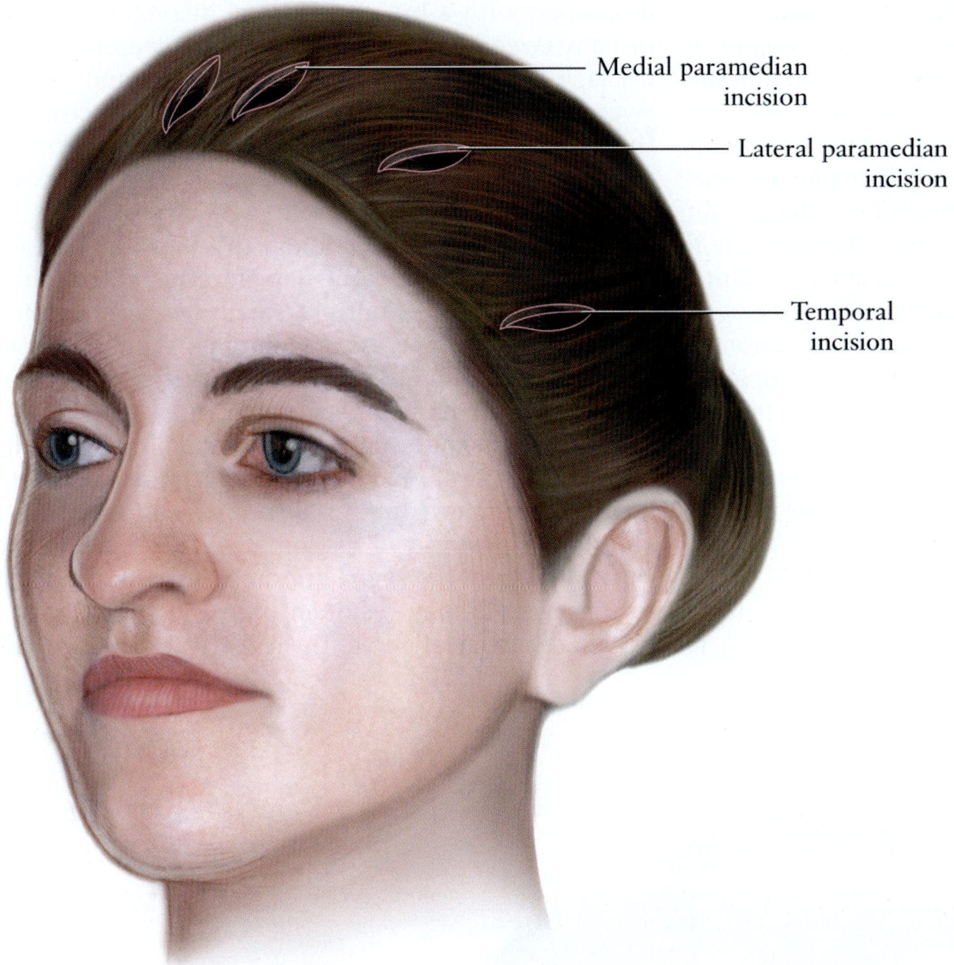

Figure 10–5 Placement of the incisions. (Courtesy of Karl Storz Endoscopy-America, Inc., Culver City, California.)

endoscopic dissection is performed. The course of the temporal branch of the facial nerve is marked by connecting the following points: one on the facial skin 1 cm anterior to the inferior ear lobule, another 3 cm anterior to the superior external auditory canal, and the third at 1.5 cm lateral to the lateral brow.

Six incisions are marked (Fig. **10–5**): two medial paramedian incisions each 2 cm lateral to the midline, 1.5 cm long, and 5 mm behind the anterior hairline; two lateral paramedian incisions, centered on the lateral canthus, 1.5 cm in vertical length, just behind the anterior hairline; and two temporal incisions 2 cm long and ~2 cm behind the temporal hairline. If greater access is needed to the forehead in the patient with a high curved forehead, additional paramedian vertical incisions can also be marked behind the anterior hairline. One should not forget to modify the incisions in patients with male pattern baldness to effectively hide the incisions. However, even in bald patients the incision scars are minimal and endoscopic forehead lift can be effectively used for forehead rejuvenation.

Dissection

General endotracheal anesthesia may be used, but we prefer monitored intravenous anesthesia in conjunction with supplemental local anesthetics; 1% lidocaine with 1:100,000 epinephrine is our standard local anesthetic, and we inject in the following order: (1) into the region of the supraorbital and supratrochlear nerves to provide a regional nerve blockade; (2) the marked parietal scalp incision sites; (3) the surrounding parietal, frontal, and glabellar soft tissues in a periosteal plane; and (4) the temporal incisions and surrounding soft tissue in a subcutaneous plane. Care is taken to prevent injury to the superficial temporal artery and vein.

Prior to making the anterior scalp incisions the superior forehead and brow are manually depressed into their natural ptotic position with the surgeon's nonactive hand. The four parietal scalp incisions are made with a #15 scalpel blade and are carried down to and through the underlying periosteum. Control holes are drilled into the calvarium at the anterior extent of each vertical incision with a hand drill fitted with a 1.7 mm diameter drill bit and a 4 mm stop. Using a millimeter caliper, the premeasured desired distance for brow elevation is marked on the calvarium posterior to the four control holes. Fixation holes are then drilled into the calvarium at these points.

Next, a wide subperiosteal undermining of the parietal scalp is accomplished with a lateral dissection to each temporal crest. Posterior dissection is completed with a large curved elevator to the superior and midoccipital scalp. Anterior dissection is carried over the forehead with a sharp down-turned elevator staying 2 cm above the superior orbital rims. In the area of the glabella a sharp, large, curved elevator is used to elevate the soft tissue down to the superior nasal bones (Fig. **10–6**).

The temporal incisions are made and a plane of dissection deep to the superficial temporal fascia is developed with a broad periosteal dissector. A front-to-back sweeping motion exposes the deep temporal fascia, which is not penetrated. A superior and medial sweeping motion with the elevator allows for incision of the tightly adherent temporal fascia and periosteum at the temporal crest. This maneuver connects the temporal pocket to the parietal pocket.

Continuing the dissection in an anterior to inferior directed motion carries the flap elevation down to the lateral orbital rim. Multiple small vessels including the sentinel vein may be encountered at this point of the dissection and are cauterized medially to the elevated flap with a bipolar cautery forceps. Additionally, caution here is important. The dissection must stay lateral to the canthal tendon to not detach this important anatomic structure. Inferior dissection continues in an anterior to posterior direction staying just along the superior edge of the zygomatic arch. Dissecting inferior to the zygoma may result in injury to the temporal branch of the facial nerve. The soft tissues are elevated

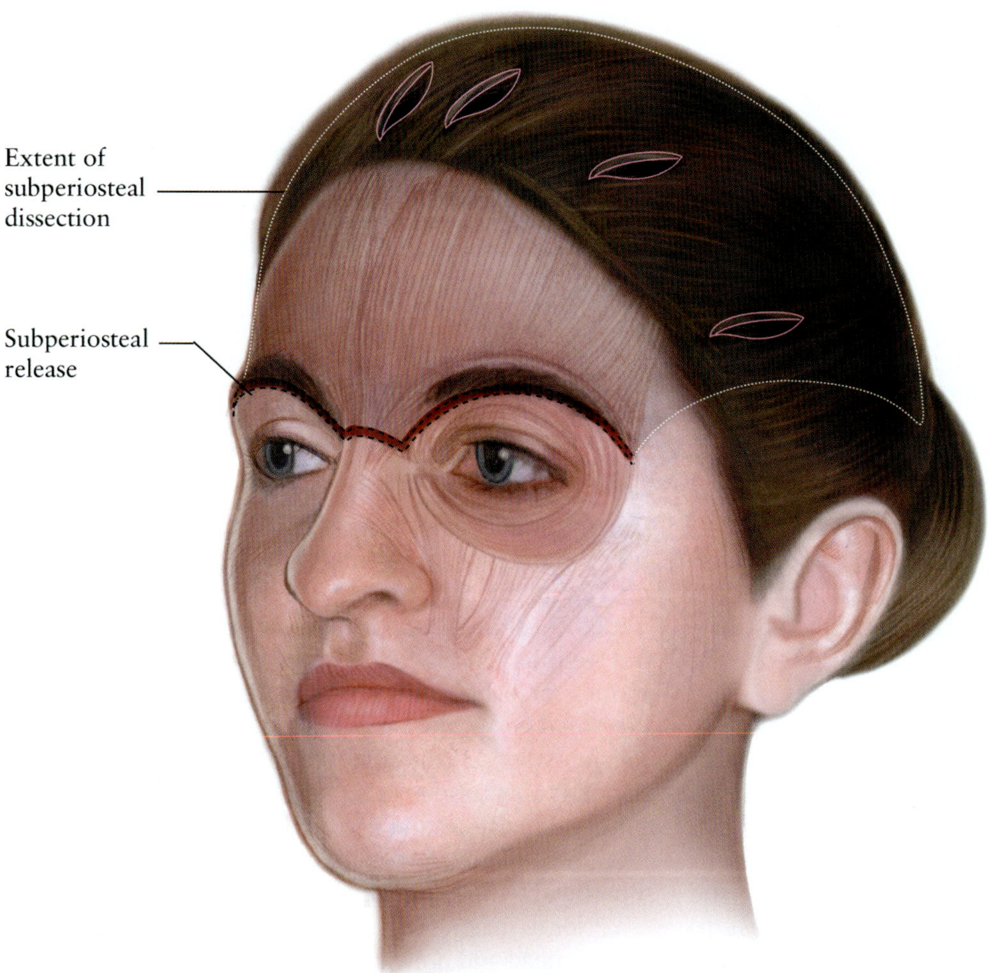

Figure 10–6 Extent of subperiosteal dissection. (Courtesy of Karl Storz Endoscopy-America, Inc., Culver City, California.)

back to and in front of the anterior helix and then carried above and behind the auricle into the mastoid region. Care must be noted here not to proceed too posterior or the mastoid vein may be injured resulting in severe bleeding.

With endoscopic visualization through a lateral paramedian incision, the curved sharp dissector is inserted through the temporal incision on the same side of the head, and a lateral to medial dissection of the periosteum from the supraorbital rim is performed. The supraorbital and supratrochlear neurovascular bundles are identified and preserved.

An upturned periosteal spreader is used along the supraorbital rim in a lateral to medial direction. This dissection provides for further periosteal release that exposes the underlying retroorbicularis oculi fat pad and produces limited myotomies in the overlying orbicularis oculi muscle (Fig. **10–6**).

Next a thin nerve dissector is introduced to further incise the medial supraorbital periosteum. The neurovascular bundles and the depressor supercilii muscle, corrugator supercilii muscle, and procerus muscle are identified with this dissection. The endoscope is then inserted through the medial paramedian incision down to the level of the glabella. A curved endoscopic forehead punch or grasping forceps is inserted through a paramedian incision and then utilized to perform myotomies of the procerus, corrugator, and depressor supercilii muscles. Myotomy of the corrugator muscle is performed both medial and lateral to the supratrochlear bundle. Hemostasis is controlled with bipolar electrocautery applied to insulated forceps. A 10 French fluted drain is routinely placed across the supraorbital brow and brought out through the right superior posterior scalp.

The release of the brow and forehead soft tissues allows intrinsic elevation of the brow with posterior pull of the occipital–galea–frontalis complex.

Permanent Fixation

Medial and central brow fixation is performed by placement of a 2 mm diameter (3.5 mm length) Mitek tacit titanium anchor (Ethicon, Westwood, Massachusetts) in each of the four holes. These small screws are fitted with a 2–0 Ethibond (Ethicon) suture. The free end of the suture is threaded through the eyelet of a free needle. Next, the needle is passed through the periosteal/galeal soft tissue at the anterior extent of each incision and brought out of the incision. The sutures are tied down under direct vision so that the anterior extent of the incision lies over the titanium anchor (Fig. **10–7A,B**). This provides exact elevation and fixation at the desired brow

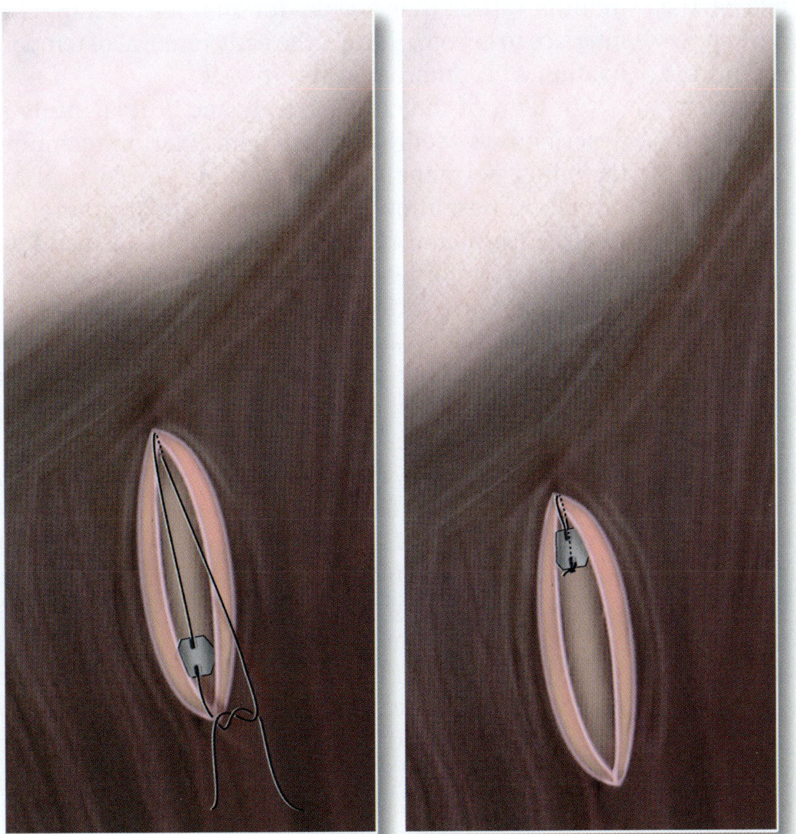

A B

Figure 10–7 **(A,B)** Precise elevation and fixation of the brow utilizing a titanium anchor with a fixed suture. (Courtesy of Karl Storz Endoscopy-America, Inc., Culver City, California.)

height. The parietal incisions are closed with 3–0 Prolene in a vertical mattress manner and supplemented with stainless steel staples.

Using the measured desired amount of brow elevation for the lateral canthus and temporal region, a fixation point is identified superior and posterior to the inferior edge of the temporal incisions. Two 2–0 polygalactin sutures are placed in the deep temporal fascia at this point and are then passed through the dermis and temporoparietal fascia of the edge of the inferior temporal flap. Manual advancement of the inferior temporal flap by an assistant is performed as the two polygalactin sutures are tied down and secured. This provides elevation of the lateral brow. The edges of the temporal incisions are approximated with a 3–0 Prolene suture in a vertical mattress fashion and then closed with stainless steel staples.

A soft, mildly compressive circumferential head dressing is placed and removed along with the drain on the first or second postoperative day. The patient is instructed to place antibiotic ointment on the scalp suture lines two or three times per day. On the fifth postoperative day gentle hair washing is allowed. The sutures and staples are removed on the second postoperative week.

Fixation Techniques: Temporary versus Permanent

One of the controversies surrounding the use of the endoscopic foreheadplasty technique concerns the postoperative brow position. Many authors have reported loss of some forehead elevation in the early postoperative period, and some surgeons advocate overcorrection to compensate for this loss. The reasons for this loss of elevation are unclear. One possibility is that technical errors in the elevation procedure (e.g., incomplete transection of the brow depressor muscles) contributed to this phenomenon. This may have been particularly relevant in the early period after surgeons adopted the endoscopic technique, but probably ceased to be a factor with increasing experience. A more likely explanation lies in the balance of forces exerted by the muscles surrounding the brow. Immediately after subperiosteal elevation and sectioning of the depressor musculature, unopposed tonic contraction of the frontooccipitalis causes the brow to rise. Significant readhesion of periosteum to cortical bone is essential in stabilizing the elevated frontooccipital complex. If the frontooccipitalis relaxes and the upward force on the brow abates before the periosteal–cortical junction is stable, the brow may relapse to a greater than expected degree.

Ensuring that the brow will settle into the correct position postoperatively requires that the periosteum be fixed to the bone during the immediate postoperative period. However, the duration of fixation required has remained a matter of debate. Numerous fixation techniques have been developed, including biodegradable screws, fibrin glue, K-wire fixation, transcalvarial suturing, and temporary titanium screws. Temporary fixation, with removal of the fixation device early in the postoperative period (several days to a few weeks), has been advocated by some authors as the technique of choice. Brodner et al[14] reported that periosteal readhesion of the surgically elevated periosteum in an animal model is virtually complete by the seventh postoperative day. However, many cases of partial loss of brow elevation in the early postoperative period associated with temporary fixation have been reported. De la Fuente et al[15] noted a 2 to 4 mm relaxation in brow position 1 month postoperatively, with the fixation screws having been removed at 2 weeks.

A clinical study by Romo et al[16] compared the long-term outcomes of patients who underwent foreheadplasty with temporary versus permanent fixation. The group with temporary fixation was found to be more likely to have postoperative partial loss of brow elevation as compared with the group with permanent fixation. Romo et al[17] investigated periosteal readherence in an animal model and found that significant stability in the periosteal–cortical junction could require as long as 6 to 12 weeks of healing. If, as suggested by this work, it takes months rather than weeks for the periosteum–cortex interface to become secure, the early removal of temporary fixation will compromise its efficacy.

In light of the clinical study and animal study just described we feel that permanent fixation techniques, including permanent fixation screws or cortical bone tunneling, best allow for stable periosteal adherence to the calvarium and result in the most precise and optimal long-term brow positioning.[9] Yet the disadvantages of permanent fixation, including the relatively higher expense of the fixation appliance and some patients' hesitance to accept permanent hardware incorporated into the cranium, cannot be ignored. Thus the optimal fixation technique does not yet exist. The choice between temporary and permanent fixation techniques would likely be resolved to everybody's satisfaction by the development of a semipermanent, absorbable fixation device that would remain for several months before dissolving, allowing adequate time for periosteal readherence. This assumes that such a device could be produced at a nonprohibitive cost. Until such a device is available, we believe that because the permanent fixation of the elevated brow gives the more predictable, long-lasting results, it should be the preferred technique (Fig. **10–8A–F**).

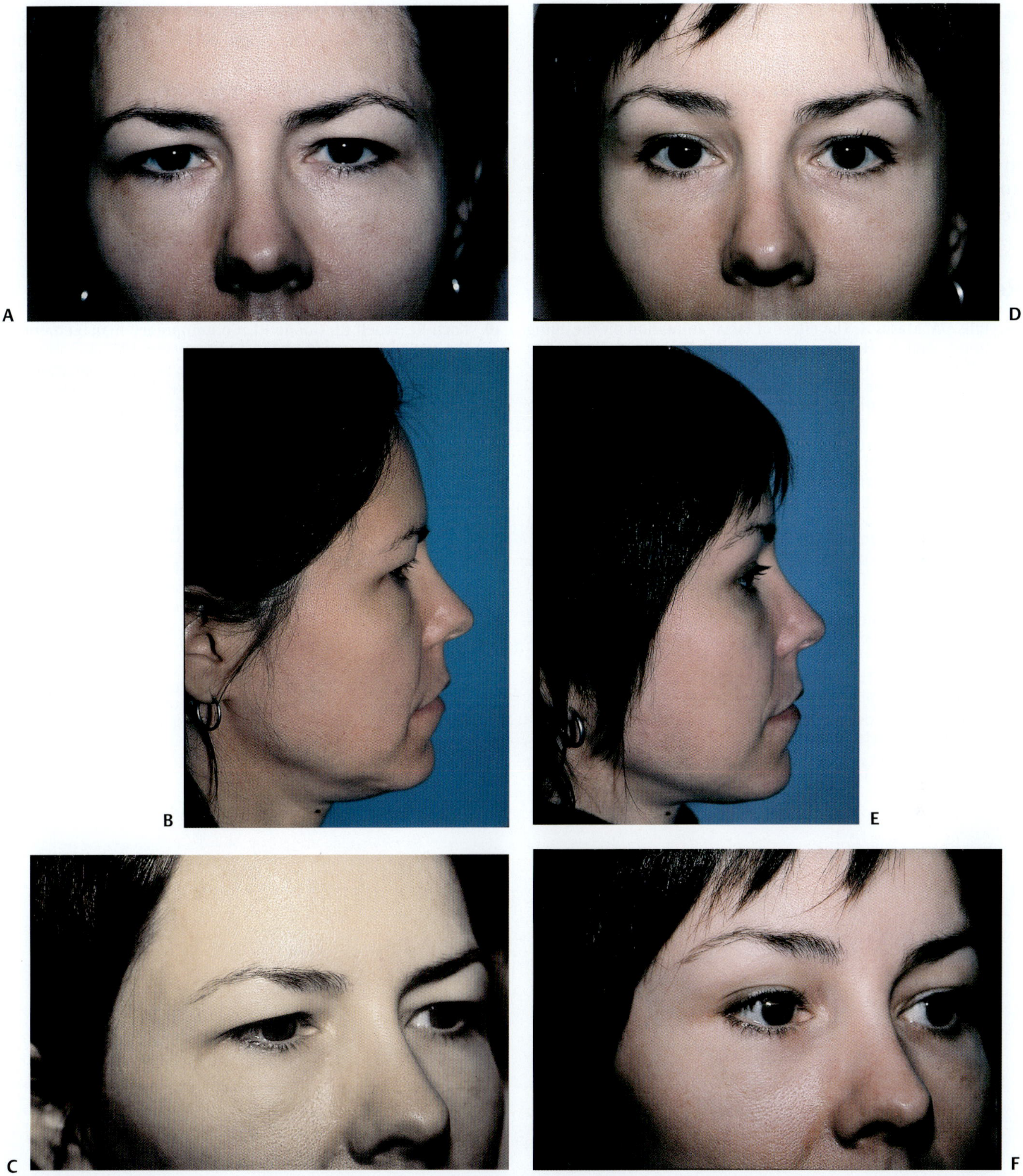

Figure 10–8 (**A–C**) Preoperative and (**D–F**) postoperative views of a patient with brow ptosis. The brow has descended and flattened with prolapse of the infrabrow tissue, leading to medial and lateral hooding of the upper eyelid. The appearance of chronic fatigue is resolved following endoscopic forehead lift with a much more alert and engaging face.

◆ Conclusions

The application of the endoscope to forehead rejuvenation surgery has provided a powerful new tool for addressing the effects of aging in the upper third of the face. With a firm understanding of the surgical anatomy in conjunction with an appreciation for aesthetic ideals and meticulous patient evaluation and selection, the aesthetic surgeon may offer the patient excellent, long-term results without many of the morbidities associated with traditional, open forehead and brow lift procedures. Although some debate exists regarding which type of fixation should be used, we feel that the permanent fixation technique offers more dependable results and should remain the method of choice until an affordable, semipermanent, absorbable fixation device becomes available.

References

1. Ellis DA, Masai H. The effect of facial animation on the aging upper half of the face. Arch Otolaryngol Head Neck Surg 1989;115:710–713
2. Mitz V, Peyronie M. The superficial musculoaponeurotic system in the parotid and cheek area. Plast Reconstr Surg 1976;58:80–88
3. Stuzin JM, Wagstrom L, Kawamoto HK, et al. Anatomy of the frontal branch of the facial nerve: the significance of the temporal fat pad. Plast Reconstr Surg 1989;83:265–271
4. Abdul-Hassan HS, von Drasek Ascher G, Acland RD. Surgical anatomy and blood supply of the fascial layers of the temporal region. Plast Reconstr Surg 1986;77:17–28
5. Narnazie AR, Keller GS. Current practices in endoscopic brow and temporal lifting. Facial Plast Surg Clin North Am 2001;9:439–451
6. Keller GS, Hutcherson RW. Browlift: a facial plastics surgeon's perspective. In Romo T, Millman AL, eds. Aesthetic Facial Plastic Surgery. New York: Thieme Medical Publishers; 2000:225–235
7. Ellenbogen R. Transcoronal eyebrow lift with concomitant upper blepharoplasty. Plast Reconstr Surg 1983;71:490–499
8. McKinney P, Mossie RD, Zukowski ML. Criteria for the forehead lift. Aesthetic Plastic Surg 1991;15:141–147
9. Romo T, Jacono AA, Sclafani AP. Endoscopic forehead lifting and contouring. Facial Plast Surg 2001;17:3–10
10. Koch RJ, Troell RJ, Goode RL. Contemporary management of the aging brow and forehead. Laryngoscope 1997;107:710–715
11. Ramirez OM. Endoscopic techniques in facial rejuvenation: an overview, part 1. Aesthetic Plastic Surg 1994;18:141–147
12. Kim IG, Oh JK, Baek DH. Personal experiences and algorithm of endoscopically assisted subperiosteal face lift in Orientals for 5 years. Plast Reconstr Surg 2001;108:1768–1779
13. Brennan HG. Correction of the ptotic brow. Otolaryngol Clin North Am 1980;13:265–273
14. Brodner DC, Downs JC, Graham DH. Periosteal readhesion after brow-lift in New Zealand white rabbits. Arch Facial Plast Surg 2002;4:248–251
15. De la Fuente A, Santamaria AB. Facial rejuvenation: a combined conventional and endoscopic assisted lift. Aesthetic Plastic Surg 1996;20:471–479
16. Romo T, Sclafani AP, Yung RT. Endoscopic foreheadplasty: temporary vs. permanent fixation. Aesthetic Plastic Surg 1999; 23:388–394
17. Romo T, Sclafani AP, Yung RT, et al. Endoscopic foreheadplasty, I: a histological comparison of periosteal refixation after endoscopic versus bicoronal lift. Plast Reconstr Surg 2000; 105:1111–1117

11

Transconjunctival Subperiosteal Cheek Lift with and without Malar Augmentation

Mark Duffy

Cosmetic and reconstructive subperiosteal cheek lifting has become more popular and controversial over the past few years. Although it can be performed through several approaches, this chapter will describe the technique that I prefer—the transconjunctival blepharoplasty approach as described by Putterman,[1] with several modifications. One of these modifications is the augmentation of either or both the inferior orbital rim and the malar soft tissue with the aid of standard prefabricated porous polyethylene implants. Augmentation just below the inferior orbital rim has several benefits. In cases of previous maxillectomy with loss of the inferior rim it can restore the support structures and cosmetic contour of the entire midface. Soft tissue and periosteum can be directly fixated to the implant itself. In cases of bony or soft tissue hypoplasia (i.e., iatrogenic lid retraction, exophthalmos, pseudoexophthalmos from a hypoplastic inferior orbital rim, congenital euryblepharon, childhood radiation therapy, etc.) the implant can be fashioned to maximize volume directly where it is needed. In cases of focal lid or cheek anomalies, the periosteal flap can be directed where it is needed and easily fixated to the implant for greater support.

A second modification (or series of modifications) deals with lateral bunching of redundant soft tissue. One of the most common criticisms of the technique from patients and surgeons is bunching and dimpling of tissue in the lateral lower lid and lateral canthal area. This seems particularly prevalent in faces with significant subcutaneous fat or those requiring excessive lift. Although patients commonly complain about this it generally resolves in 6 to 12 weeks. Despite this fact, simple attention to detail during closure can greatly diminish this problem.

◆ Background and History

Various techniques for safe and efficacious midfacial rejuvenation or augmentation are continually argued in the literature. Hester et al were instrumental in advancing the subperiosteal midface lift among oculoplastic and facial plastic surgeons.[2] However, Ramirez et al were probably among the first to describe a subperiosteal approach to midfacial rejuvenation performed in combination with cervicofacial rejuvenation.[3] When malar augmentation is performed in conjunction with other facial techniques, we perform a cheek lift as a separate procedure rather than performing extended dissections through endoscopic brow and cervicofacial dissections.

In 1989 Binder described a "new" technique of midfacial rejuvenation using a silastic implant to augment malar tissues during facial rejuvenation.[4] Following this, Mladick subclassified variations in malar hypoplasia and described two implants that could be placed in different "pockets" during various facial surgical procedures.[5] These implants included Silastic and Proplast implants and were reported associated with minimal complications. I prefer the use of preformed porous implants directly fixated in the subperiosteal pocket. The porous implants integrate well and are easily contoured for specific needs. If one desires, a variety of porous polyethylene malar implants are also available. Both types of implants (malar and inferior orbital rim) augment a hollow midface. In my experience the majority of patients with malar hypoplasia require elevation and augmentation to minimize the nasojugal trough and midface.

Although McCord emphasized the importance of incorporating lid-tightening procedures to prevent postoperative ectropion,[6] authors have also described

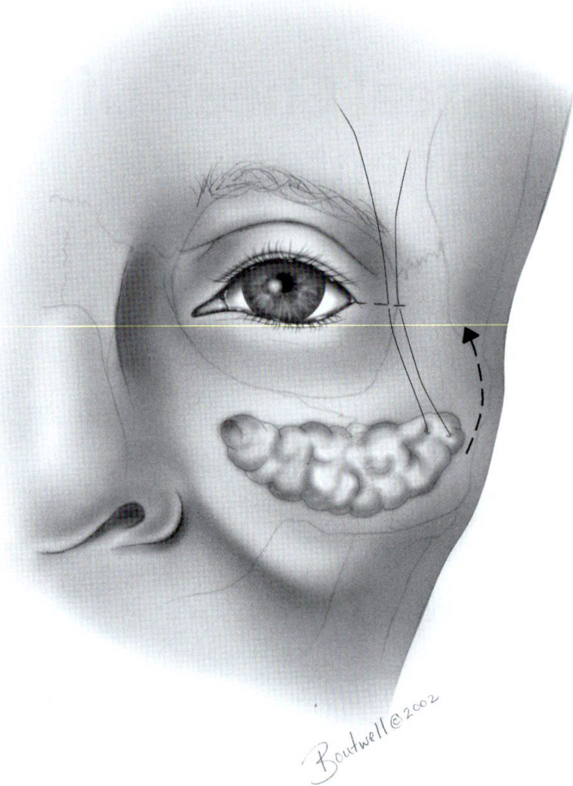

Figure 11–1 Illustration of canthotomy, descended or ptotic suborbicularis oculi fat, and principle of suture fixation of SOOF.

techniques with minimal complications without lid tightening.[3,7,8] The technique that will be described here includes lid tightening. The dramatic amount of tissue that is brought into the lower lid by this technique can have a profound effect on stabilizing vectors in the lower lid. The addition of a malar implant increases the effects on these vectors. I advocate a lateral tarsal strip procedure in each case for several reasons. It affords complete control of the shape of the palpebral fissure, prevents the occasional ectropion due to undiagnosed laxity, and allows direct access to the orbicularis muscle, suborbicularis oculi fat (SOOF), and periosteum for flap elevation and manipulation (Figs. **11–1; 11–2**).

◆ Patient Selection and Indications

Transconjunctival subperiosteal cheek lifting has many functional and aesthetic indications. It probably affords the safest and most effective access to mobilize the entire midfacial unit. Reliance on periosteal refixation to support the soft tissues provides long-lasting and effective effacement of midfacial folds, deficits, and lid retractions. In patients with mild malar hypoplasia a simple cheek lift can bring fullness to a hollow-appearing infraorbital area, simulating a small implant. In cases where there is a more substantial volume deficit, augmentation can be achieved by subperiosteal placement of an implant. The indications listed here are for standard subperiosteal cheek lifting. Each one of these cases can be further augmented with a malar implant if desired. In addition to these primary indications, this technique can be combined with other facial rejuvenation procedures including cervicofacial rhytidectomy, endoscopic brow lifting, and upper lid blepharoplasty.

◆ Common Indications for Midface Lifting

1. Cicatricial ectropion
2. Lower eyelid retraction (from lack of anterior lamellae)
3. Hollowness of lower eyelid and/or cheek (congenital or postsurgical)
4. Deep nasojugal trough

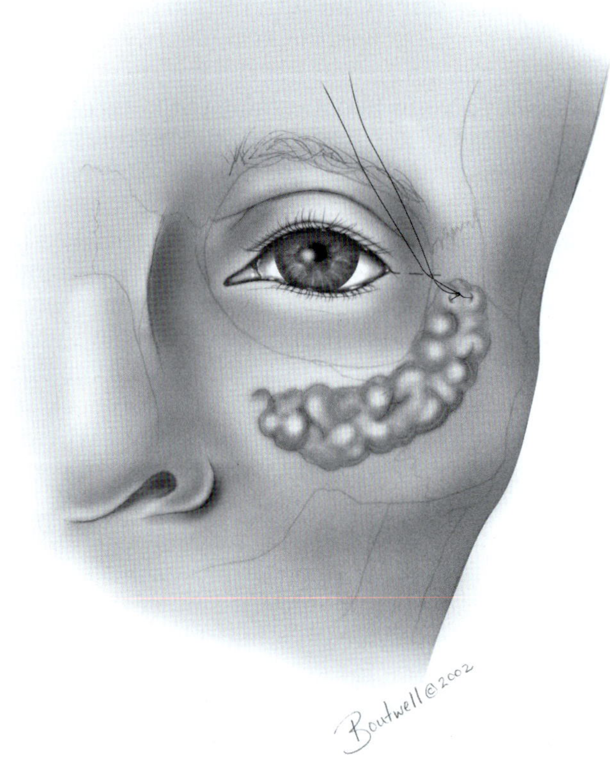

Figure 11–2 Conceptual illustration of relationship of lifted suborbicularis oculi fat and periosteum performed through standard lateral canthotomy incision with fixation to lateral periosteum or temporalis fascia.

5. Prominent nasolabial fold
6. Malar festoons
7. Midfacial and lower eyelid deficit
8. Facial palsy (with or without facial rhytidectomy)

◆ Surgical Technique

Patient Preparation and Local Anesthetic

This technique can be performed under general anesthesia or local anesthesia with sedation. The patient is laid supine on the table and the entire face is prepped with 10% Betadine solution. Betadine soap is avoided and 10% solution is kept out of the eye to avoid chemical irritation of the conjunctiva and cornea. I prep the nasal cannula or endotracheal tube to the level of the chin (if there will be other procedures performed, the prep is done as indicated for those procedures). The top of the head and forehead are also draped according to surgeon preference and additional procedures. I place a split bodysheet below the chin and out around the ear, which allows draping without any tension on the cheek or lateral periorbital tissue. This is particularly important if the patient is placed in a sitting position intraoperatively to judge symmetry.

Protective scleral shells are placed for comfort and protection, after instilling a topical anesthetic drop for patients not under general anesthesia. A normal-length (~1 cm) lateral canthal incision is drawn out. It is unnecessary to make an extended incision. The eyelids are infiltrated with a mixture of 0.5% lidocaine with 1:200,000 epinephrine (40 mL) and 0.5% bupivacaine (4 mL) in the lateral canthus, lateral one third of the upper lid, and anterior lower lid lamellae, and transconjunctivally into the fat pads. The infraorbital nerve foramen is palpated and marked. If it cannot be palpated secondary to excess malar fat, the foramen is located by making a plumb line directly inferior from the supraorbital notch to the superior fold of the external ala of the nose. Once marked, the infraorbital nerve and the cheeks are infiltrated with the dilute mixture down to the nasolabial fold and the superior gum line.

Transconjunctival Approach

The approach is the same as used for a transconjunctival blepharoplasty with a lateral tarsal strip or to reach the orbital rim in floor fracture repair. A 4–0 silk traction suture is placed centrally in the lower lid. The lid is everted over a Desmarres retractor. A transconjunctival incision is made from the caruncle to the lateral canthus staying ~5 mm below the inferior border of the tarsus. I prefer a Colorado needle tip cautery on cutting mode. The two edges of the incision are retracted and stretched apart. A combination of cutting and blunt dissection is used to expose the infraorbital rim in the plane between the orbicularis and the septum. This can be aided by placing the Desmarres inside the superior wound edge and pulling the lid down and over the orbital rim. Excision of fat or preparation for fat repositioning can be performed at this time in standard fashion. Attention is then directed to the lateral canthus. A canthotomy and cantholysis are performed, connected to the conjunctival incision and the lateral orbital rim exposed. The muscles of the cheek are bluntly dissected from the arcus marginalis with either cotton-tipped applicators or a smooth periosteal elevator. A 3 to 5 mm wide strip is cleared from the lateral canthus to just above the infraorbital nerve medially.

Subperiosteal Dissection and Release

The periosteum is incised outside the arcus marginalis for the length of the cleared rim. If direct superior elevation is needed for medial lid defects, it is important to leave enough periosteum to anchor the elevated cheek tissues. If an implant is going to be used, the periosteum can be incised closer to the rim without violating the septum. A MacKenty or sharp elevator is used to raise a periosteal flap (Fig. **11–3**). Green, Senn, or Army–Navy retractors are used to assist in enlarging the subperiosteal pocket under direct visualization. Dissection is carried down just over the ridge at the superior gum line. Nasally the infraorbital nerve is avoided but dissection can be carried nasal to it (if an implant is to be used, the preformed porous polyethylene implant [Porex Corporation, College Park, Georgia] has a notch that can fit around the nerve). The subperiosteal dissection must be carried inferior and nasal to the nasolabial fold for improvement. Laterally the periosteum is dissected for ~1 cm lateral to the lateral orbital rim. Once the desired dissection is achieved, a #11 Bard-Parker knife is used to incise the periosteum to release the entire cheek flap. The incision is begun under the nasolabial fold inferomedially and taken around to meet the initial periosteal incision laterally.

Great care is taken to insure that only periosteum is incised and not any deep neurovascular structures. A Ramirez reverse periosteal spreader or equivalent tool is then used to dissect the periosteum in an upward sweeping motion to spread and further release the flap. Finally a finger dissection is performed to feel any residual adhesions. At this point the periosteal edge (or SOOF itself) can be grasped with a forceps to judge the amount of release and decide on the best direction of elevation. In general, superotemporal elevation provides the best relief of nasolabial folds, elevation of the corner

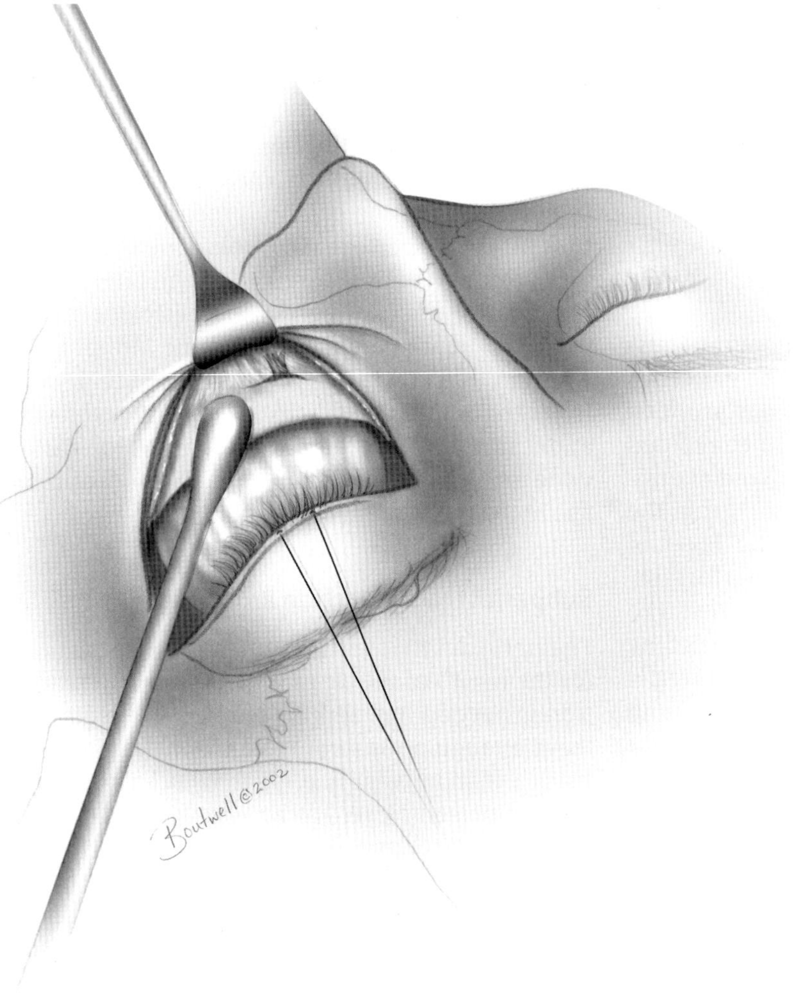

Figure 11–3 A periosteal flap is elevated with a dissector. Care is taken to preserve the periosteum and not shred it. Small dehiscences are acceptable. Great care is taken not to injure the infraorbital nerve. Laterally the zygomaticofacial foramen (with attendant nerve and vessel) may be encountered and can be cauterized.

of the mouth, and even mandibular fullness. At this point, gauze soaked in 1% lidocaine with 1:100,000 epinephrine can be placed under the flap for hemostasis and the same procedure repeated on the opposite side.

Malar Orbital Rim Implant

If an inferior rim or malar implant is to be employed, it is fixated in the subperiosteal pocket at this time. I prefer the Medpor infraorbital rim implant (Porex Corporation). Currently two types of Medpor implant are available. One is large and is designed for onlay (or orbital rim substitution) up to near the zygomaticofrontal suture. This size is rarely needed. A newer implant is designed to fill in below the inferior orbital rim where it is more often desired (in addition, myriad porous polyethylene malar implants also are available). The porous polyethylene material can be heated in warm saline and molded. In addition, it can be easily sculpted with a #10 blade for custom contouring.

Once the implant is trimmed to fit the desired subperiosteal space, it is fixated to bone. Initially I had used microplates and screws to fixate, but I have found that longer screws (4–6 mm) can be used directly through the implant and into the bone (Fig. **11–4**). This yields a smooth surface and patients are unable to palpate or feel the plates and screws. I tend to place approximately four screws through the tapered thinner portion near the edges. To assure fixation where desired, the drill bit is first placed through the implant material and into the bone. Once the screws are placed flush with the implant, the implant is grasped and tested for stability. If there is any doubt, more screws or a microplate is used.

Once the implants are fixated, the periosteum of the cheek flap is raised to the desired height. If there is significant tension or if the flap slips inferiorly, periosteum can be directly sutured to the implant using a double arm 4–0 polypropylene suture with a highly curved cutting needle. If the patient is seated in the upright position for cheek contour adjustment, the suture is tied over a loose piece of 4–0 silk. Symmetry in midface elevation as well as malar fullness is checked. If adjustment is necessary, the silk is lifted straight up untying the polypropylene suture. If no adjustment is necessary, the patient is laid back and the tarsal strip is performed.

Lateral Tarsal Strip

In general most surgeons perform a lateral tarsal strip. This cheek lifting procedure elevates so much tissue that lid stabilization is necessary. It will also aid in the contouring of the eyelid and lateral tissues. There are many variations in performing a tarsal strip, but the method described by Putterman[9] is a safe and secure method. In general, I place the tarsal strips so they are symmetric and create the desired postoperative palpebral fissure angle. Before permanently tying the tarsal strips, conjunctiva is closed with three buried interrupted 6–0 plain gut sutures and the lateral canthal angle is reformed with a 5–0 polyglycolic acid (chromic) suture from gray line to gray line with a buried knot.

Lateral Elevation and Fixation of Flap

A toothed forceps (Bishop or Adson type) is then used to grasp the SOOF through the lateral canthotomy incision (Fig. **11–5**). Where it is grasped, with respect to its medial or lateral aspect, will determine where the majority of the lift occurs. In addition, the angle of elevation will also influence the lifting vectors and postoperative appearance. The combination SOOF and associated orbicularis flap is dissected away from the dermis. This eliminates dimpling and bunching associated with flap elevation. Hemostasis is meticulously achieved with a disposable handheld cautery. The dissected flap is imbricated with a double-arm 4–0 polypropylene suture and fixated to the lateral periosteum or the temporalis fascia lateral to the orbital rim.

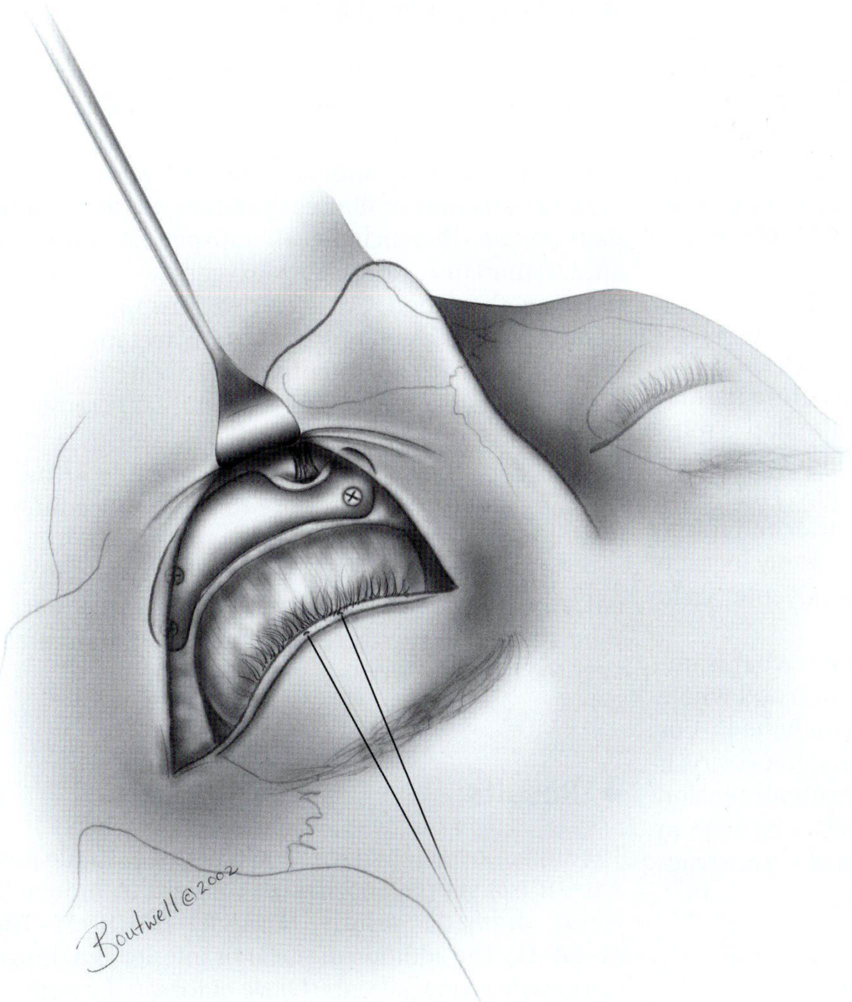

Figure 11–4 Malar or inferior orbital rim augmentation with artificial implant. Once the desired position and contour are achieved, the implant is permanently fixated using microplates or screws. The completely released periosteal flap can then be elevated over the implant. The flap can then be sutured directly to the implant if necessary.

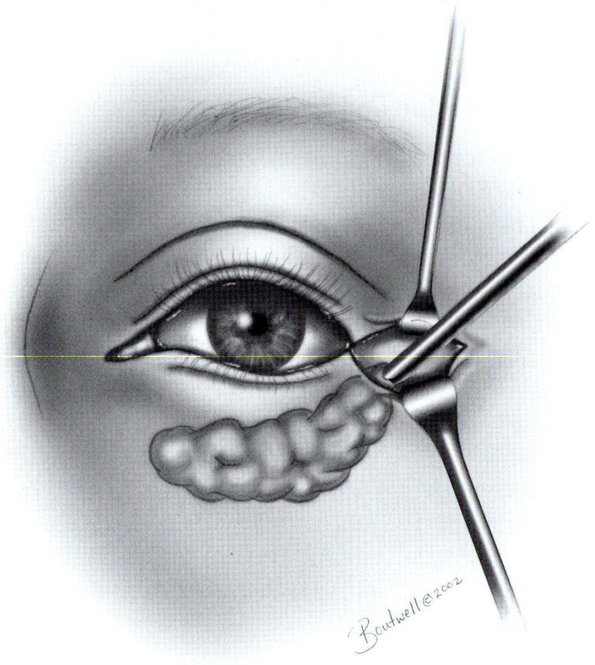

Figure 11–5 The suborbicularis oculi fat (SOOF) (or periosteum) is grasped through the lateral canthotomy incision and elevated. It is imbricated with a 4–0 polypropylene suture and then secured over a 4–0 silk tie to the lateral rim periosteum. The same is performed on the opposite side and symmetry of flaps is adjusted. Once symmetry is achieved the flaps are securely tied down. Several reinforcing 4–0 polypropylene sutures to SOOF and orbicularis can be placed to help support the cheek flap as well as contour the eyelid separately from the cheek.

This is tied over a 4–0 silk tie to allow refixation if necessary. Once again this is performed on both sides (if a bilateral case) and symmetry is adjusted before permanently tying the polypropylene sutures. The flap is reinforced with two single-armed sutures and excess flap tissue is trimmed to reduce lateral bunching. Finally the trimmed edge of orbicularis is directly attached to the orbicularis at the upper edge of the canthotomy incision using interrupted polyglactin or polyglycolic acid sutures (4–0 or 5–0).

Note that the soft tissue flap is actually what is imbricated and used to elevate the periosteum and whole cheek. Because periosteum will refixate to bone in 1 or 2 weeks, direct suturing of periosteum is unnecessary. It can be done, however, if there is concern about tension on the flap and early flap descent. This can be seen in cases of moderately large tissue defects in reconstructive surgery.

Multistep Closure

The lower lid and lateral tissues are inspected for dimpling or retraction. If any is present, the dermis is further dissected away from underlying orbicularis. Attention is then directed to any bulging or overriding orbicularis in the temporal lower lid. A subciliary incision can be performed for the length of the bulge. This is typically one quarter or one third of the lid. I do not excise any skin from here unless it is excessive (or a subciliary approach was used for this procedure). Rather, a strip of orbicularis is excised. The skin is then redraped over the lid and lateral incision. Excess lateral skin is then resected. A 5–0 polyglycolic acid suture is placed to fixate the skin flap at the lateral edge of the lower lid margin. A separate suture is then used to approximate the upper border of the incision to the lateral edge of the lower margin. Skin incisions can be closed with running or interrupted sutures. I prefer a running 6–0 nylon suture for ease of removal. If a limited subciliary incision was performed, it can be closed separately from the canthotomy incision or as one continuous running suture—again for ease of removal.

◆ Postoperative Care

Care for an isolated midface lift consists of cleaning and drying the face and applying an ophthalmic antibiotic ointment (without steroids) to the sutures and eyes. Cold compresses are applied to the face and eyelids. Any medications that inhibit coagulation are avoided for 5 days postop. This includes all nonspecific nonsteroidal antiinflammatory drugs. Cyclooxygenase-2 inhibitors do not thin the blood, are effective postoperative analgesics, and work synergistically with acetaminophen or opiates. Standard postblepharoplasty care instructions are followed, especially when orbital fat is removed. If other procedures were performed in concert with this such as cervicofacial rhytidectomy or brow lifting, the dressing and care appropriate to those procedures are instituted.

Patients are seen 5 to 7 days later, when the external nonabsorbable sutures are removed. Patients are then allowed to slowly resume more strenuous activity over the next few weeks.

◆ Results

The subperiosteal midface cheek lift is a versatile procedure. It is a simple and straightforward technique that yields dramatic results (Figs. **11–6A-D; 11–7A–C; 11–8A–D**). The addition of malar or inferior rim implants can benefit many patients. I have quite satisfactorily performed this procedure in young adults who were irradiated for rhabdomyosarcoma with resultant hypoplasia of

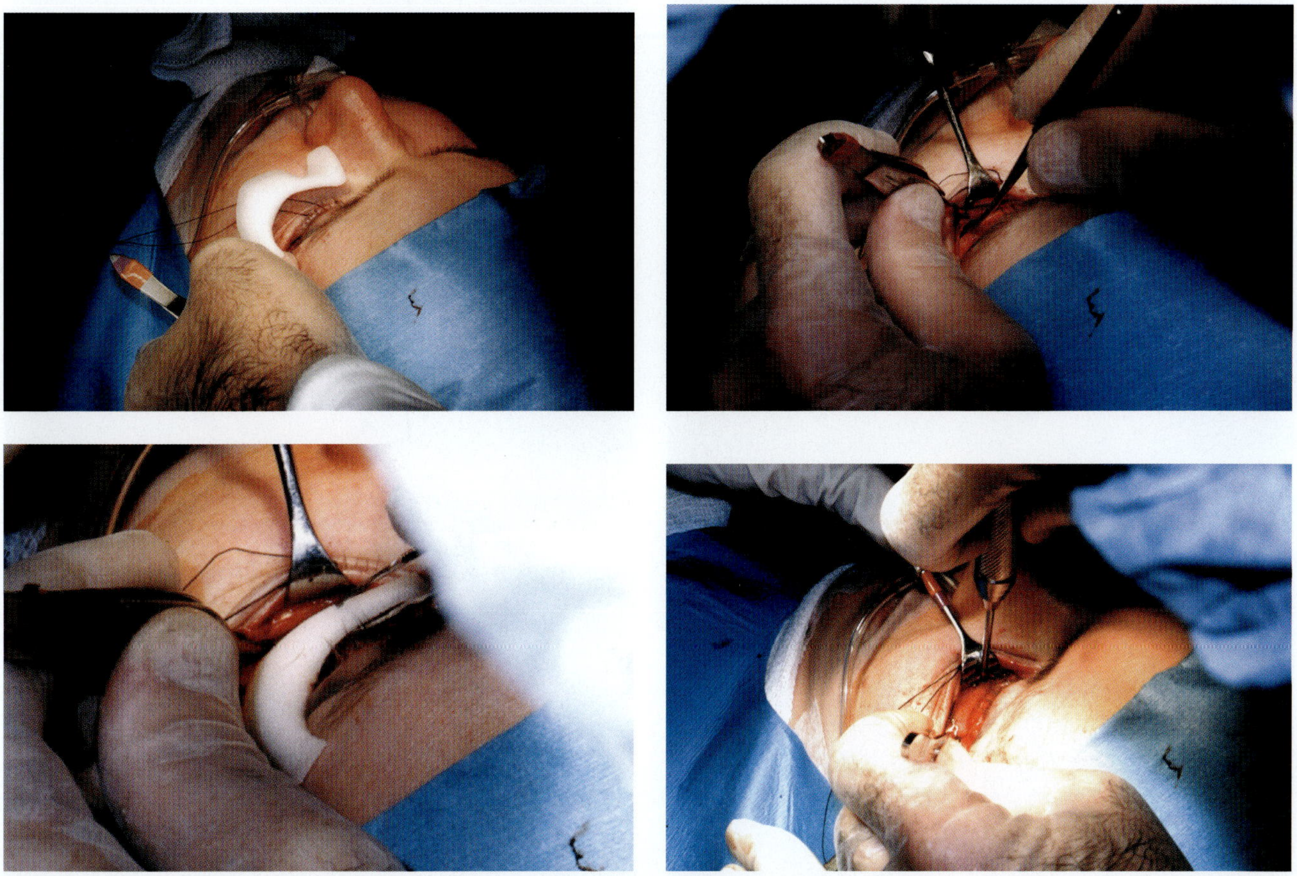

A B C D

Figure 11–6 Young female patient with unilateral midfacial hypoplasia (bone and soft tissue deficit) secondary to childhood radiation therapy for rhabdomyosarcoma. (**A**) Implant is overlaid in the desired area. General size and contour are sculpted and the implant is placed on a nonfibrous surface until it is needed. (**B**) The periosteal flap is raised. The periosteal flap is completely freed and released before implant placement and fixation. (**C**) Fine trimming allows a snug fit into the pocket. (**D**) The implant is fixated utilizing microplates for stability to support the weight of the cheek, eyelid, and midface.

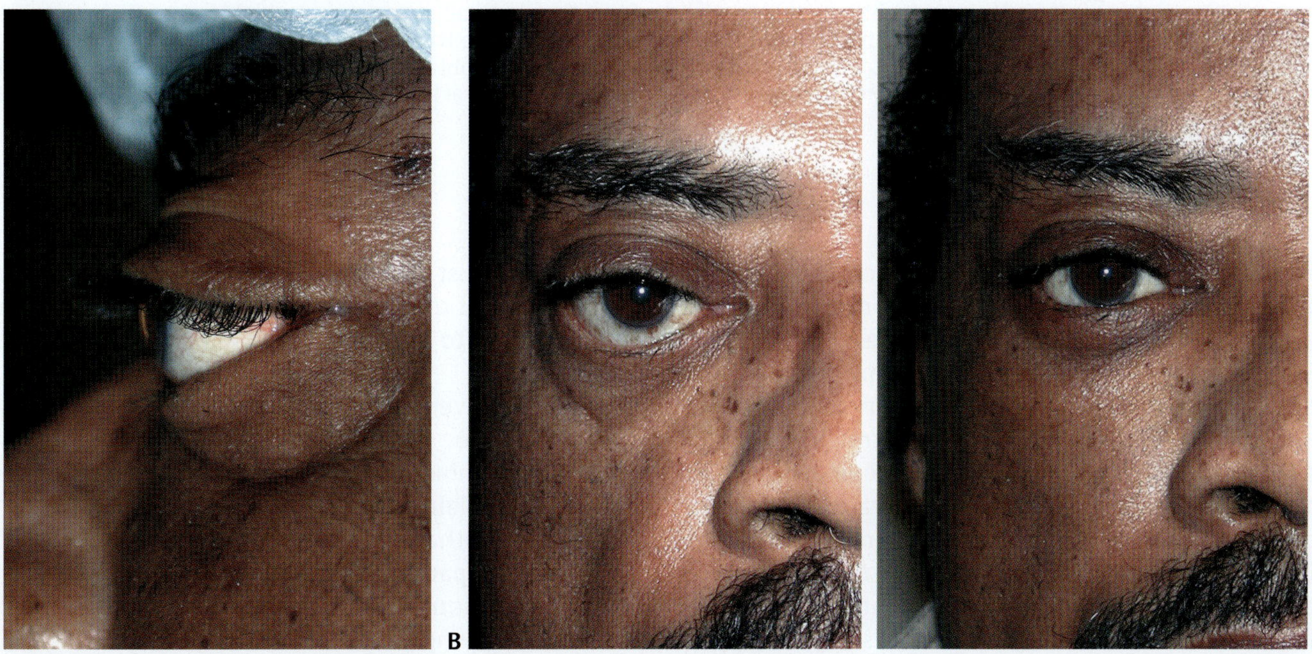

A B C

Figure 11–7 (**A**) Male patient with moderate thyroid-related exophthalmos and lid retraction greatly exaggerated by inferior orbital rim hypoplasia. (**B**) Preoperative frontal view showing relative malar hypoplasia, lid retraction, and hollow nasojugal trough. (**C**) Two-month postoperative appearance. Patient underwent bilateral subperiosteal cheek lift with Medpor inferior orbital rim implants, lateral tarsal strips, and recession of lower lid retractors with dermal allograft spacers. Notice the dramatic improvement in the contour and general appearance of the midface, nasojugal trough, and lower lid contour.

A B C D

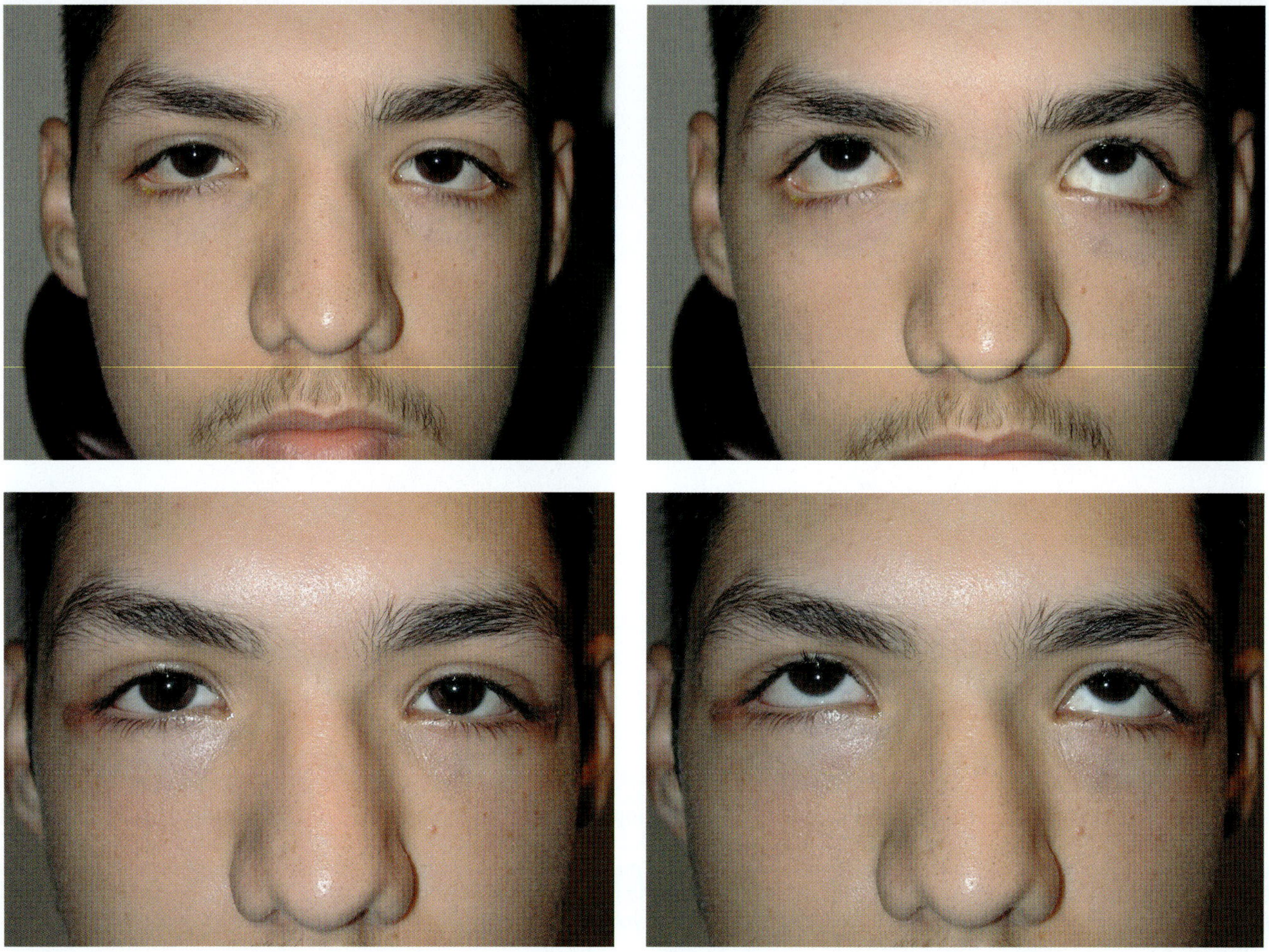

Figure 11–8 (**A**) Young male with congenital euryblepharon and lack of anterior lower lid lamellae. Note the lid retraction in primary gaze. The patient suffered from lagophthalmos, exposure keratopathy, and inability to wear contact lenses. (**B**) Accentuated lid retraction in upgaze. (**C,D**) One-week postoperative appearance following simple transconjunctival subperiosteal cheek lift. No malar augmentation was performed. Significant cosmetic benefit would have been obtained with malar implants; however, patient and family were concerned about drastically changing his appearance. Simple lateral tarsal strips would have been insufficient to support any eyelid elevation.

the midfacial soft tissue and bony structures. The most common indications in my practice for this procedure have been inferior orbital rim hypoplasia with real or perceived exophthalmos and the unhappy postblepharoplasty patient with lid retraction or periorbital hollowness. In cases of simple thyroid lid retraction, one can usually perform a recession of the retractors with a hard palate or alloplastic human dermis graft to the lower lids—with or without a permanent lateral tarsorrhaphy. In cases where malar hypoplasia coexists with either or both significant lid retraction and exophthalmos, a cheek lift with a malar implant is often necessary to support the lids and assist elevation to the inferior limbus. A simple recession of retractors and spacer graft would often be insufficient to achieve the desired amount of lid elevation.

I myself have not seen any cases of ectropion, infraorbital nerve, or facial nerve injury as a result of this procedure, although such cases are possible. The most common complaint from patients is bulging and bunching laterally. Although this resolves spontaneously over 6 to 12 weeks, patients are nonetheless frequently concerned. Attention to detail during closure can alleviate or lessen this temporary inconvenience.

References

1. Putterman AM. Cheek and midface lift combined with full-thickness temporal lower eyelid resection. In Putterman AM, ed. Cosmetic Oculoplastic Surgery: Eyelid, Forehead and Facial Techniques. Philadelphia: WB Saunders; 1999:235–247
2. Hester T, Codner MA, McCord CD Jr. Subperiosteal malar cheek lift with lower lid blepharoplasty. In McCord CD Jr, ed. Eyelid Surgery: Principles and Techniques. Philadelphia: Lippincott-Raven; 1995:210–215
3. Ramirez OM, Maillard GF, Musolas A. The extended subperiosteal face lift: a definitive soft-tissue remodeling for facial rejuvenation. Plast Reconstr Surg 1991;88:227–238
4. Binder WJ. Submalar augmentation: an alternative to face-lift surgery. Arch Otolaryngol Head Neck Surg 1989;115:797–801
5. Mladick RA. Alloplastic cheek augmentation. Clin Plast Surg 1991;18:29–38
6. McCord CD Jr. Lower lid blepharoplasty. In McCord CD Jr, ed. Eyelid Surgery: Principles and Techniques. Philadelphia: Lippincott-Raven; 1995:196–209
7. Byrd HS. The extended browlift. Clin Plast Surg 1997;24: 233–246
8. Hobar PC, Flood J. Subperiosteal rejuvenation of the midface and periorbital area: a simplified approach. Plast Reconstr Surg 1999;104:842–851
9. Putterman A. Tarsal strip procedure combined with lower lid blepharoplasty. In Putterman AM, ed. Cosmetic Oculoplastic Surgery: Eyelid, Forehead and Facial Techniques. Philadelphia: WB Saunders; 1999:211–220

12

Midface Restoration with Hand-Carved e-PTFE Orbital Rim Implants

Kenneth D. Steinsapir

This chapter provides details on a midface surgical technique that places a hand-carved expanded polytetrafluoroethylene (e-PTFE) implant on the orbital rim and malar face to replace lost bone volume at these locations. The implant is fixed to the orbital rim with titanium microscrews and serves as a fixation site for vertically lifted ptotic midface soft tissue reestablishing more youthful midface anatomic relationships. In reconstructive situations, the surgery is used to reestablish functionally appropriate anatomic relationships. Obviously this requires an invasive surgery. The method is discussed in a book on minimally invasive surgery because it accomplishes something that has proven elusive with less invasive methods. It should be noted that this surgery can and should be accomplished with just a 5 mm skin incision at the lateral canthus. A longer transconjunctival incision carried behind the lower eyelid and a flexible implant makes this surgery possible. As such, this technique has the virtue of creating an almost undetectable scar and achieving an even more important goal of creating a very powerful and natural midface restoration.

◆ Anatomical Considerations

A youthful midface is full. It is filled by the malar fat pad, which in youth is firmly held in place by the zygomatic and orbitomalar osteocutaneous ligaments. This soft tissue is also supported by a properly projected orbital rim and malar face composed medially by the maxilla and laterally by the zygoma. The malar fat is a subcutaneous fat pad that is 6 to 8 mm thick and can be conceptualized as a base-up triangle that originates along the lower eyelid crease 4 to 6 mm below the lower eyelid margin.

The midface from a practical standpoint is the facial area around the lower eyelids that is neither improved by the lower facelift nor by the upper facelift. Anatomically, the midface is a triangular zone bound medially by the nose, laterally by a line that extends from the angle of the mouth to the inferior aspect of articular tubercale on the zygomatic arch, and superiorly by a line that extends from the medial canthus to the superior aspect of the articular tubercale on the zygomatic arch. As such, the midface includes the entire lower eyelid complex, the malar fat pad, the lip elevators, and the zygomaticus major and minor.

Over time, the malar fat pad falls. Ptosis of the malar fat pad contributes to a prominent nasolabial fold. In the lower eyelid complex, malar fat pad ptosis contributes to the nasojugal or tear trough hollow under the eye. This hollow can also be exacerbated by a deep canine fossa. Aesthetically, patients are bothered by these anatomic changes including a related condition commonly referred to as "dark circles." Functionally, midface ptosis and inadequate orbital rim projection contribute to inferior scleral show, entropion, ectropion, and adverse outcomes following a variety of lower eyelid surgeries.[1,2] The growing understanding of the importance of the midface is also forcing a reappraisal of the lower blepharoplasty.[3]

Many cosmetic surgeons embrace lower eyelid surgery as one of the best cosmetic procedures. However, in many cases it simply makes the tear trough hollow more evident. Something is clearly missing in our analysis of the problem. Herniation of orbital fat into the lower eyelid is at most a minor cause of the prominence of the inferior orbital fat pad. The most significant change is the long-term remodeling of the bony orbital rim and malar face. Studies have shown that the facial skeleton remodels during adulthood. The inferior orbital rim and malar face falls and retrudes. Not surprisingly, the next most important change is ptosis of the malar fat pad in association with laxity of the osteocutaneous ligaments of the midface, in particular, the orbitomalar ligament. These changes expose the inferior orbital fat. Lower blepharoplasty is surgery on an epiphenomenon.

The descent or absence of subcutaneous fat anterior to the orbicularis oculi muscle is responsible for the appearance of the dark circle. In youth, the leading edge of the malar fat pad originates anterior to the orbicularis oculi muscle and contributes to the fullness that defines the inferior aspect of the lower eyelid crease. Subcutaneous fat has a much higher light reflectivity than muscle. Light incident to the facial skin can be reflected, absorbed, or scattered. Light that is absorbed may be reflected, absorbed, or scattered by the deeper tissues. Where this light is scattered or absorbed less light is reflected back through the skin producing an area of darkness compared with areas where more of the light is reflected back out of the skin. The dark circle is an area of the lower eyelid that has little or no subcutaneous fat. Instead, light that is transmitted through the skin strikes the orbicularis oculi muscle where it is primarily absorbed by the muscle. In contrast, the adjacent cheek skin contains relatively abundant subcutaneous fat. Here the transmitted light is reflected back through the skin making the cheek look less dark than the dark circle. Midface surgery by lifting the subcutaneous fat back into the eyelid helps to decrease the appearance of the dark circle.

Our understanding of the soft tissue changes associated with midface ptosis has also changed with our increasing understanding of the midface superficial musculoaponeurotic system (SMAS). Recent studies by Lucarelli and coworkers have elucidated the role of orbitomalar ligament laxity in midface ptosis.[4] Along the orbital rim the orbitomalar ligament is a well-defined facial condensation that extends through the orbicularis oculi to insert into the dermis.[5] This ligament helps to support the malar fat pad. Malar fat pad ptosis is associated with laxity of this ligament. This laxity is superimposed on the bone changes noted above. These studies also demonstrate that the suborbicularis oculi fat (SOOF) is relatively fixed and as such does not contribute to midface ptosis. Therefore, approaches that emphasize the advancement of the SOOF over the entire cheek soft tissue mass are likely to be unsatisfactory.

◆ Review of Prior Approaches

It could be argued that flattening the fullness in the lower eyelid is better than having the double convexity deformity described by Hamra.[3] Certainly lower blepharoplasty does have a role as a compromise procedure in patients who are unwilling to have midface surgery. Our patients may be happy with an improvement or a changed appearance, but a critical surgeon will recognize that this approach does not restore "youthfulness" to the midface. It does nothing to address the remodeling of the orbital rim and malar face. It does not correct the descent of the malar fat pad. In fact, lower blepharoplasty wastes an important tissue volume represented by the anterior orbital fat.

Advocates of arcus marginalis release open the orbital septum and preserve and reposition the inferior anterior orbital fat along the external edge of the inferior orbital rim. Arcus marginalis release was first described in 1981 by Loeb who correctly understood that there was more going on in the midface than just herniation of orbital fat.[6,7] He noted that patients who underwent lower blepharoplasty failed to have improvement of the nasojugal groove. Rather, surgery seemed to worsen its appearance. He theorized that the ideal midface morphology was a flat surface essentially from the lower eyelid lashes into the cheek. To address the nasojugal groove, he proposed advancing the lower eyelid fat pads over the inferior orbital rim and onto the malar face to fill in the nasojugal groove. Hamra popularized the preservation of inferior orbital fat.[3,8] Revisiting Loeb's concepts, he pointed out that with age there is an increasing skeletonization of the orbits and that a youthful midface is associated with soft contours and an absence of bone contours. Although arcus marginalis release provides a moderate improvement of the orbital rim soft tissue relationships, it is inadequate to replace the volume from the inferior rotation and retrusion of the bony malar face or the situation where there is an abnormally deep canine fossa. An anatomically correct approach is the replacement of the volume lost by bone remodeling and a vertical midface soft tissue lift. When these two factors are controlled, the advanced midface soft tissue meets the lower eyelid orbital fat in continuity to reestablish a more youthful midface contour.

Flowers was one of the first surgeons to address midface ptosis.[9] He conceptualized the tear trough deformity to be the result of a soft tissue deficiency between the orbicularis oculi and the levator labii alequae nasi muscle in some and a static lack of bone projection in others. His surgical correction relied on the placement of a small comma-shaped silicone "Flower's tear trough" implant (Implant Tech, Van Nuys, California). This implant has a notch to accommodate the infraorbital neurovascular bundle and could be placed via an infraciliary incision or laterally through a facelift approach. Other authors have also described placing this implant via a transconjunctival approach.[10] However, the Flower's implant provides a limited amount of increased orbital rim projection, which is not adequate for many individuals. Options for fixation of the implant are limited. It has been this author's approach to suture the implant to the diaphanous arcus marginalis. Others have advocated direct vertical SOOF lifting with fixation to the arcus marginalis.[11,12] However, published reports of these methods provide no long-term follow-up to assure midface surgeons that the site is adequate for long-term tissue fixation. It is highly likely that the arcus marginalis is not adequate to support the weight of the midface. For these reasons, methods that rely on a superior lateral lift for elevating midface tissue, even though they do not provide an anatomically correct vector of support, are more popular.[13–15]

The Goldberg implant produced from porous polyethylene (Porex Surgical, Newnan, Georgia) is another option for midface augmentation.[10] This implant was developed as an alternative to split rib and calvarial onlay bone grafting as a means to increase the projection of the inferior and lateral orbital rim without the necessity of craniofacial midface advancement. It is thicker than the Flowers tear trough implant. The implant can be trimmed with difficulty and it is fixed to the bone with microscrews. The rigidly fixed implant can then be used as a fixation site for advanced soft tissue. Given the difficulty in carving this implant for individual patients and the desire to have a material that is softer and more elastic, an alternative material was sought for augmenting the malar face and orbital rim.

The material selected for orbital rim augmentation was e-PTFE reinforced sheets (W. L. Gore & Associates, Flagstaff, Arizona). This material is readily available and U.S. Food and Drug Administration (FDA) approved for deep augmentation in the face. It has been used clinically since 1971 as a vascular graft and has been used in millions of patients.[16,17] The material is available in several thicknesses up to 7 mm and in sheets up to 3 × 10 cm. The implant is shaped to replace volume in the nasojugal groove and along the inferior and lateral orbital rim. These implants are easily carved and have significant strength so that they can be fixed to the orbital rim with microscrews where they are used as a site for supporting advanced midface soft tissue. The remainder of this chapter discusses the method of performing this surgery as well as other clinical considerations.

◆ Surgical Approach

Patient Assessment

Preoperatively the patient is assessed to identify the degree of malar and orbital rim retrusion. At present there is no reliable systematic method for making this assessment. However, a caliper can be used to measure the relative depth of the tear trough hollow. This determines the use of a 4.5 or 7 mm thick e-PTFE reinforced sheeting. It is also helpful to assess the degree of preoperative asymmetry between the two sides of the face. Some of the asymmetry can be compensated by the appropriate adjustment in implant size. Patients should also be assessed preoperatively for the need for vertical lengthening of the lower eyelid. This requires some experience in judging the degree of vertical inadequacy of the lower eyelid margin position. When there is greater than 1 to 2 mm of inferior scleral show and significant tethering in the middle lamella of the lower eyelid, a spacer graft in the lower eyelid is usually necessary.[18–20] Smaller degrees of inferior scleral show can be addressed at the time of midface lifting with the lateral canthoplasty, which completes this surgery. Typically, a hard palate graft is chosen for spacer graft material. Under these circumstances, the lower eyelid is resuspended on a Frost suture to the eyebrow so the eyelid can heal in an immobilized position. Surgery is then done in stages with the second surgery on the contralateral side performed at least a week after the first side.

Surgical Procedure

Surgery is performed under intravenous sedation. This permits the patient to sit up and open and close the eyes during the procedure. This degree of cooperation is needed to adjust the lateral canthal angle when it is resuspended. Once the skin is prepped and the patient draped, the lower eyelid deficit is marked with a methylene blue marking pen (Fig. **12–1**). A sheet of sterile x-ray film is pressed firmly over these marks transferring the marking to the film to create a template.

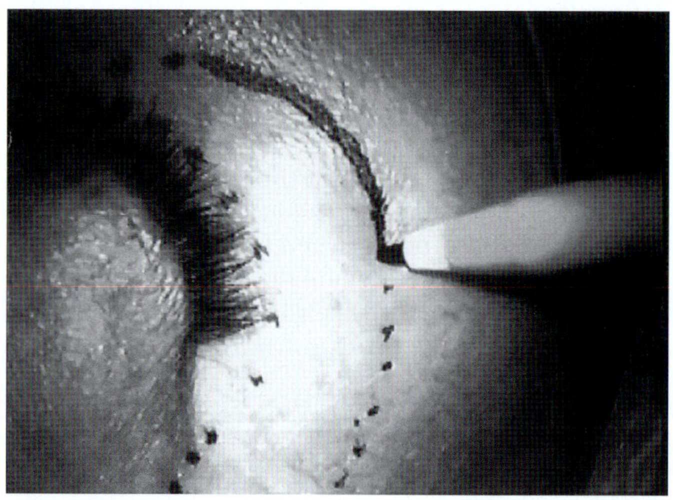

Figure 12–1 Area of midface deficit is marked with methylene blue on the skin surface.

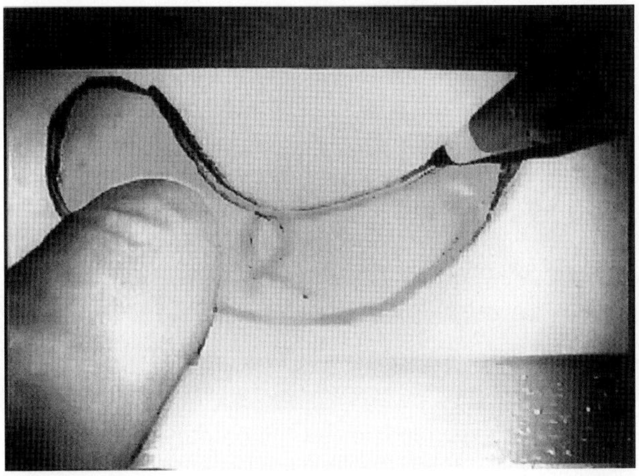

Figure 12–2 The marks are transferred to sterile dental film that is cut to create a template for the expanded polytetrafluoroethylene sheet.

Local infiltration of the cheek and lower eyelid is then performed. Typically 10 to 15 mL of lidocaine 1% with 1:100,000 epinephrine is infiltrated on each side. This includes field infiltration of the lower eyelid, lateral canthal structures, and cheek complex to the superior gingival sulcus. Additionally, the zygomatic temporal nerves, zygomatic facial nerves, and infraorbital neurovascular bundles are also blocked.

While the epinepherine is taking effect, the orbital rim implants are fabricated on a back table. The template is usually a crescentic or comma-shaped object (Fig. **12–2**). Because augmentation needs vary in the two sides of the face, separate templates are created for each side. The template is laid over the rectangular sheet of e-PTFE. Operator experience is required to determine the extent of the implant and the appropriate thickness. The shape is outlined with a marking pen. Typically, an implant is 3 cm tall and 6 cm wide. Generally, only one implant can be obtained from a 3 × 10 cm sheet. When the midface deficit is small, however, two implants may be cut from one block. A #10 blade is used to cut the implant from the sheet. It is then carved with a #11 blade to the desired shape (Fig. **12–3**). The anterior aspect of the implant is shaped and the posterior surface is left flat. The completed implant is soaked in a solution of gentamicin (80 mg in 100 mL of normal saline) for use later in the case.

A lateral canthotomy is performed with the skin incision limited to 5 mm. All attachments of the inferior limb of the lateral canthal retinaculum and orbitomalar ligaments are severed along the orbital rim. At this point, the lateral aspect of the lower eyelid is freely mobile. A Westcott scissors is used to make an incision 6 to 8 mm below and parallel to the lid margin across the conjunctiva and lower eyelid retractors from the lateral canthus laterally to a point just below the inferior puncta medially.

If a spacer graft is planned, the transconjunctival incision is made just below the inferior edge of the lower eyelid tarsus. Upward traction is then placed on the lower eyelid retractors at the proximal aspect of the incision with a toothed forceps. This allows the proximal inferior cul de sac conjunctiva to be pulled up and over the corneal surface. Generally a metal corneal shield is used to protect the cornea. The lower eyelid margin is retracted inferiorly with a lacrimal rake. A combination of blunt and sharp dissection is used to define a bloodless plane anterior to the inferior orbital fat pads and posterior to the orbital septum to the orbital rim. White glistening connective tissue at the orbital rim is the insertion of the arcus marginalis and the proximal aspect of the orbitomalar ligament.

With the orbital rim defined, a needle cautery is used to incise the soft tissue covering 3 mm beyond the orbital rim. The incised soft tissue covering at this point is constituted by the leading edge of the SOOF pad and the periosteum. A subperiosteal dissection over the malar face is then performed with a periosteal elevator. Centrally, one encounters the levator labii superioris muscle, which inserts just superior and drapes over the infraorbital neurovascular bundle. As this muscle is disinserted, care is made to avoid damaging the infraorbital nerve. Below this, the levator anguli oris muscle is also disinserted. Medially, the dissection is continued to the cartilaginous nose and superior on the frontal process of the maxilla. Laterally, the dissection encounters the zygomatic facial nerve, which is sacrificed. Inferolaterally the insertions of the zygomatic minor and major muscle are encountered. The origin of zygomatic cutaneous ligament is just superolateral to the insertion of the zygomaticus major. The subperiosteal dissection is continued over the zygomatic arch, superiorly along the orbital rim to the level of the frontozygomatic suture. When necessary, dissection is performed above the zygomatic arch. It is well to remember that the most

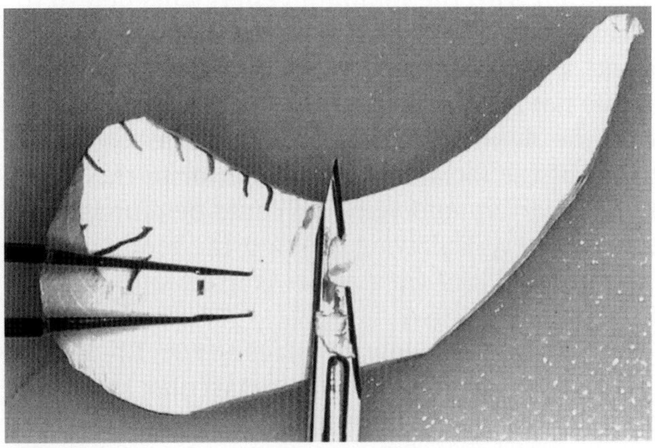

Figure 12–3 The expanded polytetrafluoroethylene implant is trimmed to shape with a #11 blade.

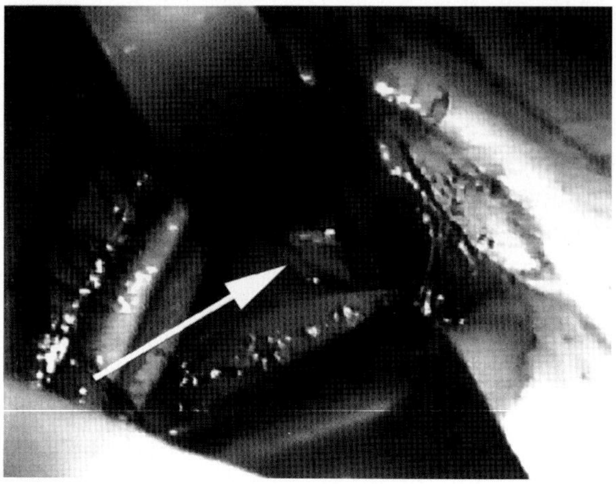

Figure 12–4 A long, insulated, cutting cautery needle with a right-angle bend is used to cut the periosteum (arrow). This step is needed to fully mobilize the overlying cheek soft tissue.

anterior branches of the frontal branch of the facial nerve are located 19 mm posterior to the lateral aspect of the orbital rim. Below the zygomatic arch care is taken to maintain the dissection in a subperiosteal plane. At the inferior edge of the zygoma, the plane is extended onto the masseter fascia. Above the zygomatic arch, the dissection plane is deep to the intermediate temporal fascia. By respecting these dissection planes, the facial nerve is avoided. This dissection defines a midface subperiosteally based flap that includes the midface periosteum, the SOOF pad, the malar fat pad, the lip elevators, the zygomaticus major and minor, the orbicularis oculi muscle, and the overlying skin.

The periosteum is incised and released to permit the permanent advancement of these tissues superiorly. A long insulated needle tip cautery (Colorado Microdissection Needle, Stryker Corp., Kalamazoo, Michigan) is used on a cutting setting to incise the overlying periosteum along the inferior edge of the zygoma (Fig. **12–4**). This periosteal incision is made under direct visualization with the minimum energy needed to incise the periosteal tissues. The use of loupe magnification and a headlight facilitates this dissection. It is advisable not to extend the tip of the dissection needle beyond the depth of the periosteum. The zygomatic branches of the facial nerve run inferior to the transverse facial artery and vein and could be damaged by excessive cautery. Following this step, the gentle spreading action of a blunt tip scissors is used to obtain the necessary tissue release.

The implant can now be placed (Fig. **12–5**). The position of the infraorbital neurovascular bundle is marked on the skin. These marks are transferred to the implant and a notch is trimmed so the implant fits around the nerve. The superior edge of the implant should be aligned along the orbital rim so that it acts as an extension of the orbital rim. If the implant is carried around the lateral aspect of the orbital rim, it should also extend to the rim in this location with an appropriate feathering of the implant so that it blends with the facial contours. When necessary or appropriate, the implant is cut to extend slightly above the orbital rim. Properly positioned in a pocket of adequate size, the implant should lay flat with no buckling. The implant is then fixed with three 1.3 mm titanium microscrews of 6 to 8 mm length. Longer microscrews are used on implants carved from 7 mm thick e-PTFE. Three microscrews are placed laterally, centrally, and medially for fixation. An 18-gauge needle is used with a twisting motion to core a path through the implant where the microscrews are to be placed. A power drill with the appropriate drill bit creates guide holes in the bone (Fig. **12–6**). The microscrews are tightened

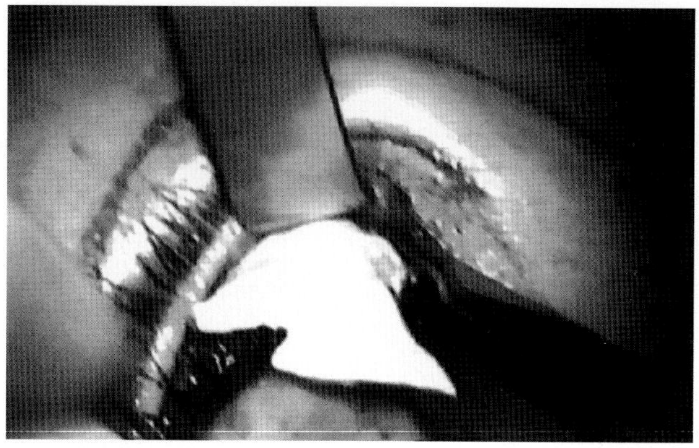

Figure 12–5 The expanded polytetrafluoroethylene implant is inserted into the dissected midface pocket prior to fixation to the orbital rim.

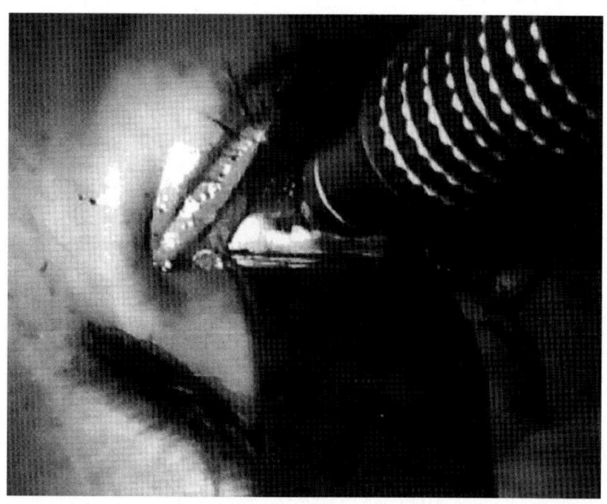

Figure 12–6 A power drill is used to place a guide hole for the titanium microscrews used to fixate the expanded polytetrafluoroethylene implant to the orbital rim.

until their heads are embedded in the implant material. Alternatively, self-drilling screws can be used.

The implant fixed to the orbital rim with microscrews creates the ideal site for substantial fixation of the advanced cheek soft tissue. A 3–0 polyethylene monofilament suture on a reverse cutting needle is passed in a horizontal mattress fashion from the superior edge of the implant and through the cheek soft tissue and then back through the implant where the suture is tied. At least three horizontal sutures are placed to provide adequate suspension of the cheek soft tissue along the orbital rim from medial to lateral.

To resuspend the lower eyelid, a small tarsal strip is created in the lateral aspect of the cut lower eyelid. The lower eyelid margin is denuded laterally for a few millimeters to expose the tarsal tissue. A double-armed 4–0 permanent suture on a spatulated semicircular needle (Supramid Extra, S. Jackson Inc., Alexandria, Virginia) is passed though the exposed tarsal strip to resuspend the lateral element of the lateral canthal tendon on the lateral orbital rim. Once this suture has been placed, the patient is placed in an upright sitting position to permit an accurate judgment of the repositioned lateral canthal angle. Generally, this point should be no higher than 1 mm above the medial canthal position. The placement of the lateral canthal angle should be bilaterally symmetric. Small differences in the placement of the lateral canthal angle are readily apparent postoperatively. Once a satisfactory placement is found this suture should be loosened and one or two absorbable chromic sutures are placed to reapproximate the conjunctiva. Alternatively if a spacer graft of hard palate is to be sutured between the inferior cut edge of the lower eyelid tarsus and the proximal cut edge of the conjunctiva it is sutured into position at this point in the surgery.[18,20] Finally, the inner lateral canthal angle is reformed with an absorbable mattress suture and the lateral canthal resuspension suture is permanently tied. The lateral raphe of the orbicularis oculi muscle and overlying skin is closed with a running absorbable suture.

Typically, both sides are operated on during the same operative session unless a spacer graft is needed. When a spacer graft is needed, the lid is sutured closed with multiple temporary Frost sutures and patched closed for 5 to 7 days. The second side is scheduled at least a week later and the first eye is opened before surgery is performed on the second side to avoid depriving the patient of vision. Postoperative management includes icing for the first 2 days and a 7-day course of prophylactic antibiotics. Steroids are not routinely given.

◆ Results

Patients are swollen postoperatively for several months. However, within 7 days the bruising and swelling are sufficiently diminished so that most individuals are able to return to their daily activities. Typically a restriction on heavy aerobic exercise is maintained for 3 weeks. In the immediate postoperative period there may be eye irritation that is addressed with artificial tears and bland ophthalmic ointment. The chromic sutures used to close the skin over the lateral orbicularis oculi raphe are removed at 1 week to minimize scarring.

Motor injury has been a very rare complication with just one patient experiencing transient weakness in the pretarsal orbicularis oculi muscle of one upper eyelid. This resulted in minor lagophthalmos addressed with ocular lubrication. The problem resolved spontaneously within a few weeks of surgery. The reader should be aware that the facial nerve is at risk in the surgical dissection. This includes zygomatic branches of the facial nerve and the frontal branches. The status of these nerves is assessed and documented preoperatively and postoperatively. Cutaneous anesthesia is a relatively common but minor complication. Typically anesthesia is transient. Temporary anesthesia in the distribution of infraorbital nerve is seen in 12% of cases. By careful dissection, and by preventing the implant from impinging on the nerve, permanent nerve injury is avoided. Interestingly, the zygomatic facial nerve is sacrificed with the dissection, yet it is unusual to find cutaneous anesthesia in the distribution of this nerve postoperatively.

Infections have been very rare. In the last 100 cases, the only infection was in a patient with a history of recurrent squamous cell carcinoma and prior radiation therapy. Fifteen months after his reconstructive midface surgery a fistula developed over the implant. The infected implant was removed and a frozen section from the edge of the fistula revealed recurrent squamous cell carcinoma. The patient elected radiation therapy with resolution of the fistula.

Other complications have included asymmetry of the lateral canthal angles requiring revisional surgery in one case. In another case, the medialmost tip of an implant folded onto itself resulting in a skin irregularity. This was corrected as a minor procedure in the office setting. A small incision was made over the tip of the folded implant. A simple dissection allowed the tip to be unscrolled, resolving the problem. It is anticipated that despite extensive preoperative discussion, there will be patients requiring alterations in implant volume. Although this has not happened, experience has shown that removing e-PTFE implants is straightforward. Although they do not seem to develop the same type of

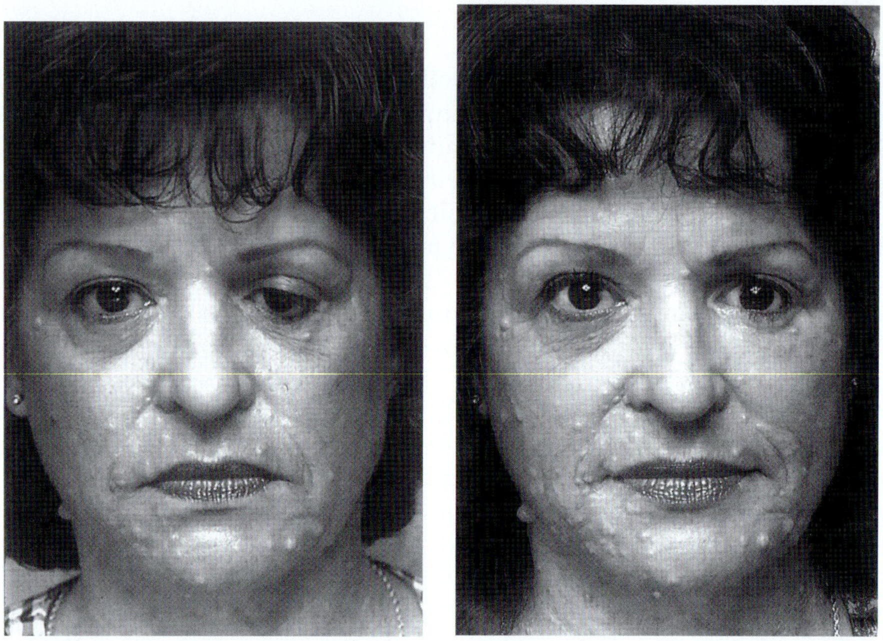

A B

Figure 12–7 (**A**) A 52-year-old woman with neurofibromatosis. The left socket is anophthalmic following resection in childhood of an optic nerve glioma. Prior orbital surgery with the placement of glass beads into the orbital cavity has caused a near loss of the left interior conjunctival cul de sac. (**B**) The patient has had the benefit of staged surgery including replacement of the intraconal implant and removal of the majority of the glass beads. Her second surgical stage was midface surgery with a porous polyethylene orbital rim implant that became infected. It was removed and replaced with a hand-carved expanded polytetrafluoroethylene midface implant. Ptosis surgery was performed as a final stage of surgery.

fibrotic capsule as seen with silicone implants, the soft tissue enclosing these implants is easily separated from the implant.

◆ Indications for Patients

This midface procedure may effectively be used for both reconstructive and purely cosmetic indications. Generally these indications overlap because an eyelid/midface that functions well to protect the eye has an overall morphology that is also aesthetically pleasing. The cases presented here are representative examples to provide the reader with an overview of the results of these surgeries.

Case Studies

Case 1 is a 52-year-old woman with neurofibromatosis who had her left eye and optic nerve resected for a benign optic nerve glioma in childhood. As a young adult, further surgery compromised the inferior conjunctival cul de sac. She had staged surgery. The first stage included replacement of her original intraconal implant with a 22 mm porous polyethylene spherical implant. Following this, left midface surgery was performed with the placement of a porous polyethylene orbital rim implant and reconstruction of the conjunctival cul de sac with a hard palate graft. She developed an atypical mycobacterial infection in the implant 4 months after surgery necessitating its removal. Six months later the midface surgery was revised with a hand-carved e-PTFE orbital rim implant. Fig. **12–7A,B** demonstrate the patient before and 1 year after her procedures, which included left upper eyelid ptosis surgery as the final stage of reconstruction.

Case 2 is a 41-year-old woman who desired aesthetic rejuvenation. She had an endoscopic forehead lift followed approximately 8 months later with bilateral midface lifting with hand-carved e-PTFE midface implants. Fig. **12–8A,B** show her before and 6 months after her midface surgery.

◆ Summary

This technique of midface surgery addresses both the soft tissue and bone changes associated with midface ptosis. Surgery is performed through a small lateral canthal incision with the remainder of the incision hidden behind the eyelid. The e-PTFE implant is customized for the needs of each patient and provides a means for both correcting the changes in bone projection and securely anchoring the vertically lifted cheek soft tissue. The surgery is associated with very few complications.

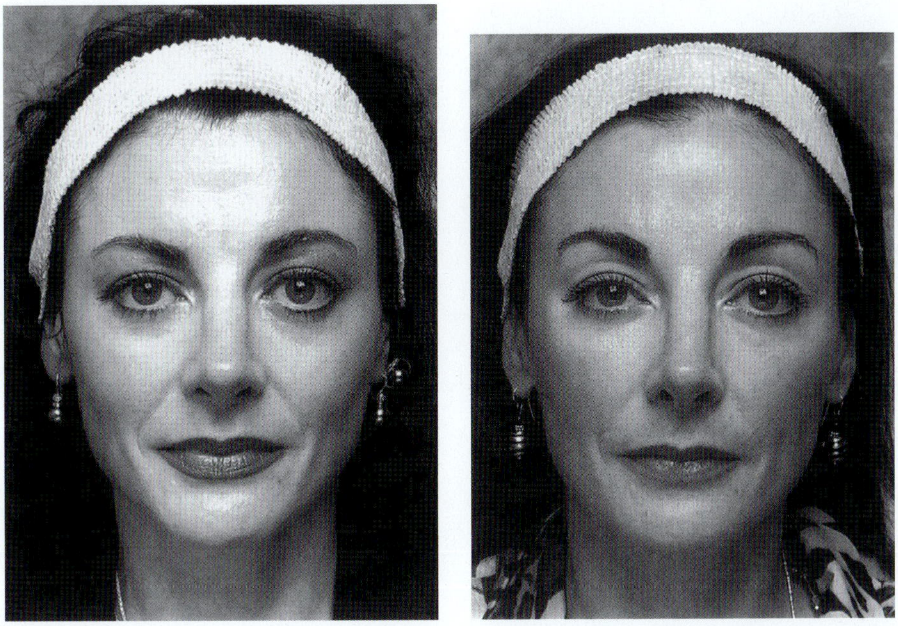

A B

Figure 12–8 (**A**) A 41-year-old woman looking for facial rejuvenation. (**B**) Her surgery was performed in two stages. Initially she had endoscopic forehead surgery. Approximately 8 months following this, she had bilateral midface surgery with hand-carved expanded polytetrafluoroethylene implants.

References

1. Goldberg R, Relan A, Hoenig J. Relationship of the eye to the bony orbit, with clinical correlations. Aust N Z J Ophthalmol 1999;27:398–403
2. Pessa JE, Desvigne LD, Lambros VS, Nimerick J, Sugunan B, Zadoo VP. Changes in ocular globe-to-orbital rim position with age: implications for aesthetic blepharoplasty of the lower eyelids. Aesthetic Plast Surg 1999;23:337–342
3. Hamra ST. The role of orbital fat preservation in facial asethetic surgery: a new concept. Clin Plast Surg 1996;23:17–28
4. Lucarelli MJ, Khwarg SI, Lemke BN, Kozel JS, Dortzbach RK. The anatomy of midfacial ptosis. Ophthal Plast Reconstr Surg 2000;16:7–22
5. Kikkawa DO, Lemke BN, Dortzbach RK. Relations of the superficaial musculoaponeurotic system to the orbit and characterization of the oribtomalar ligament. Ophthal Plast Reconstr Surg 1996;12:77–88
6. Loeb R. Fat pad sliding and fat grafting for leveling lid depressions. Clin Plast Surg 1981;8:757–776
7. Loeb R. Nasojugal groove leveling with fat tissue. Clin Plast Surg 1993;20:393–400
8. Hamra ST. Arcus marginalis release and orbital fact preservation in midface rejuvenation. Plast Reconstr Surg 1995;96: 354–362
9. Flowers RS. Tear trough implants for correction of tear trough deformity. Clin Plast Surg 1993;20:403–415
10. Steinsapir K, Shorr N. Suborbital augmentation. In Bosniak S, ed. Principles and Practice of Ophthalmic Plastic and Reconstructive Surgery. Vol 1. Philadelphia: WB Saunders; 1996:484–503
11. Hoenig JA, Shorr N, Shorr J. The suborbicularis oculi fat in aesthetic and reconstructive surgery. Int Ophthalmol Clin 1997;37:179–191
12. Patipa M. Transblepharoplasty lower eyelid and midface rejuvenation: part 1. Avoiding complications by utilizing lessons learned from the treatment of complications. Plast Reconstr Surg 2004;113:1459–1468
13. Hester TR, Codner MA, McCord CD, Nahai F, Giannopoulos A. Evolution of techique of the direct transblepharoplasty approach for the correction of lower lid and midface aging: maximizing results and minimizing complications in a 5-year experience. Plast Reconstr Surg 2000;105:393–406
14. Keller GS, Nanazie A, Blackwell K, Rawnsley J, Khan S. Elevation of the malar fat pad with a percutaneous technique. Arch Facial Plast Surg 2002;4:20–25
15. Collawan SS, Vasconez LO, Gamboa M, Guzman-Stein G, Carriquiry C. Subcutaneous approach for elevation of the malar fat pad throught a prehairline incision. Plast Reconstr Surg 1996;97:836–841
16. Lewis RP, Schweitzer J, Odum BC, Lara WC, Edlich RF, Gampper TJ. Sheets, 3-D strands, trimensional (3-D) shapes, and sutures of either reinforced or nonreinforced expanded polytrtraflouroethylene for facial soft-tissue suspension, augmentation, and reconstruction. J Long Term Eff Med Implants 1998;8:19–42
17. Lagneau P, Michel J, Charrat J. Use of polytetrafluoroethylene grafts for renal bypass. J Vasc Surg 1987;5:738–742
18. Patel B, Patipa M, Anderson R, McLeish W. Management of postblepharoplasty lower eyelid retraction with hard palate grafts and lateral tarsal strip. Plast Reconstr Surg 1997;99:1251–1260
19. Patipa M. The evaluation and management of lower eyelid retraction following cosmetic surgery. Plast Reconstr Surg 2000;106:438–459
20. Shorr N. Madame butterfly procedure with hard palate graft: management of postblepharoplasty round eye and scleral show. Facial Plast Surg 1994;10:90–118

13

The S-Lift Rhytidectomy

Steven B. Hopping and Ziya Saylan

The wish of many patients seeking facial rejuvenation is for a limited procedure, devoid of complications, with a natural, nonoperated result and a rapid return to regular activities. Patients will often demonstrate their aesthetic desires by lifting the skin of their face with their fingers from the angle of the mandible vertically upward toward the tragus of the ear, a maneuver many of them have repeated endless times in the mirror prior to presenting for consultation (Fig. **13–1**). It is important to remember that there is no surgical procedure more elective than facelift surgery. Consequently, cosmetic surgeons must continually strive to maximize results while, at the same time, minimizing complications and postoperative recovery. Patients' wishes, as just outlined, may not always be shared by cosmetic surgeons, many of whom often prefer a more aggressive surgical facial rejuvenation program. The S-lift procedure as described by Saylan[1] can in the properly selected patient achieve many of our patients' wishes for facial rejuvenation, providing a limited operation with minimal risks and a short recovery period.

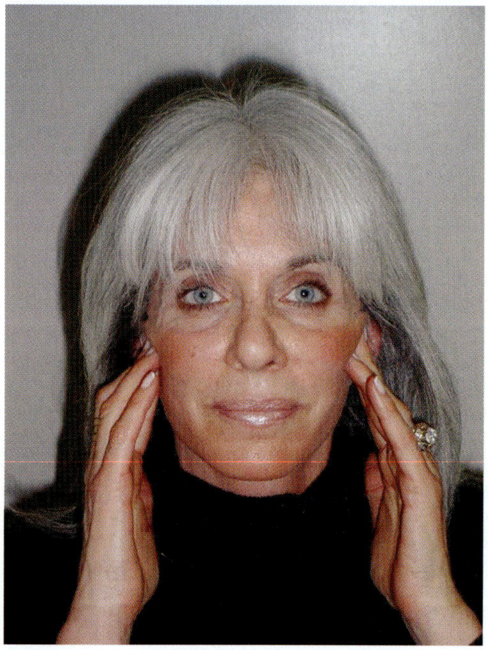

Figure 13–1 Patient demonstrating the results she would like to achieve from facelifting. Note the primarily vertical vector of this mock rejuvenation.

The S-Lift facelift, as popularized by Dr. Ziya Saylan, has received much attention around the world. The S-Lift is a conceptually new approach to facelifting and is particularly applicable to younger patients and patients requiring secondary facelifts. It is important to note that the S-Lift is not a simple "mini-lift" skin excision, but is rather an advanced superficial musculoaponeurotic system (SMAS) multiplane rhytidectomy. In this chapter, we also describe what is referred to as the S-Plus Lift. This procedure combines aspects of the technique of lateral SMASectomy described by Baker[2,3] and malar fat pad suspension utilizing a purse-string suture, suspending the ptotic malar fat pad from the temporalis fascia (M-suture), described by Tonnard et al.[4] The S-Plus Lift extends the efficacy of S-Lift in those patients who have significant midfacial ptosis. The S-Lift is generally a "short flap" facelift procedure, whereas the S-Plus with its midface extension is a "long flap" rhytidectomy.

◆ Advantages of the S-Lift

- Limited incisions and scars
- A primarily vertical vector rejuvenation
- No postauricular scar (ponytail friendly)
- Excellent neck and jowl rejuvenation

- Reduced surgical time
- Can be combined with platysmaplasty or minimal incision brow lift or buccal fat reduction for further enhancement
- SMAS procedure
- Short recovery period

◆ Disadvantages of the S-Lift

- Limited access to the neck
- Posterior dog ear that can last 1 to 3 months and can often require revision surgery
- Pain over the zygomatic arch secondary to the "O" and "U" suture
- Limited improvement on severely ptotic necks
- Limited improvement in patients with ptotic midface

◆ Key Technical Points

- Retrotragal incision, both in men and women, except for smokers in whom a pretragal incision is recommended (Fig. **13–2**)
- Preexcision of a limited skin ellipse (always be conservative, especially in secondary facelift cases). Skin only. Stay superficial.
- A #15 blade to create thick flaps and demarcate the dissection plane just superficial to the parotid fascia
- Complete flap elevation under direct vision with facelift scissors
- Extent of undermining determined by extent of midface laxity (the greater the midfacial laxity, the greater the undermining)
- Closed and open liposuction only after elevation of flap to maximize flap viability

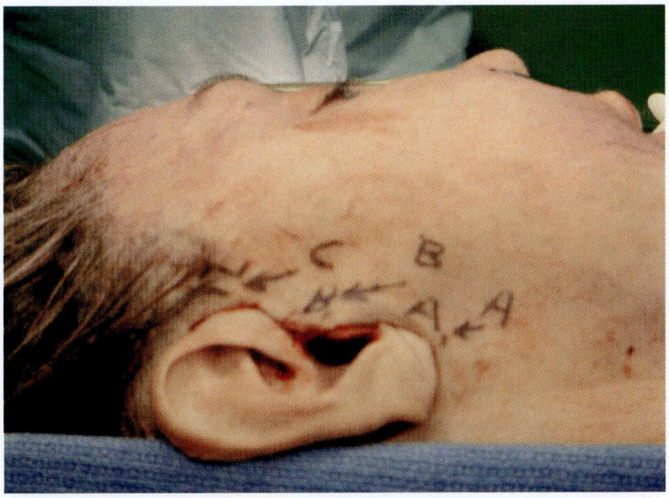

Figure 13–2 S-Lift incision demonstrating three key vectors: A to A_1, B to B_1, and C to C_1.

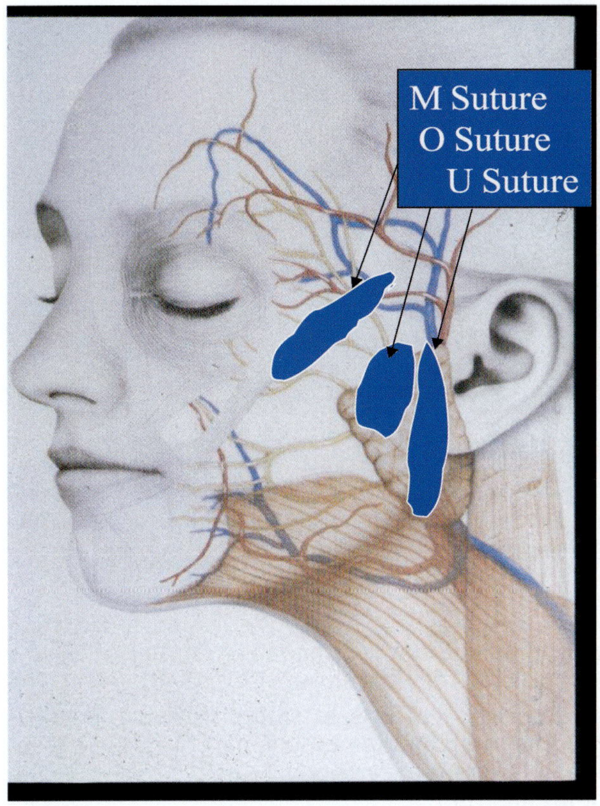

Figure 13–3 Diagramatic depiction of U suture, O suture, and M suture.

- Identify the extended SMAS platysma (ESP). Grasp the ESP with a long forceps and evaluate the ideal location for elevation and rotation with the U suture.
- Placement of the U suture (from the zygomatic arch vertically inferior to a point ~1–2 cm inferior to and posterior to the angle of the mandible) (Fig. **13–3**)
- Placement of the O suture (again from the zygomatic arch toward the jowl to tighten the jowl and achieve some midface tightening) (Fig. **13–3**)
- Placement of the M suture for midface lifting from the temporalis fascia to the malar fat pad (purse-string suture) (Fig. **13–3**)
- SMASectomy for enhanced midface elevation in patients with excessive midface ptosis (Fig. **13–4**)
- Flap demarcation to accurately measure the amount of skin that can be safely excised (Fig. **13–5**)
- Complete hemostasis. A "second look" technique is recommended before closure.
- Flap rotation achieving a primarily vertical vector lift
- Closure C to C_1 initially as the key closure, followed by A to A_1 and B to B_1 (Fig. **13–6**)
- Close the posterior and temple "dog ear" redundancies first.
- The S-designed horizontal temporal incision and excision preserves the temporal hairline, while removing the temporal dog ear (Fig. **13–7**).
- Two-layer closure (4–0 Vicryl in subcutaneous layer and 5–0 fast-absorbing plain or intracuticular 5–0

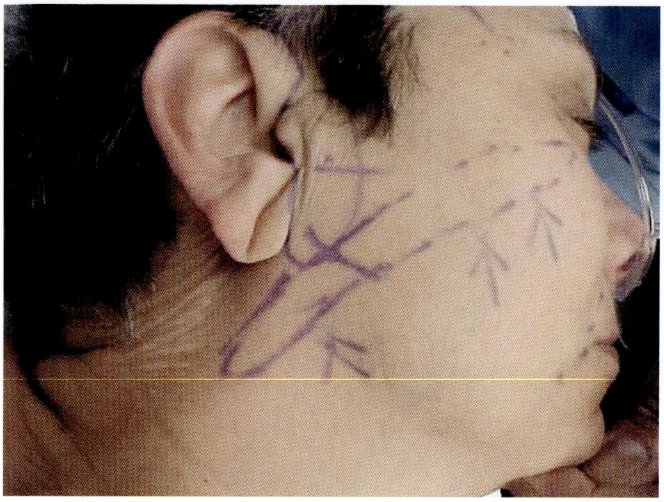

Figure 13–4 S-Plus Lift with planned U suture and SMASectomy outlined.

Monocryl for the skin) (Ethicon Inc., Somerville, New Jersey) provide the final closure (Fig. **13–8**).

- Autogenous fat grafting to smile, frown, and marionette lines and lips. Remember, part of aging is gravity, but a large part is atrophy. Effective rejuvenation must lift and fill.

◆ Indications

S-Lift (short flap) is indicated in patients who have mild-to-moderate neck laxity, without platysma banding at rest, and mild-to-moderate jowl laxity. Often the S-Lift will also require neck and jowl liposuction and/or chin augmentation.

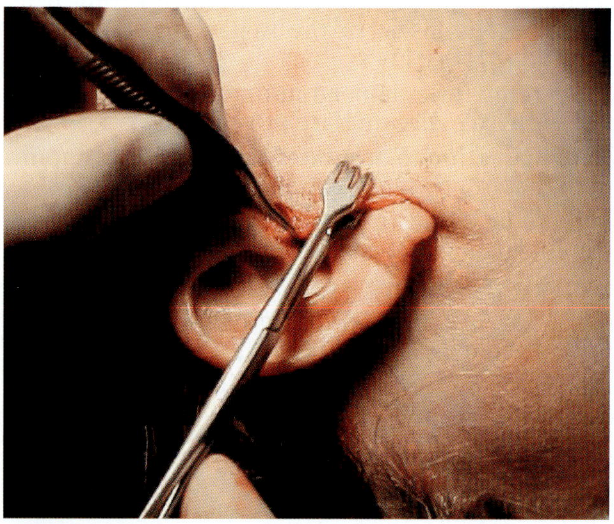

Figure 13–5 Flap demarcator is used for precise measurement of flap excision.

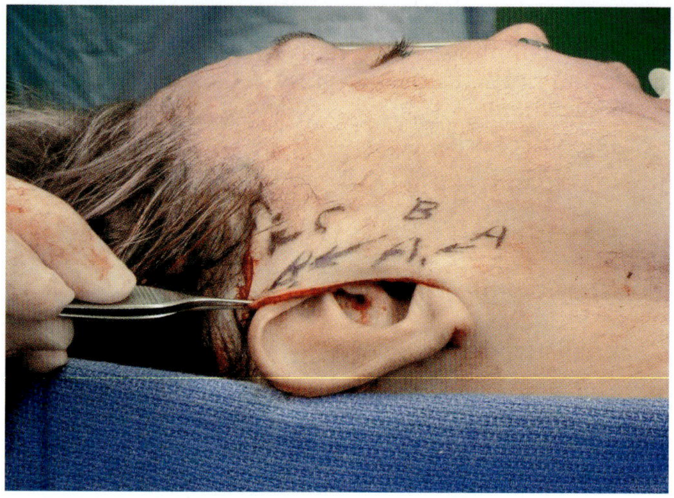

Figure 13–6 The initial key suture is placed by advancing C to C_1 in a primarily vertical vector.

S-Plus Lift (long flap) with midface extension is indicated in patients who have moderate to severe midface laxity/ptosis and malar insufficiency. The M suture or SMASectomy or both give midface elevation and rejuvenation.

S-Lift or S-Plus Lift with platysmaplasty is indicated in patients who have platysma banding at rest (Table **13–1**).

◆ Retrospective Review of Cases

A retrospective review of 100 consecutive S-Lift and S-Plus Lift rhytidectomies performed from December 2000 to December 2002 was undertaken. All procedures

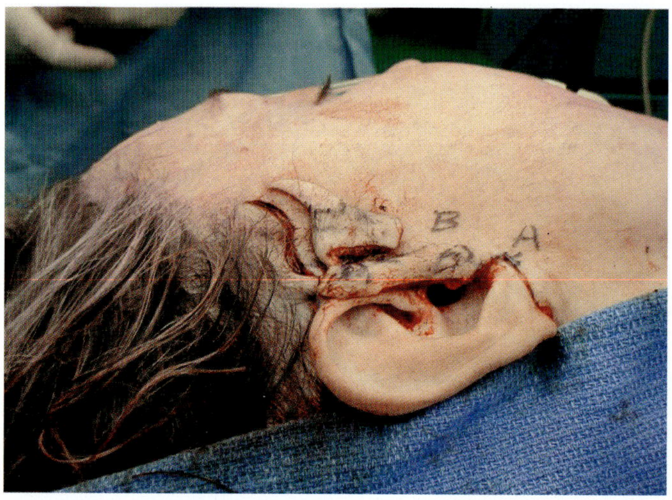

Figure 13–7 A horizontal S incision preserves the temporal hair tuft while correcting the superior “dog ear.”

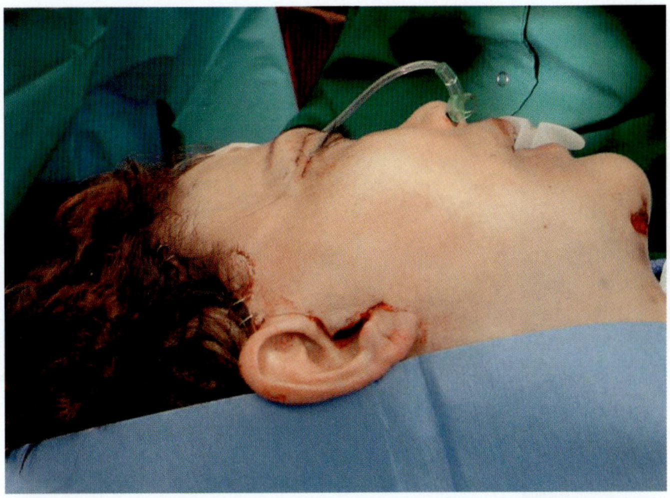

Figure 13–8 Final closure. Note the skin redundancy over the tragus to prevent tragal contracture and deformity.

Table 13–2 Patient Satisfaction Survey at 6 Months[a]

Very Satisfied	Satisfied	Unsatisfied	Total
58%	36%	6%	100%

[a]In 100 consecutive S-Lift, S-Lift, S-Plus Lift patients.

were done in a private Accreditation Association for Ambulatory Health Care (AAAC) accredited cosmetic surgical office operating suite under IV sedation anesthesia. Modified tumescent anesthesia was utilized (1000 mg of normal saline mixed with 50 mg of 1% xylocaine plain and 2 mg of epinephrine). The satisfaction index of these patients was tabulated from postoperative questionnaires evaluated at 6 months. Fifty-eight percent indicated that they were "very satisfied" with the results. Thirty-six percent were "satisfied," giving an overall satisfaction rate of 94%. Six percent of patients indicated that they were "not satisfied" with their aesthetic results. Patients not satisfied with the results at 6 or 12 months were offered secondary surgeries. In most cases, this involved a secondary S-Lift, with or without a posterior limb. Such a secondary enhancement can be readily performed in 90 minutes. Comparatively, the author's revision rate for standard rhytidectomy is similar, 5 to 7% (Table **13–2**).

A retrospective review of complications from these 100 cases revealed hematoma in two cases (2%). Both were S-Lift procedures and required return to the operating room, with opening of the flaps, control of bleeding, and drainage. Two cases (2%) of facial nerve palsies, one of the buccal and one of the ramis mandibularis branches, were noted. Both resolved spontaneously within 3 months. One case (1%) of parotid fistula was noted, which resolved with drainage and pressure dressings after 3 weeks. There was persistent pain over the zygomatic arch in two patients (2%), related to the U and O sutures, which resolved with dilute Kenalog injections (5%) and time. There were three cases (3%) of hypertrophic preauricular scarring, treated with intralesional Kenalog (5%) injections. There were six cases with unsatisfactory results (6%), requiring secondary surgeries. Three of these were due to concern with earlobe redundancy or irregularities, necessitating a posterior flap. There were no cases of infection (0%) (Table **13–3**).

◆ Discussion

Following Hamra's publication of composite rhytidectomy in 1992,[5] the sophistication and technical challenge of facelift surgery rose significantly. This was followed by an increase in serious postoperative sequelae, including temporary and permanent dyskinesias and facial nerve injuries. As alluded to earlier, facelifting is perhaps the most elective of all surgical procedures. Patients do not anticipate and, even if warned, do not accept long-term recovery or permanent adverse sequelae following facelift surgery. Today, the majority of patients, regardless of informed consent, expect an excellent aesthetic result without complications and with a rapid return to normal activities.

Table 13–1 Clinical Indications for S-Lift Rhytidectomy

Clinical Findings	Procedure
Mild to moderate neck laxity, mild to moderate jowling	S-Lift (short flap)
Moderate to severe neck laxity, moderate to severe jowling, midfacial laxity	S-Plus Lift (long flap)
Platysmal banding at rest	S-Lift, S-Plus Lift with midline platysmaplasty

Table 13–3 Percentage of Complications[a]

Hematoma	2%
Facial nerve palsies	2%
Parotid fistula	1%
Persistent pain at zygomatic arch	2%
Hypertrophic preauricular scarring	3%
Unsatisfied aesthetic results	6%
Infections	0%

[a]In 100 consecutive S-Lift, S-Plus Lift patients.

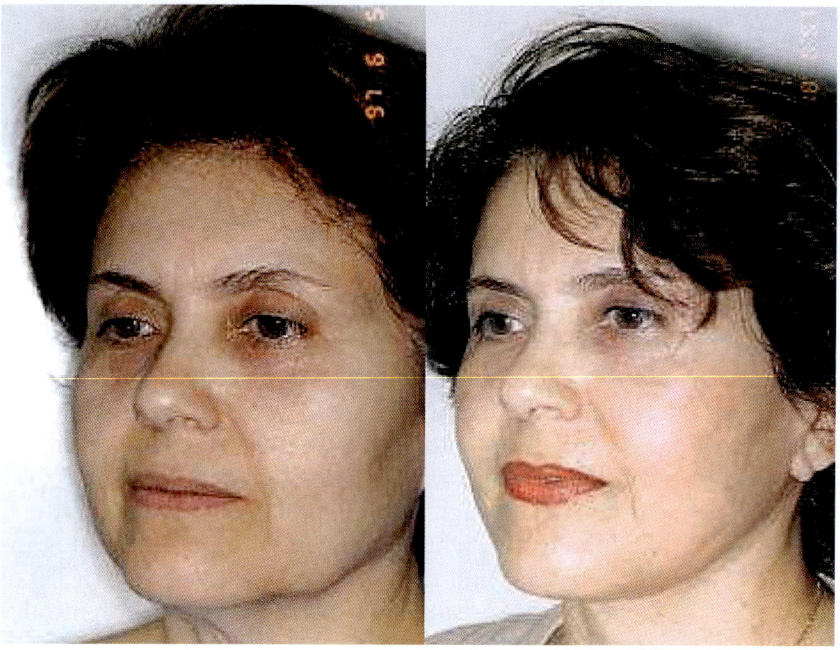

Figure 13–9 S-Lift. (**A**) Before and (**B**) after 6 months. Note improved contour of neck and jowl line.

The S-Lift and S-Plus Lift represent a return of the pendulum in the direction of less aggressive and less complicated rhytidectomy procedures. These procedures can provide the aesthetic results that patients desire, while achieving their wishes for limited risks and an acceptably short recovery period. In our series, 94% of patients were either satisfied or very satisfied with their surgical outcome. The most common problem with the procedure is inadequate correction in patients who have excess skin laxity or poor skin elasticity, necessitating a secondary "tuck-up" procedure at 6 to 12 months. This is an easy procedure to offer patients and they readily accept a secondary procedure, particularly if their first experience was a positive one. Persistent earlobe redundancy or deformity is another cause for revision surgery.

S-Lift and S-Plus Lift should not be construed as simple, skin excision "mini-lifts." They are complex facelifts that incorporate SMAS lifting techniques and principals. Surgeons performing S-Lifts must possess an intimate knowledge of facial nerve anatomy, must be able to control bleeding, and must know how and when to convert to the more classical rhytidectomy techniques if necessary. In our series, we encountered hematomas, facial nerve palsies, parotid fistulas, hypertrophic scars, and persistent neuralgias. The use of tumescent anesthesia and direct rather than blind dissection is strongly encouraged to preserve tissue planes and prevent facial nerve injuries. This is particularly true for secondary rhytidectomies where tissue planes have been altered, making blind dissection particularly risky.

Not all patients are good candidates for S-Lifts or S-Plus Lifts and it behooves the cosmetic surgeon to carefully select patients who are well-suited for this procedure. In our experience, this includes the younger patient who would like to be proactive in maintaining a youthful appearance (Fig. **13–9A,B**), the patient who does not want an overpulled classical rhytidectomy stigmata (Fig. **13–10A–D**), patients who have had previous facelift surgery and who now require a secondary procedure, and patients with a smoking history or who have medical problems dictating a short anesthetic and surgical procedure.

The S-Lift, as described by Saylan, is a short-flap SMAS facelift that is safe, even in patients with a history of smoking, hypertension, controlled diabetes, or other medical problems.[1] The vector of lift is vertical, which gives a natural appearance while at the same time providing rejuvenation to the neck and jowls. Careful attention must be given to creating and closing the temporal hair-sparing incision superiorly and the infralobular redundancy below the earlobe. The initial key suture is C to C_1, placed in a principally vertical rotation rather than A to A_1 as originally proposed by Saylan[1] (Fig. **13–6**).

The S-Plus Lift with midface extension utilizing SMASectomy or malar fat pad suspension utilizing the M suture is better suited for patients with moderate to severe midface laxity/ptosis. The incision for the S-Lift and S-Plus Lift is exactly the same but the latter is a long flap technique that requires dissection nearly to the myelolabial fold to perform the SMASectomy and malar fat pad elevation. The malar fat pad is not undermined, but rather is suspended vertically from the temporalis fascia as a vascular pedicle utilizing the purse-string M suture. S-Lift with or without midface extension combined with platysmaplasty is best for patients who demonstrate platysma bands at rest (Table **13–1**).

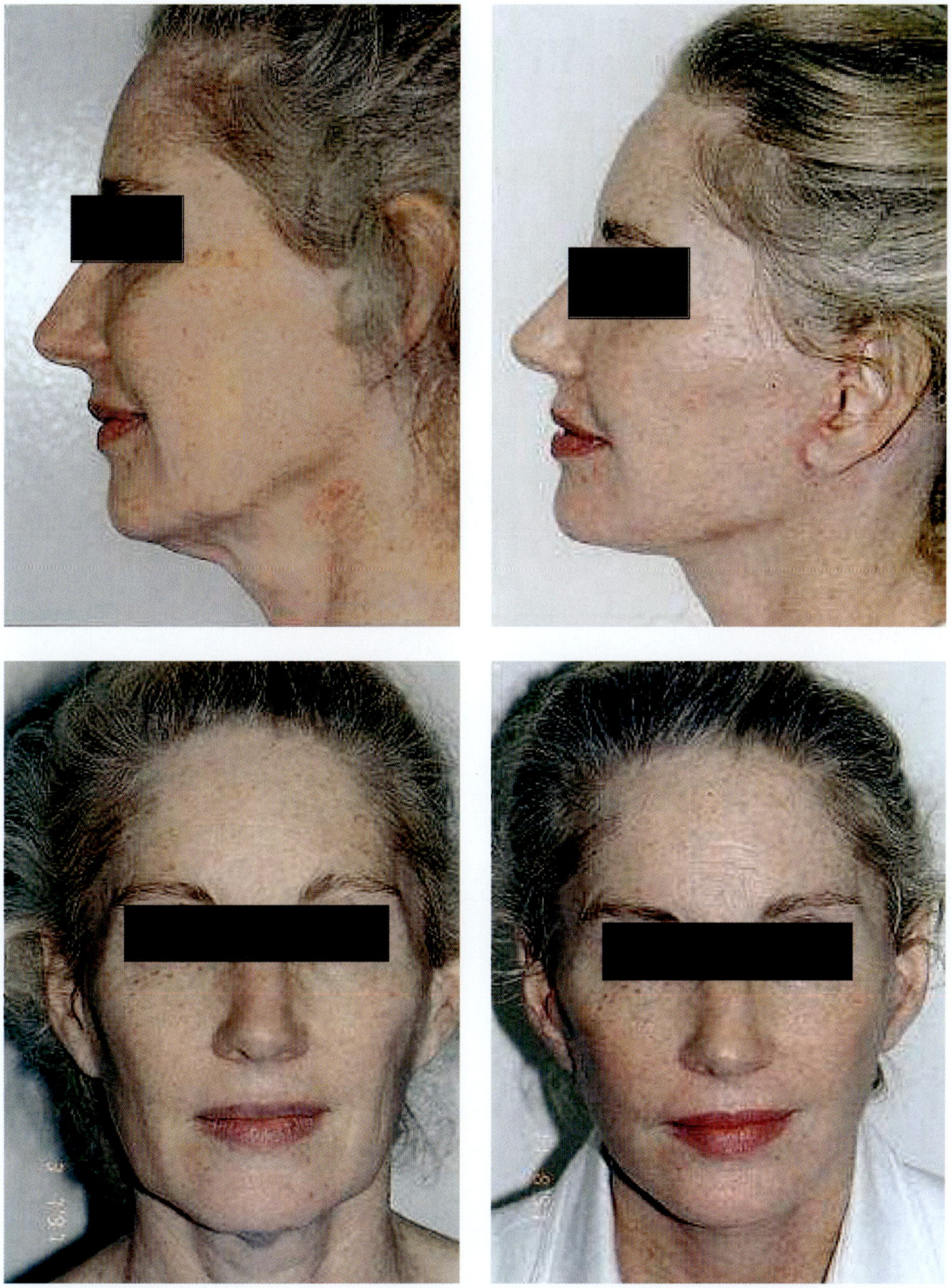

A B C D

Figure 13–10 S-Lift. (**A,C**) Before and (**B,D**) after. Note improvement in neck and jowl with preservation of temporal hair, and the natural-looking results.

◆ Conclusion

Utilizing the S-Lift and the S-Plus Lift for the indications outlined here has resulted in a high overall patient satisfaction rate (91%), while at the same time achieving patients' desires for a limited procedure, minimal complications, natural-looking results, and a rapid return to normal activities.

References

1. Saylan Z. The S-Lift: less is more. Aesthetic Surg J 1999;19:406–409
2. Baker DC. Lateral SMASectomy. Plast Reconstr Surg 1997;100: 509–513
3. Baker DC. Minimal incision rhytidectomy (short scar facelift) with lateral SMASectomy: evolution and application. Aesthetic Surg J 2001;21:14–20
4. Tonnard P, Verpaele A, Monstrey S, et al. Minimal access cranial suspension lift: a modified S-Lift. Plast Reconstr Surg 2002;109:2074–2086
5. Hamra ST. Composite rhytidectomy. Plast Reconstr Surg 1992;90:14–22

Section III

Perioral Rejuvenation

14

Defining the Principles of Perioral Rejuvenation

Stephen Bosniak

Rejuvenation of the perioral area is inadequately addressed with soft tissue facial surgical procedures. Restoration of the internal architecture and compensation for the loss that results from diminishing of the midfacial bone volume and dental support is a prerequisite for rejuvenation of the perioral contours and the lips. These changes are not always age related. They can be enhanced and fine-tuned with neuromodulation and soft tissue filling. Lip volume can be enhanced with filling agents and faded pigment restored with micropigmentation.

◆ Approach to Perioral Rejuvenation

We use a five-step approach to perioral rejuvenation:

1. Intraoral compensation for midfacial bone volume loss
2. Establishment of dental support
3. Neuromodulation plus soft tissue filling
4. Laser resurfacing of the upper lip skin (when indicated)
5. Augmentation and micropigmentation of the lips

Steps 1 and 2 are discussed in Chapters 15 and 16, respectively. Steps 3 through 5 are discussed below.

Neuromodation Plus Soft Tissue Filling

After the reestablishment of the midfacial volume and dental contours, the perioral soft tissue can be addressed. In the perioral area, Botox neuromodulation sets the stage and prolongs the results of effective filling and recontouring of the soft tissues. Placement of the injection sites and dosages must be precise to avoid imbalance of mouth movements. Two units to each depressor anguli oris muscle at the mandibular angle will subtly elevate the corners of the mouth and soften the oral commissures,[1–3] (Fig. **14–1A,B**) facilitating filling. Perlane (Q-Med, Uppsala, Sweden), more viscous

A

B

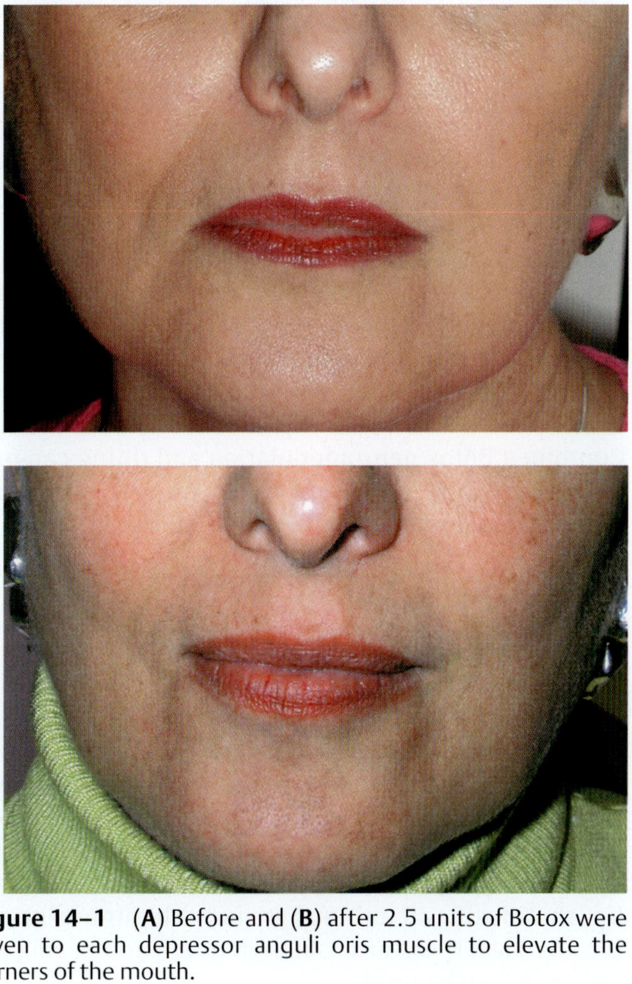

Figure 14–1 (**A**) Before and (**B**) after 2.5 units of Botox were given to each depressor anguli oris muscle to elevate the corners of the mouth.

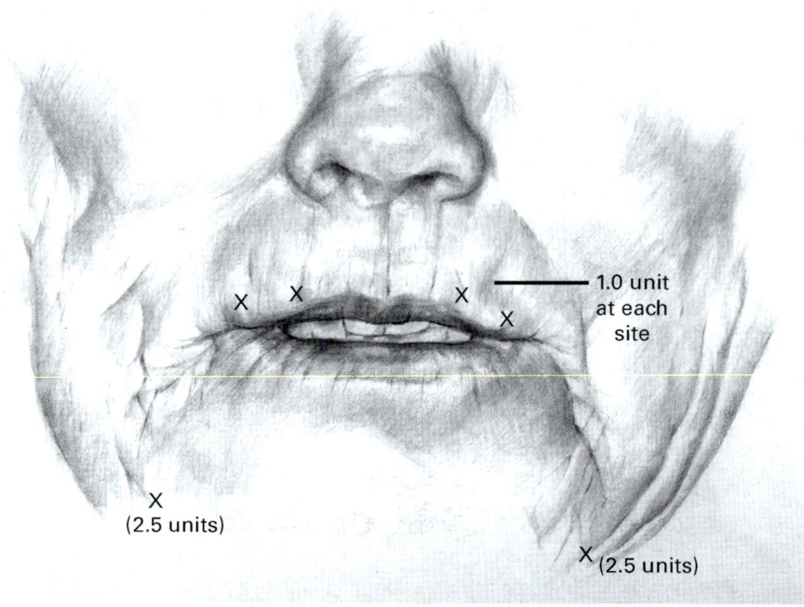

Figure 14–2 Neuromodulation of the depressor anguli oris muscles can augment the use of filling agents to improve oral commissures contours. Cautious neuromodulation of the orbicularis oris muscle can augment the use of filling agents to improve upper lip rhytidosis and contour deficiencies.

than Restylane (Medicis, Scottsdale, Arizona), effectively fills the oral commissures and can further support the angles of the mouth[4] (Figs. **14–2; 14–3A,B**). When loss of skin tone and resilience is apparent, results can be further enhanced with skin tightening and collagen-stimulating procedures using Thermage (Thermage, Hayward, California), nonablative lasers, and intense pulsed light (IPL) (Fig. **14–4A,B**).

Minute vertical rhytids adjacent to the upper lip vermilion border can be reduced with Restylane or Cosmoplast (INAMED Corporation, Santa Barbara, California) used to augment the upper lip border. Deeper, longer vertical upper lip rhytids can be filled with Restylane or Restylane Fine Lines (Q-Med Uppsala, Sweden), and flattened with four 1-unit injections of Botox across the upper lip mucocutaneous border. Combined Botox neuromodulation and filling can provide effective resolution of upper lip vertical rhytids without downtime.

Laser Resurfacing of the Upper Lip Skin (When Indicated)

Upper lip carbon dioxide laser resurfacing following neuromodulation provides the most effect long-term results but requires at least 1 week of healing before it can be camouflaged and protected with makeup. Power settings between 200 and 300 mJ using pattern 3, size 6 to 8, densities 4 to 6, and two to three passes are typically used[5] (Fig. **14–5A,B**). For less pronounced upper lip rhytidosis, an erbium:yttrium-aluminum-garnet (Er:YAG) laser, pattern 3, sizes 6 to 8, 1 to 2 J, three to six passes can be used.

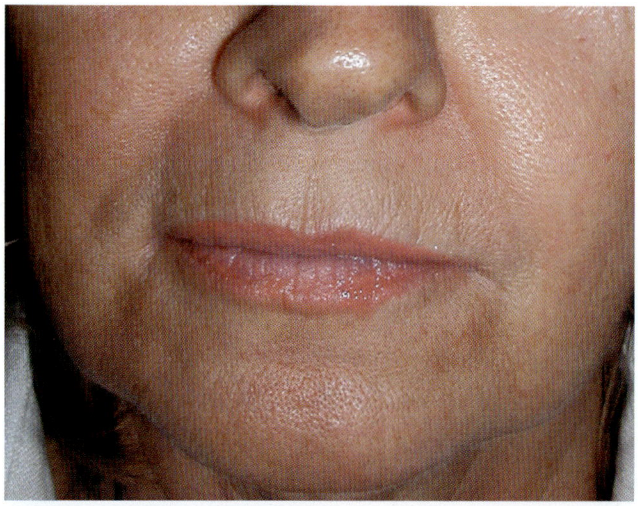

A

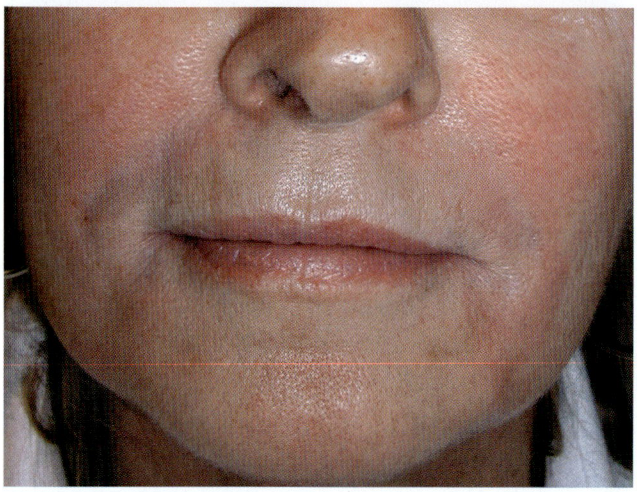

B

Figure 14–3 (**A**) Before and (**B**) after photos show improvement of perioral and upper lip contour following Botox neuromodulation of depressor anguli oris muscles; Perlane filling of the nasolabial folds, oral commissures, and perioral depressions; and Restylane layered onto Cosmoplast in the upper lip vermilion border and vertical perioral rhytids.

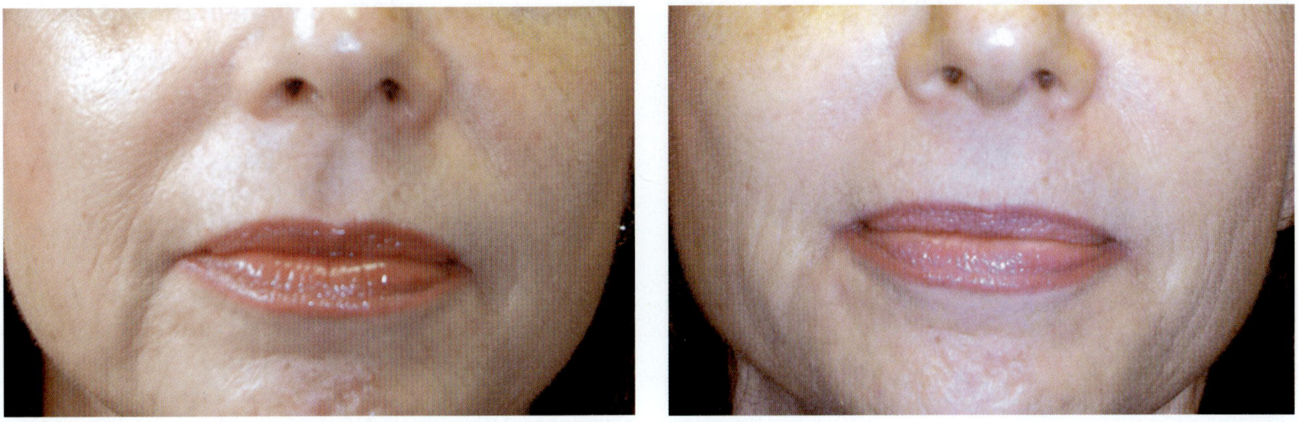

A B

Figure 14–4 (**A**) Before and (**B**) after combination therapy to soften the oral commisures: facial Thermage, 2.5 units of Botox to each depressor anguli oris, layered Restylane on Perlane.

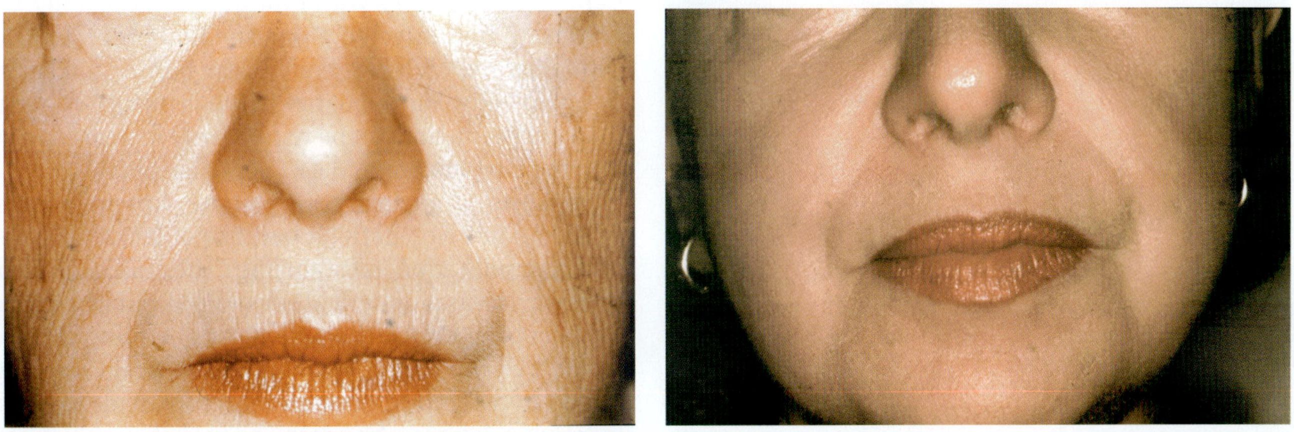

A B

Figure 14–5 (**A**) Before and (**B**) after full-face carbon dioxide (CO_2) laser resurfacing (three passes of 300 mJ, pattern 3, size 8, density 6) shows a restored smooth surface to this patient's upper lip and an everted vermilion border, giving the appearance of an augmented upper lip.

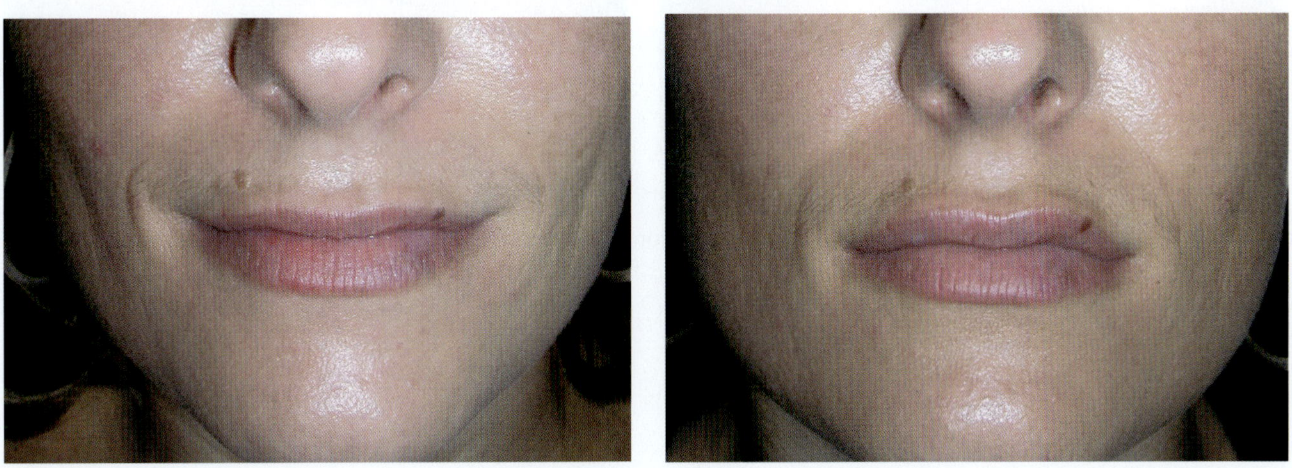

A B

Figure 14–6 (**A**) Before and (**B**) after Restylane was used to augment her upper lip border and to accentuate the contour of her upper lip.

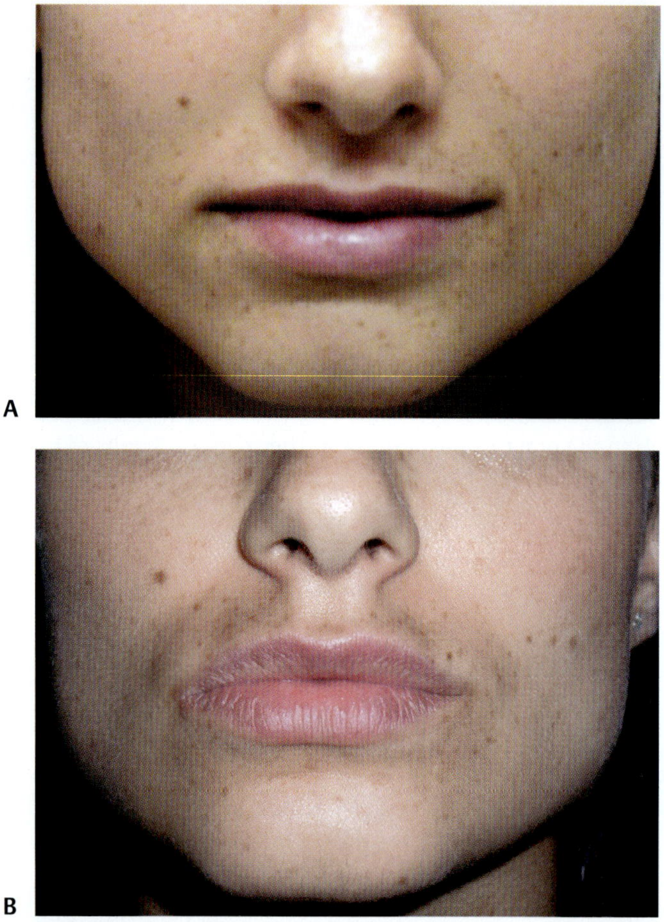

Figure 14–7 (A) Before and (B) after upper lip position and volume were augmented following orthodontic treatment and Perlane injections.

Augmentation and Micropigmentation of the Lips

The final step in perioral rejuvenation after reestablishing soft tissue volumes and contours is restoring lost lip volume and pigment.[6] Lip volume is augmented with Restylane or Cosmoplast to the lip borders (Fig. **14–6A,B**). Cosmoplast flows more easily and is mixed with anesthetic solution, but Restylane has increased longevity of result. Perlane, more viscous and longer lasting, is used to augment lip body volume (Fig. **14–7A,B; 14–8A,B**). We use dental blocks to anesthetize these patients only on rare occasions. We prefer topical anesthesia enhanced by a Natragel lip mask (Gel Concepts, Whippany, New Jersey) because we can more accurately ascertain the lip volume and contours with complete, unrestricted lip movement. The combined use of Cosmoplast (mixed with anesthetic), Restylane, and Perlane is effective and may be a superior alternative to the use of dental blocks in the rare patient who is intolerant of lip injections with topical anesthesia only. Cosmoplast is first injected along the lip border and then supplemented with Restylane to the border and Perlane to the lip body. For the patient who is unsure of her defined endpoint, lips can be temporarily increased in size with the Lip Plumper II Mask (Gel Concepts).

In spite of adequate lip volume, lips may appear small and not well defined because of lack of pigment. Micropigmentation reestablishes the mucocutaneous junction. Natural understated colors should be chosen, avoiding bright reds. The patient's underlying skin tone should be taken into consideration to avoid creating a muddy brown effect. Because this is a vascular area, the underlying color is a blue-red—a cool color—which must

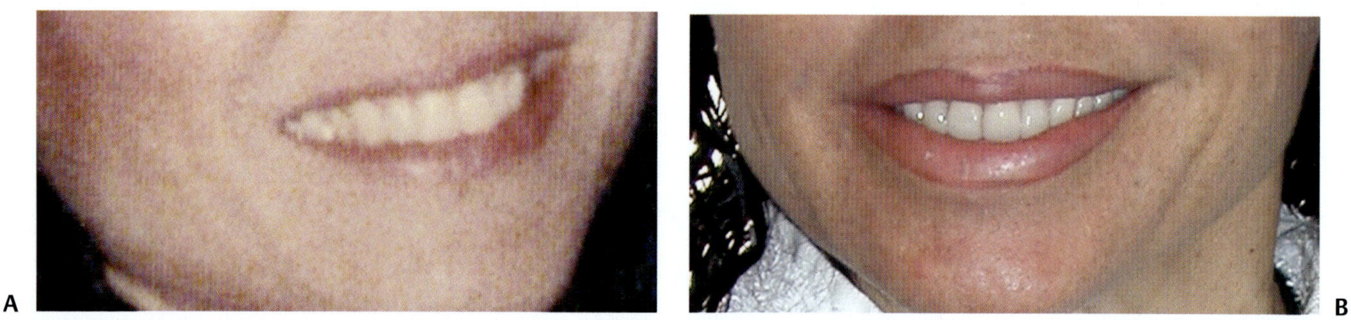

Figure 14–8 (A) Before and (B) after the height of the vermilion border was expanded with micropigmentation and the volume enhanced with Perlane and cosmetic dentistry.

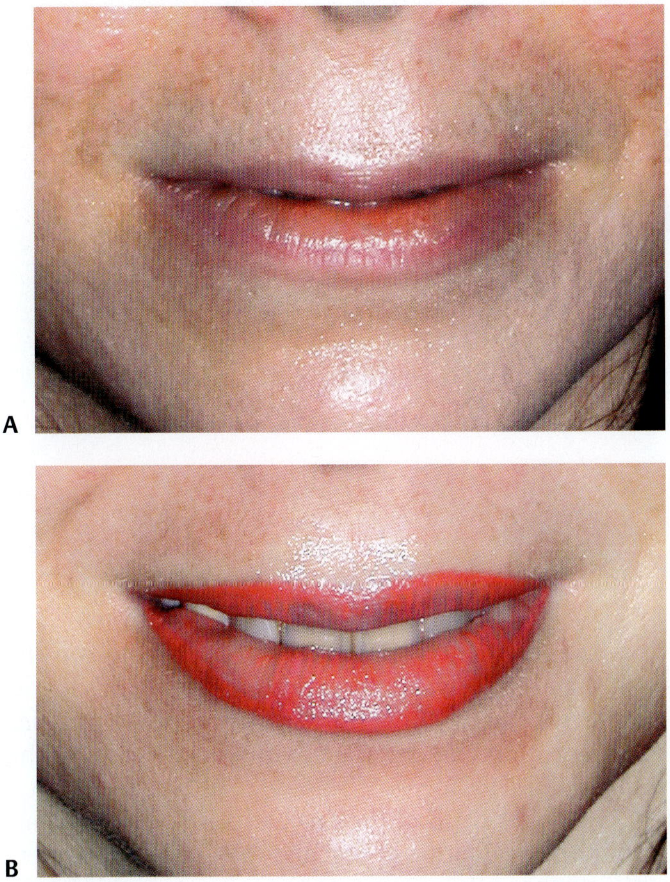

Figure 14–9 (A) Before and (B) after full lip micropigmentation with feathering over the body of the lip compensates for lack of pigment.

be neutralized before warm colors can be added to the lip. A trial with makeup is performed before the procedure to confirm patient acceptance.

A clean, sharp, and well-defined lip border can be created using #1 or #3 needles. And a flat #5 or flat #7 can be used to feather the pigment over the lip surface (Fig. **14–9A,B**). Initially the colors will be too intense, but they will fade after the first week. We prefer to use a sturdy, stable, powerful machine that utilizes a foot pedal and has a pigment cartridge (Harmonix, Boca Raton, Florida).

A postprocedure care regimen is essential to preserve the longevity of the effect. The pigmented area must be lubricated four to six times daily for 1 week and not washed with water during that time. Skin care products containing retinoids and alpha or beta hydroxy acids must also be avoided. A touch-up is performed in 1 month.

◆ Summary

Our approach to the perioral area can be briefly summarized. The midfacial and perioral bony architecture is first reestablished with oral surgical and dental rejuvenation. The perioral soft tissue can then be enhanced with combined neuromodulation and filling. And finally lip volume is restored with injectable fillers while lip pigmentation is restored with micropigmentation.

References

1. Bosniak S, Cantisano-Zilkha M. Botox: a 22-year experience. Operative Techniques in Oculoplastic, Orbital, and Reconstructive Surgery 2001;4:74–80
2. Carruthers J, Carruthers A. Botox use in the mid and lower face and neck. Semin Cutan Med Surg 2001;20:85–92
3. Hexsel D, Trindade de Almeida A. Uso Cosmetico da Toxina Botulinica. Porto Alegre, Brazil: Leandro Augusto dos Santos Limka Publisher; 2002
4. Bosniak S, Cantisano-Zilkha M. Restylane and Perlane: a 6-year clinical experience. Operative Techniques in Oculoplastic, Orbital, and Reconstructive Surgery, Vol. 4, No. 2, Amsterdam: Swets & Zeitpinger; 2001: 89–93
5. Bosniak S, Cantisano-Zilkha M. Cosmetic Blepharoplasty and Facial Rejuvenation. New York: Lippincott-Raven; 1999
6. Meneuzes. The principles of permanent facial makeup. Operative Techniques in Oculoplastic, Orbital, and Reconstructive Surgery 1999;2:182–187

15

Dental and Bony Architecture in Perioral Rejuvenation

Tracey J. Rosenberg

Facial beauty is achieved when there is harmony between the size, shape, and position of all the elements in the face. Orthodontists and oral and maxillofacial surgeons use orthognathic principles based on lateral cephalometric radiographic evaluation to determine ideal facial proportions and bony positions. Orthognathic norms have been developed based on clinical and radiographic interpretation of the most aesthetically pleasing facial features of North Americans. Data obtained from patients with disproportionate facial components are compared with accepted orthognathic norms. Based on the deviation of the patient's values from accepted norms, diagnoses of aesthetic deficiencies may be determined. Detailed evaluation from both profile and frontal views is always necessary for accurate assessment. All profile photographs and radiographs are taken with the patient in "natural head position." A patient is considered to be in natural head position when the patient's visual axis is parallel to a true horizontal plane (HP). This may be achieved by having patients look at the reflection of their eyes in a mirror. Alternatively, a line on the lateral cephalometric radiograph connecting porion (the external auditory canal) to orbitale (the infraorbital rim), commonly referred to as the Frankfurt horizontal (FH), may be used as true horizontal (Fig. **15–1**).[1] After the soft tissue and skeletal problems are identified, either orthodontic treatment, surgery, or a combination of both may be necessary to address the aesthetic needs of the patient.

The most beautiful face exhibits approximately equal vertical proportions of the upper, middle, and lower thirds of the face. The superior third is defined as the vertical distance from the trichal line (hair line) to nasion, which is the bony point separating the nose from the forehead. The middle third lies between the nasion and subnasale, the point where the nasal columella meets the upper lip. The inferior third lies between subnasale and the most inferior point on the chin.[2]

The lower third of the face, which is of most concern in the evaluation of oral and maxillofacial cosmetics, is further subdivided into the lower two thirds and the upper one third. The lower two thirds is composed of the lower lip and chin, and the upper one third consists of the upper lip.

The straight profile is considered most aesthetically pleasing according to arthropometric data obtained by Farkas and his colleagues from a population of young, North American adults.[3] The profile is determined by the anterior–posterior positions of the maxilla, mandible, chin, and nose. If these bones are either too far behind or in front of a vertical line drawn through the nasion, the soft tissue profile appears either concave or convex, respectively, due to skeletal disproportions. In addition to being unaesthetic, a skeletal discrepancy may cause functional problems as a result of the teeth not fitting together properly. This discrepancy may cause difficulty with articulating speech, masticating food, or airway patency. Although some patients seek surgical correction of discrepancies of the facial bones for cosmetic reasons, others seek correction because of the resulting functional problems.

Harmony between the lower facial third and the rest of the face is achieved when the size, shape, and position of the teeth and bones underlying the facial soft tissues is balanced. Recognition of aesthetic abnormalities in the lower face will be discussed, and the link will be made to the etiology of the underlying dental and skeletal anomaly. Either or both surgical and orthodontic correction of these deficiencies based on accurate diagnoses will also be presented.

◆ Profile

Lip Projection

Determinants of the facial profile in the perioral region include the anterior–posterior position of the lips, mandible, and chin. Many methods have been described in the literature to illustrate the ideal lip position. One method is by using Rickett's E-line. The E-line is a line drawn from the nasal tip to the anterior chin on soft tissue profile. Ideally, the lower lip should be 2 mm behind this line, and the upper lip should be 2 to 4 mm behind it.[4] This method of evaluating lip position is limited because an excessively small chin or large nose can falsely predict abnormal lip position. Alternatively, we can use a vertical line perpendicular to FH through subnasale. Ideally, the upper lip should lie 1 mm anterior to, and the lower lip on the vertical line through subnasale (Fig. **15–1**).[1]

Many factors influence lip projection. Lip thickness varies with age, gender, and ethnicity. Thick lips will be more prominent whereas thin lips will be less prominent. Protrusion of the teeth and jaws may cause the lips to be more projected whereas retrusion of the teeth, maxilla, or mandible may give the appearance of very thin lips. Size of the nose and chin on profile influences the perception of lip projection. Deficient chin projection may falsely give the perception of excessive lip protrusion. In addition, a large nose may falsely give the impression of deficient lip projection.

Clinical evaluation of the face, cephalometric analysis, and dental models are all helpful in determining the etiology of the lip projection problem and to distinguish true from perceived lip projection anomalies. Abnormal flaring of either or both the upper and lower teeth may cause excess lip protrusion. Teeth are considered flared when their inclination exceeds ideal. The ideal angulation of the upper incisors on profile is determined cephalometrically to be ~110 degrees from the palatal plane. The ideal angulation of the lower incisors is ~90 degrees to a line parallel to the inferior border of the mandible, or mandibular plane, on profile (Fig. **15–2**).[1] Excessive lip protrusion due to dental flaring with normal skeletal relationships may be reduced with orthodontic retraction of the anterior teeth combined with dental extractions of upper and lower premolars. Severe cases of bimaxillary (upper and lower jaw) protrusion that cannot be corrected with dental extractions and orthodontics alone may require maxillary and mandibular osteotomies to set back the jaws, in conjunction with orthodontic treatment

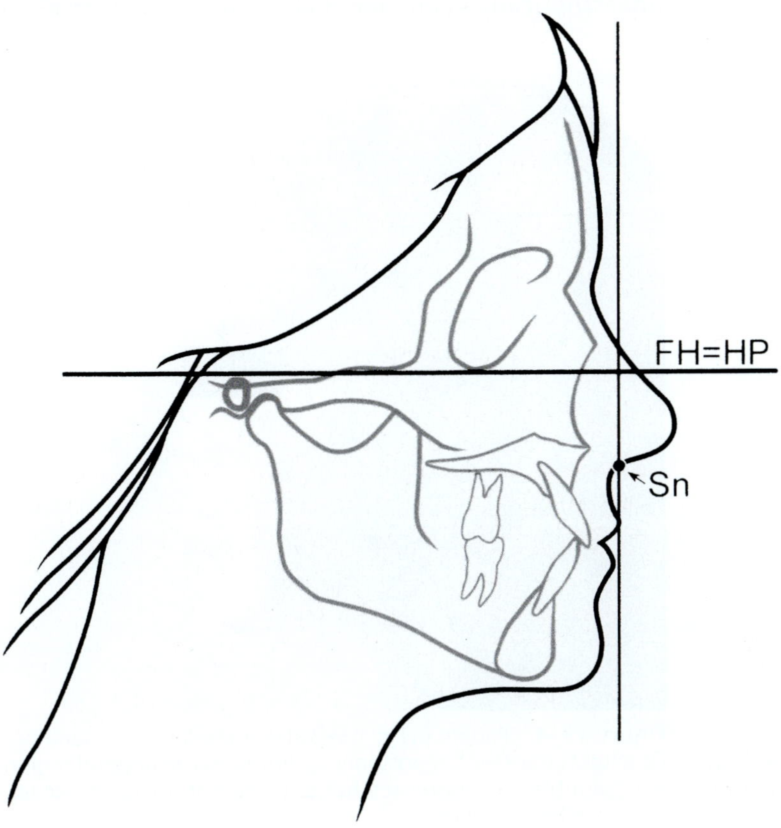

Figure 15–1 Lateral cephalometric tracing of facial bones and soft tissue profile. Frankfurt horizontal (FH), a line through the porion and orbitale is parallel to the true horizontal plane (HP). A vertical line perpendicular to the FH through the subnasale (Sn) demonstrates the soft tissue relationship of the lips and chin.

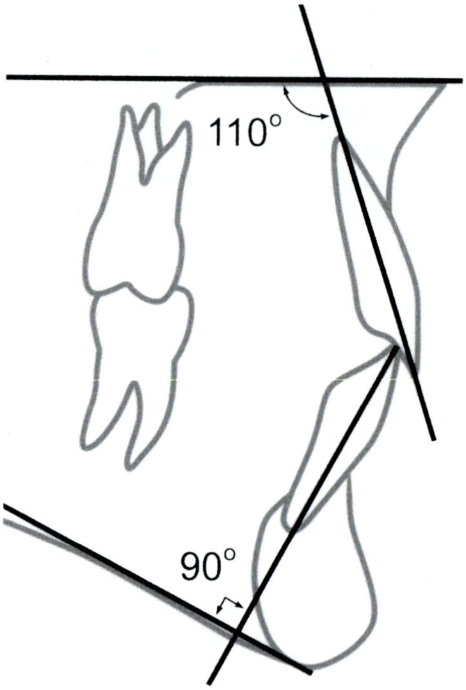

Figure 15–2 Ideal angulation of the upper and lower incisors. The angle between the palatal plane and upper incisor is 110 degrees. The angle between the mandibular plane and lower incisor is 90 degrees.

(Figs. **15–3; 15–4**). The surgically assisted movement of the jaws to achieve a straighter profile, in conjunction with orthodontics, is referred to in the oral and maxillofacial literature as orthognathic surgery.

Patients with inadequate lip projection due to retrusion or severe crowding of the teeth may undergo orthodontics to flare, level, and align the teeth, which will improve lip projection. When lip projection is severely inadequate due to maxillary or mandibular skeletal hypoplasia, maxillary and/or mandibular osteotomies with advancement will improve lip projection and create a more harmonious profile. Patients who perceive subtle deficiencies in lip projection and whose teeth and jaws are in the appropriate positions may be candidates for lip augmentation procedures using fillers. These techniques are beyond the scope of this chapter, and are discussed elsewhere in Chapter 6.

Labiomental Sulcus

The labiomental sulcus is defined as the fold of soft tissue between the lower lip and chin. Form and depth of the labiomental sulcus may vary depending on the inclination of the lower and upper incisors, as well as chin projection. Cephalometric principles dictate that the ideal position of the most anterior point on the bony chin, the pogonion, should be about 2 mm behind a vertical line perpendicular to the FH through nasion.[1] Position of pogonion and inclination of the incisors should both be measured when determining the etiology of labiomental sulcus anomalies.

For example, a prominent chin with severely proclined upper and lower incisors can create an unaesthetically deep mentolabial sulcus. Conversely, a

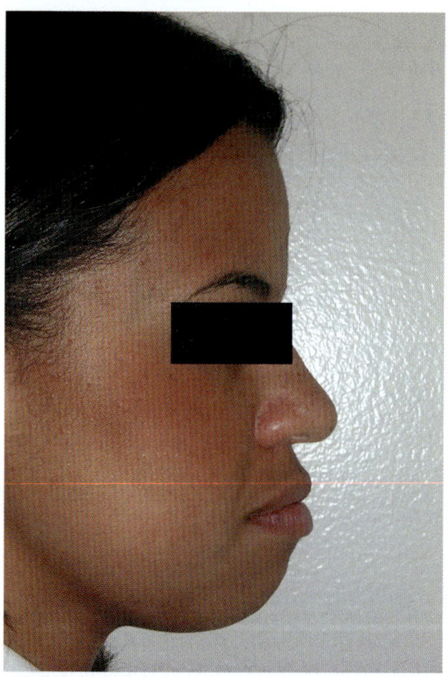

Figure 15–3 Patient with excess lip protuberance from bimaxillary protrusion. (Courtesy of Dr. S. Roser, Emory, Atlanta, Georgia.)

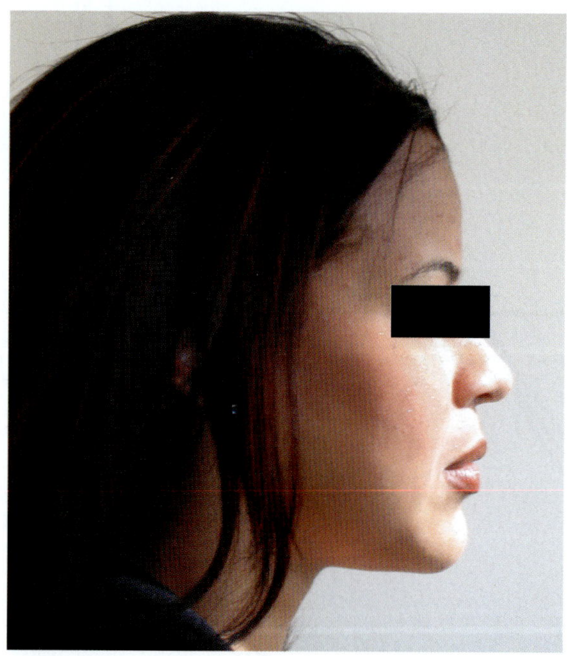

Figure 15–4 Patient in Fig. 15–3 after maxillary and mandibular osteotomies with repositioning. Profile in the perioral region is straighter and more aesthetic. (Courtesy of Dr. S. Roser, Emory, Atlanta, Georgia.)

prominent chin due to mandibular hyperplasia, or excess growth of the lower jaw, with retroclined incisors may give the appearance of a shallow labiomental sulcus.

Correction of labiomental sulcus anomalies can be achieved orthodontically, surgically, or both. In the case of a deep labiomental sulcus with normal chin projection and flared upper or lower teeth, orthodontic retraction of the teeth may successfully reduce the depth of the sulcus. However, when clinical and cephalometric analyses demonstrate mandibular hypoplasia (small lower jaw) with reduced chin projection and dental overjet causing a mismatch of the upper and lower dental arches, the result may be a deep labiomental sulcus with lip eversion. Surgical augmentation of the chin alone will deepen the labiomental sulcus giving an unaesthetic appearance and will not address the mismatched dental arches. Ideal correction for this case requires a mandibular osteotomy with advancement combined with orthodontic treatment. Matching of the upper and lower dental arches will not only improve aesthetics but will also improve the ability to chew and articulate.

The shallow labiomental sulcus may also be a cosmetic concern with some patients. This variation from normal may occur due to inadequate chin projection with ideal incisor inclination and a normal-sized mandible. When these cephalometric findings are observed, surgical augmentation of chin projection is the appropriate treatment. Methods of chin augmentation will be discussed in greater detail later in this chapter.

Chin Projection

Size and position of the mandible are major determinants of the anterior–posterior position of the bony chin and the soft tissue profile of the inferior third of the face. As previously discussed, the patient with a hypoplastic mandible and inadequate chin projection should be treated with mandibular advancement surgery combined with orthodontic treatment. However, there are other skeletal anomalies that result in inadequate chin projection. One such anomaly is an excessive vertical skeletal growth pattern of the posterior maxilla. This results in a clockwise rotation of the mandible from a profile view. Clockwise mandibular rotation results in a more inferior and posterior position of the chin, which deemphasizes its projection. This type of skeletal deformity is often accompanied by an excessively long appearance to the lower facial third and a discrepancy in the bite or occlusion; most commonly an open bite. Augmentation genioplasty alone would address neither the excessive lower facial height nor the malocclusion. To improve chin projection in this situation, a maxillary osteotomy with superior repositioning combined with orthodontic treatment would be the optimal treatment. Repositioning the maxilla superiorly allows the mandible to rotate counterclockwise to close the bite and results in improved chin projection. In some cases chin augmentation in addition to maxillary repositioning may be necessary to optimize the soft tissue profile.

Genioplasty

The most common adjunctive aesthetic procedure performed with orthognathic surgery to correct dentofacial deformities is the genioplasty. This procedure may be used to address underprojection, overprojection, excessive or deficient height, as well as asymmetries of the chin. Surgical aesthetic modification of the chin may be accomplished by two major methods. The first uses a horizontal osteotomy of the anterior inferior mandible with repositioning of the segment to achieve the desired cosmetic result.[5] The second method uses an alloplastic implant.[6] There are specific indications, risks, and benefits to each procedure. Careful evaluation, diagnosis, and treatment planning of the chin anomaly will allow the practitioner to offer the most appropriate treatment options to each patient.

Inferior Border Osteotomy

There are specific situations where the inferior border osteotomy, or sliding genioplasty may be preferable to the alloplastic implant. The inferior border osteotomy can be used to achieve greater projection than an implant for the deficient chin. The maximum amount of chin projection that can be obtained with a sliding osteotomy depends on the anterior–posterior thickness of the mandibular symphysis, angulation of the osteotomy, and preservation of anterior soft tissue attachments. Advancement greater than the symphyseal thickness would prevent the bone-to-bone contact necessary for healing of the osteotomy. Preservation of the muscle attachments in the anterior chin will improve the ratio of soft tissue to bone advancement. Angulation of the osteotomy will determine the change in height and projection of the chin.[7]

The horizontal sliding osteotomy gives the ability to shorten an excessively long chin by removing a wedge of bone. An oblique osteotomy with advancement can both shorten a long chin and provide increased projection for the deficient chin. The sliding osteotomy also allows for the correction of a chin asymmetry. Neither vertical modifications nor correction of asymmetries of the chin are possible using alloplastic chin implants.[8]

The sliding osteotomy technique has many advantages. It has excellent long-term stability due to minimal resorption of bone.[9] The soft tissue changes at nearly a one-to-one ratio with the bone when the mentalis muscle remains attached to the bone.[10] This improves the accuracy of predicting the amount of soft tissue projection gained from the procedure. The mentalis muscle is typically stripped in the alloplastic implant technique, thus making the amount of chin projection gained less predictable. Finally, due to the attachment of the geniohyoid muscles to the genial tubercles, the suprahyoid muscles are tightened when the chin is advanced, resulting in improved chin–neck contour on profile.[11]

Disadvantages of the sliding osteotomy genioplasty technique have been reported. Many of these problems are due to improper surgical technique. There is a greater chance of neuropraxia to the mental nerve, which could result in temporary or permanent numbness to the lip and chin.[7] The roots of teeth in the anterior mandible may potentially be damaged by improper positioning of the osteotomy. Posterior movement of the chin can result in an obtuse chin–neck angle due to slackening of the suprahyoid musculature. The sliding osteotomy genioplasty procedure should be avoided in the patient with an already short lower facial third height because the osteotomy usually causes some vertical height shortening. Finally, the patient's perception that an implant is less traumatic may reduce acceptance of this treatment modality, even though this may be a misconception.[11]

Alloplastic Chin Implants

Alloplastic implants are frequently used to correct chin deformities. Some of the materials that have been described in the literature include silicone, Proplast, mersilene mesh, Gore-Tex, Medpor, and Silastic.[6] Usually these are self-stabilizing without requiring pin or screw fixation. Typically, the use of alloplasts should be reserved for small, subtle augmentations in the chin area. They should not be used for large advancements due to the risk of wound dehiscence.[7] Alloplasts may be used to improve the appearance of parasymphyseal depressions in elderly patients as a result of their relaxed soft tissues, commonly referred to as "marionette groves." This is possible because the alloplastic implant has lateral projections capable of widening the parasymphyseal region.[5] Often, alloplasts are used in conjunction with other facial rejuvenation procedures such as Botox Cosmetic and filler injections for wrinkles, submental liposuction, platysmal placation, and rhytidoplasty to enhance the aesthetic outcome.

Advantages of alloplastic chin augmentation over the sliding osteotomy are well known. There may be less risk of paresthesia to the lip and chin due to the nature of the procedure. If the aesthetic result is undesirable to the patient, it is reversible by simply removing the implant. Placement of alloplastic chin implants may be considered atraumatic due to the fact that no bony cuts are necessary. Finally, lateral augmentation is helpful in reducing marionette grooves or widening the narrow chin.[11]

Problems with this method of augmentation are few but have been described. Resorption of the anterior mandibular plate may occur.[12] This can result in diminished chin projection over time, and damage to the roots of the lower incisors.

Either method of genioplasty may be performed via a conservative intraoral approach or an extraoral approach. In addition, either procedure may be performed with local anesthesia and IV sedation in the office or under general anesthesia in the operating room setting. For the most severe defects, both alloplastic and sliding osteotomy genioplasty techniques may be required.[5]

◆ Vertical Height Disproportions

Harmony between the vertical facial thirds is necessary for optimal beauty. A disproportionate vertical relationship between the lower facial third and the rest of the face may produce an unaesthetic appearance. Vertical height discrepancies may manifest as soft tissue abnormalities. When soft tissue problems are recognized, a thorough clinical exam as well as cephalometric radiographic analysis will assist in identifying the skeletal and dental components contributing to the perceived abnormality.

Mentalis Strain

In patients with normal facial proportions, the lips come together at rest, or in repose, with no gap and no redundancy. Lip closure at rest, which is referred to as lip competence, is essential for normal swallowing and speech, preservation of the periodontal structures, and optimal aesthetics. When the lips are apart at rest, or incompetent, due to abnormal positioning of the underlying jaw bones, the person must strain to close the lips to swallow and speak properly. In addition, exposed teeth and gingiva are susceptible to gingival inflammation and periodontal problems from chronic air exposure. Patients may become self-conscious about the appearance of their perioral region and strain their mentalis muscle to cover the teeth with their lips. This is referred to as mentalis strain, which causes an unaesthetic dimpling, or cobblestone appearance to the chin.[5] On profile, this results in decreased chin projection and reduced depth of the labiomental sulcus.

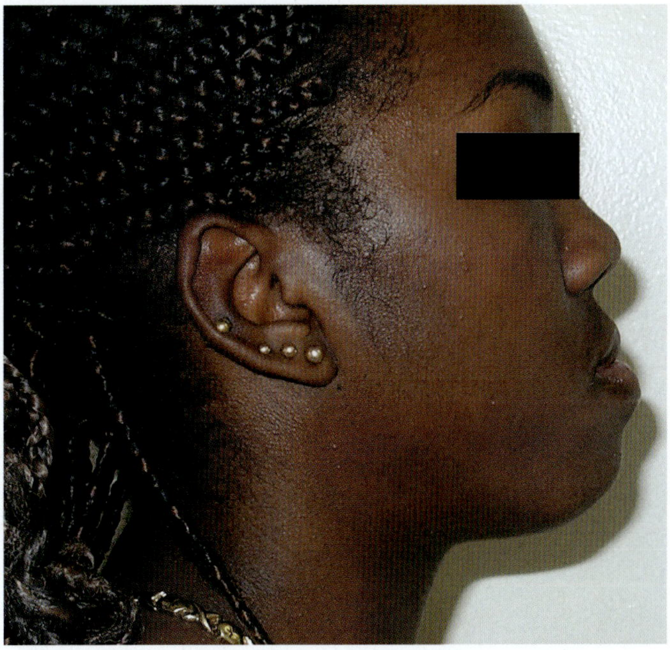

Figure 15–5 Mentalis strain on the profile of a patient with incompetent lips due to vertical maxillary excess and a protruded mandible. (Courtesy of Dr. S. Roser, Emory, Atlanta, Georgia.)

Incompetent lips can result from misalignment of the facial bones (maxilla, mandible, and/or chin), as well as inappropriate positions of the teeth. A retruded mandible with significant dental overjet could result in lip incompetence and mentalis strain. Surgically repositioning the mandible in a more forward position would bring the lips together at rest, alleviating the mentalis strain. The cobblestone appearance of the chin would then disappear and improve the profile. In some cases, chin augmentation may also be necessary to achieve the desired aesthetics.

A long lower face could also produce lip incompetence at rest and the need for mentalis strain to cover the teeth. The patient with a dental open bite, meaning space between the upper and lower incisors while teeth are in a biting position, may have incompetent lips at rest. Cephalometric evaluation usually demonstrates that the open bite is a result of posterior vertical maxillary excess. These patients may exhibit a flattened labiomental sulcus on profile when straining to cover the teeth (Fig. **15–5**). Surgically repositioning the maxilla superiorly would close the open bite, bring the lips together in the resting position, and eliminate mentalis strain (Fig. **15–6**). It is important to recognize that, although excess muscle activity in these two cases of cobblestone chin may be alleviated by neuromodulation with Botox injections,[13] this does not treat the underlying cause. In both cases, lip incompetence and lower lip eversion may result from mentalis muscle weakness, which may not be aesthetically pleasing. Careful recognition of the etiology of mentalis muscle strain cannot be overemphasized in the treatment planning of these patients.

The Smile

The smile is one of the most important aspects of facial beauty. The aesthetics of the smile may be compromised by vertical facial height disproportions. The smile may be categorized into the low, medium, or high lipline smile. A high lipline smile would show more than 5 mm of gingiva above the necks of the central incisors. This is commonly referred to as a "gummy smile." In a low lipline smile, no gingiva would be visible and the entire tooth would be covered by the lip. The medium lipline smile shows the central incisor in its entirety, and about 1 mm of gingiva above the teeth. The medium lipline smile is accepted as most aesthetic by North American standards.[14]

Gummy Smile

To treat the patient who complains of a gummy smile, the clinician must determine the source of the problem. Dental, gingival, muscular, or skeletal factors may be responsible for the gummy smile. Clinical and cephalometric exam should assist in distinguishing the problem specific to each patient. Excessive gingiva or a long maxilla due to excessive vertical growth are the most

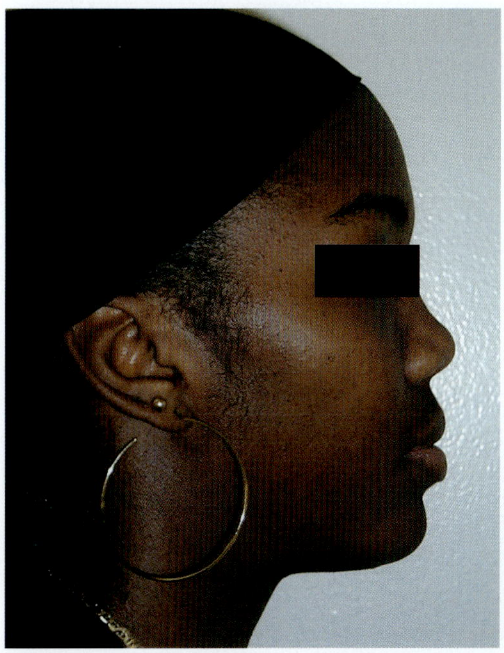

Figure 15–6 Postoperative profile of the patient in Fig. 15–5. Absence of mentalis strain and improved profile in the perioral region after orthodontic treatment, maxillary superior repositioning, mandibular setback, and sliding genioplasty. (Courtesy of Dr. S. Roser, Emory, Atlanta, Georgia.)

common contributing factors. To distinguish between dental or skeletal origin of a gummy smile, the length of the clinical crowns of the six anterior teeth should be determined, in addition to the amount of tooth showing in repose. Following this, the location of the cementoenamel junction, which is the point where the crown meets the root of the tooth, should be identified. If there is more than 3 mm of attached gingiva between the cementoenamel junction and the location where the gum meets the tooth, and there is not more than 3 mm of incisor showing at rest, then the problem is gingival excess. For this case, gingival reduction surgery is indicated to increase the length of the tooth and reduce gingival show when smiling.[14]

If there is excess gingiva showing when the patient is smiling, however, and dental evaluation reveals no gingival excess, then gingival reduction surgery is not indicated, and a skeletal etiology must be considered (Fig. **15–7**). The tooth to lip relationship in repose is the most important factor in determining skeletal etiology of a gummy smile. The ideal amount of tooth show when the lips are in repose is 2 or 3 mm. If there is more than 3 mm of incisal tip showing, and if there is any gingiva showing in repose, this suggests that the maxilla is too long in the vertical dimension. Surgically repositioning the maxilla superiorly to show 2 or 3 mm of incisal edge would be the preferred treatment to correct this case of vertical maxillary excess (Fig. **15–8**). The surgeon must be acutely aware of not "overimpacting" the maxilla because this would cause instant aging.

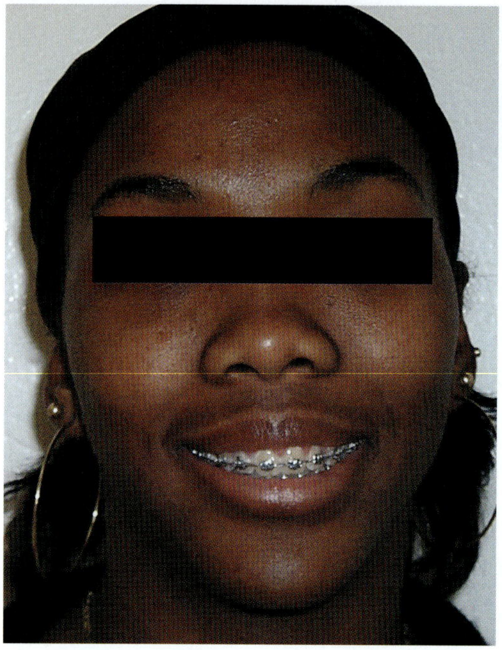

Figure 15–8 Improved smile of the patient in Fig. 15–5 after surgical repositioning of the maxilla superiorly and mandible posteriorly. (Courtesy of Dr. S. Roser, Emory, Atlanta, Georgia.)

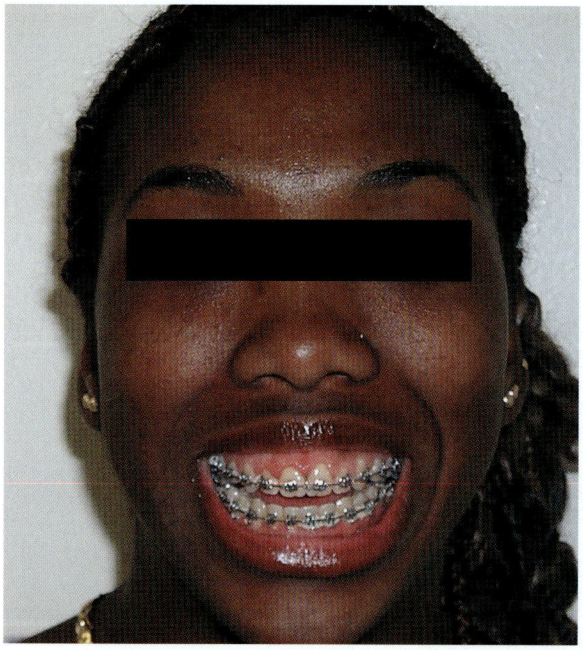

Figure 15–7 Gummy smile of the patient in Fig. 15–5 with vertical maxillary excess. More than 5 mm of gingiva is visible when she is smiling. (Courtesy of Dr. S. Roser, Emory, Atlanta, Georgia.)

Low Smile Line

Another deviation from the ideal smile is the low lipline smile. Patients with a low lipline that is not aesthetically pleasing will complain that they show too little or none of their teeth when smiling. This could mean that the maxilla is too short in the vertical dimension, which gives a more aged facial appearance. Although dental veneers may be used to lengthen teeth and camouflage inadequate maxillary height in some cases, the deficiency may be too great to fabricate aesthetically pleasing dental restorations alone. A low smile line may also result from an excessively retruded maxilla. In both cases, a maxillary osteotomy with anterior and inferior repositioning to show 2 or 3 mm of tooth in repose would improve the appearance of the smile in these patients.

◆ Conclusion

Cephalometric analysis, orthognathic surgery, and orthodontic treatment should be part of the armamentarium available to the cosmetic surgeon when treatment planning facial aesthetic cases. Advances in minimally invasive cosmetic techniques have greatly expanded the treatment options available to patients who seek facial rejuvenation. However, there are many cases where cosmetic deficiencies in the facial soft tissues, specifically in the perioral region, cannot be treated successfully by noninvasive techniques alone. It is important for the cosmetic surgeon to recognize the vertical discrepancies and projection anomalies that require surgical repositioning of the facial bones to improve facial aesthetics. Referral to an oral and maxillofacial surgeon as well as an orthodontist is encouraged when maxillofacial discrepancies appear to be due to improper positioning of the teeth and bones. Analysis of cephalometric radiographs, photographs, and dental models are essential for accurate diagnosis and treatment planning for these patients. The maxillofacial procedures described in this chapter may be useful adjuncts to other invasive as well as minimally invasive cosmetic procedures used to achieve optimal facial balance.

References

1. Schendel SA. Cephalometrics and orthognathic surgery. In Bell WH, ed. Modern Practice in Orthognathic and Reconstructive Surgery. Philadelphia: WB Saunders; 1992:84–99
2. Betts NJ, Fonseca RJ. Soft tissue changes associated with orthognathic surgery. In Bell WH, ed. Modern Practice in Orthognathic and Reconstructive Surgery. Philadelphia: WB Saunders; 1992:2170–2209
3. Farkas LG, Hreczko TA, Kolar JC, Munro IR. Vertical and horizontal proportions of the face in young adult North American Caucasians: revision of neoclassical canons. Plast Reconstr Surg 1985;75:328–338
4. Ricketts RH. Cephalometric analysis and synthesis. Angle Orthod 1961;31:141–156
5. Epker BN. The chin: genioplasty. In Epker BN, ed. Esthetic Maxillofacial Surgery. Philadelphia: Lea & Febiger; 1994:2–77
6. Choe KS, Stucki-McCormick SU. Chin augmentation. Facial Plast Surg 2000;16:45–54
7. Darab DJ. Mandibular deficiency. In Bell WH, ed. Modern Practice in Orthognathic and Reconstructive Surgery. Philadelphia: WB Saunders; 1992:2334–2517
8. Chang EW, Lam SM, Karen M, Donlevy JL. Sliding genioplasty for correction of chin abnormalities. Arch Facial Plast Surg 2001;3:8–15
9. Hoffman GR, Moloney FB. The stability of facial osteotomies, III: chin advancement. Aust Dent J 1995;40:289–295
10. Gallagher DM, Bell WH, Storum KA. Soft tissue changes associated with advancement genioplasty performed concomitantly with superior repositioning of the maxilla. J Oral Maxillofac Surg 1984;42:238–242
11. Sarver DM. Esthetic Orthodontics and Orthognathic Surgery. St. Louis: Mosby; 1998
12. Friedland JA, Coccaro PJ, Converse JM. Retrospective cephalometric analysis of mandibular bone absorption under silicone rubber chin implants. Plast Reconstr Surg 1976;57:144–151
13. American Society for Aesthetic Plastic Surgery. Botulinum toxin (btx): new cosmetic uses, expanded applications [press release]. April 2002
14. Allen AP, Bell WH. Achieving the aesthetic smile. In Bell WH, ed. Modern Practice in Orthognathic and Reconstructive Surgery. Philadelphia: WB Saunders; 1992:235–262

16

Teeth and the Perioral Area in Facial Aesthetics

Peter Rinaldi and Jon B. Marashi

Similar to the expanding diversity of aesthetic disciplines in the medical specialties, general dentistry has begun to emerge into its own subspecialty. On its own merit, aesthetic dentistry has become a mainstream for treatment alternatives, from both the functional and the purely aesthetic aspects. Biological and mechanical improvement of the oral cavity is many times a necessity. Decay, fractured teeth, and periodontal disease are all manifestations that cannot be overlooked. There is a medical and dental responsibility by the clinician to address these problems as they develop in an individual. With proper maintenance, a person can avoid many of the dental afflictions that debilitated earlier generations. Newer understandings of disease processes have made early diagnosis and treatment easier. Recent technology and material advances have made it possible to restore teeth and their supporting structures to almost their original state. This can now be termed rejuvenation dentistry. It is also these advances that have made it possible to restore a person when there is a need for only aesthetic improvement.

◆ Muscle Distribution and Innervations

From a surgeon's perspective, to have a good understanding of the perioral aesthetics, form, and function, it is important to review muscle distribution and innervations. There are 20 muscles of facial expression, each with a unique location and function. Because this chapter focuses on the perioral region, only a few of the major muscles are discussed.

Orbicularis oris originates in the maxilla above the incisor teeth and inserts in the skin of the lip. Its action is to close the lips.

Levator anguli oris originates in the canine fossa of the maxilla and inserts at the angle of the mouth. Its action is to elevate the angle of the mouth medially.

Levator labii superioris originates in the maxilla above the infraorbital foramen and inserts on the skin of the upper lip. Its action is to elevate the upper lip.

Zygomaticus major originates on the zygomatic arch and inserts on the angle of the mouth. Its action is to draw the angle of the mouth upward and backward. This action is what we most commonly refer to as a smile.

Depressor anguli oris originates on the oblique line of the mandible and inserts at the angle of the mouth. Its action is to depress the angle of the mouth. This muscle plays a major role in frowning.

Risorius originates over the masseter and inserts at the angle of the mouth. Its action is to retract the angle of the mouth laterally.

Buccinator has multiple points of origin—the mandible, pterygomandibular raphe, alveolar process. The insertion is located at the angle of the mouth. Its action is to press against the cheeks and keep them taut.

Mentalis originates in the incisive fossa of the mandible and inserts on the skin of the chin. Its action is to elevate and protrude the lower lip.[1]

Motor innervation to the muscles of facial expression is provided by the facial nerve. The facial nerve comes from cranial nerve seven. The terminal branches include the temporal, zygomatic, buccal, marginal mandibular, and cervical.

Of all these muscles, the zygomaticus major and risorius are key players in positioning the lips into a smile position. With this in mind, the surgeon can begin to appreciate how the teeth and their supporting structures are affected by these muscles, and in turn how the teeth affect the muscles. With the loss of muscle tone due to aging, the amount of tooth display will be affected, when the lips are at rest and when the patient smiles.

◆ Patient Selection

The reasons a person seeks out dental aesthetic improvement are not age dependant. There are a multitude of factors that contribute to the need for dental aesthetic and functional enhancement. Anomalies, parafunctional habits, congenital abnormalities, and trauma are some of the reasons (Fig. **16–1A,B**). Other considerations for aesthetic improvement would be tooth crowding or spacing, tooth size discrepancies, worn teeth, and color changes. All of these are non-age-related indications. These manifestations can become apparent at any age or be a part of the aging process.

More often, though, the desire for an improved smile is evoked from want rather than need. The media has played a tremendous role in promoting the concept of white teeth and what is considered a healthy smile. What was once considered too white is now not white enough, and as our patients see more television and magazine advertisements, they too want to have a beautiful smile.

It is both the old and the young patient who can benefit from a "smile makeover." The increase in self-esteem and confidence that occurs after a patient is given a new smile can be overwhelming. How patients interpret what they see when they look in the mirror dictates what they want to accomplish from an aesthetic overhaul. Both body and smile image are purely subjective perceptions. Therefore, similar to the plastic surgeon, the general dentist is confronted every day with the challenge of improving upon a patient's oral health and reconstruction. It is the correct evaluation of both the functional and the aesthetic aspects that will help to improve the debilitated dentition. Comprehensive dentistry is built upon the combination of these two disciplines. In the triad of the periodontal complex; that is, the hard and soft supporting tissues of the teeth, the teeth, and the temporomandibular joint complex, a working synergy must exist if the patient is to function without discomfort. There is a very significant relationship in that form and function are in fact dependent on one another. In the absence of one of these variables, the other will falter. Simply stated, in regard to the restoration of the human dentition, if it looks good, then it probably works well—and vice versa.

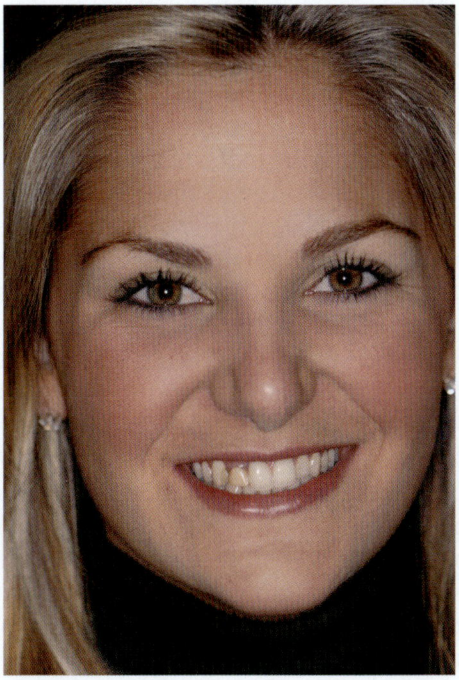
A

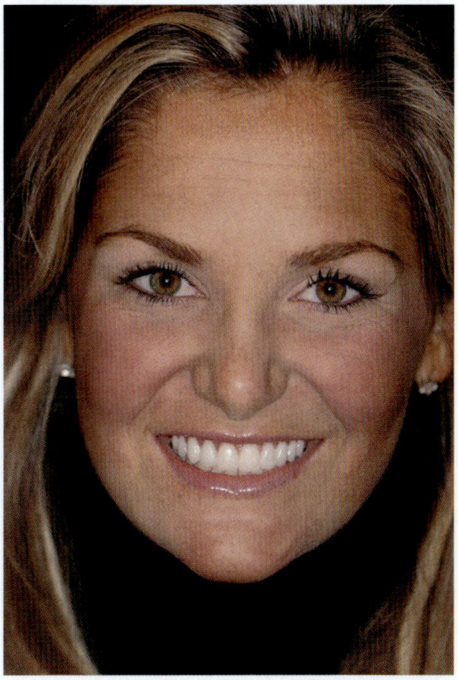
B

Figure 16–1 (**A**) A missing upper right lateral incisor not present since birth (**B**) can be replaced with high-tech materials such as pressed ceramics.

◆ The Smile

The concept of smile design has become increasingly important in the creation of a beautiful smile. The dentist must function as both a clinician, such that the appropriate diagnosis and treatment planning have been made, and an artist. Similar to the plastic surgeon, the dentist as an artist must be able to look at a project prior to starting and already know what the desired outcome is to be.

There are several key determinants in smile design. The first is establishing the proper arch form of the dentition. An ideal arch form is a U-shaped arch. This helps broaden the buccal corridors and eliminate negative space. Next is the shape and position of teeth, both individually and collectively. Each tooth has its own unique shape and position in the mouth. Each tooth has its own specific width to length ratio that provides for its own unique look and function. Most of this is related to Golden proportions. The term Golden proportion is a mathematical theorem based on the Pythagorean Theorem. It was first introduced and applied in dental aesthetics by Lombardi[2] and further developed by Levin.[3] Simply, the Golden proportion of aesthetic dentistry relates specifically to the anterior six teeth. The central, lateral, and canine should have a proportion that is 60% of the adjacent tooth. When viewed in a two-dimensional plane, in a snapshot or looking directly at the patient, the relationship between these teeth should be 1.618 to 1 to 0.618.

Individually, the central incisor is the most important tooth when it comes to anterior aesthetics. An ideal central incisor has a width to length ratio of 75 to 80%. The average central length is 10.5 to 11.0 mm long. Correct axial inclinations provide for soothing tangents that decrease stress throughout the arch.[3] To reproduce symmetry and balance throughout the arch, these parameters of tooth relationships need to be established to reflect a decrease in tension and therefore beauty.

The gingival tissues surrounding the teeth also play an important role. The apex of gingival tissue across the upper anterior teeth should have a balance that creates proper flow and transition. These tissues should also follow a pattern of gradation, where the height of each tissue gets progressively lower as we move from the anterior to the posterior portion of the mouth.

Smile design protocol and theory are applied to the diagnosis of each specific problem as it relates to each individual. A patient's wants and desires must be scrutinized to determine if it is possible to deliver what the patient is asking for in a smile makeover. A multitude of variations exist, along with causes, but there should always be a clear picture within the clinician's mind of what the final outcome will be. It is for this reason, as the scope of our understanding of facial esthetics increases, the dentist and plastic surgeon must work closely together to deliver the optimum treatment.

Dentition

Similar to the aging process itself, the aging dentition is a factor that cannot be avoided. As a part of the aging process, there are dimensional changes that occur and are unavoidable. This change can be as simple as color shifts that occur over time. All teeth will darken to some extent. The loss and thinning of enamel, the outermost layer of tooth structure, reveals more of the inner layer of tooth substrate, the dentin. It is within this dentinal layer that a tooth derives its color. The more dentin showing through a tooth, the more yellow-brown is perceived. Aesthetically, this may mean that the patient may require some method of bleaching to lighten and brighten the teeth. By doing so, the whiter teeth will in turn brighten the entire face of the patient. Vital tooth bleaching is the simplest way to improve upon a patient's smile. Brighter teeth, and therefore a whiter smile, give the perception of a younger, happier, healthier person.

The aging dentition will demonstrate a constant wear and tear from loss of tooth structure. Along with the supporting substructures, there will eventually be a need to rejuvenate these worn teeth and the resulting loss of vertical height that occurs. Structural tooth loss is more a function of occlusal dysfunction than it is an age factor. Therefore, premature tooth structure loss can be seen as easily in young adults as in older individuals. With certain forms of reconstruction and rejuvenation being performed on women and men at an earlier age than ever before, the smile outline of the individual must be taken into account. The elimination of deep labionasal folds and the enlargement of upper and lower lips are easily performed treatments via injectable solutions, but the surgeon should be aware of the influence that teeth have on the support of these structures. Lip support is highly dependent upon the orientation of the upper teeth. Correct alignment of the upper anterior teeth will aid in the elimination of accentuated lines in the perioral area. The aesthetic dentist can also help to promote a fuller upper lip by building out the negative space, or buccal corridor, in the area just distal to the canines or cuspids. On the other hand, excessive lip plumping can actually hide teeth, especially in a resting position. With more and more patients looking for a broader, whiter smile, overcompensating for a thin upper lip via injectables or permanent membranes may detract from the patient's smile. The position of the anterior teeth in both a labial and an anterior–posterior (mesiodistal) direction should be taken into consideration (Fig. **16–2A–E**).

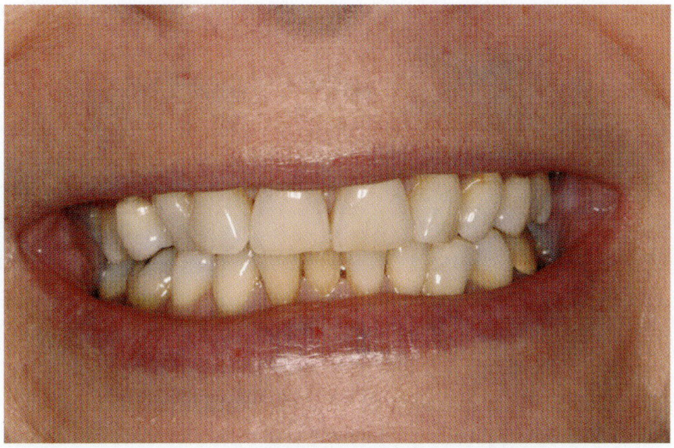
A

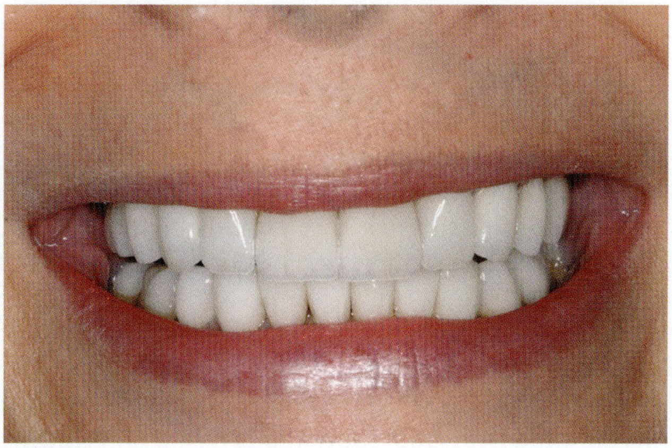
B

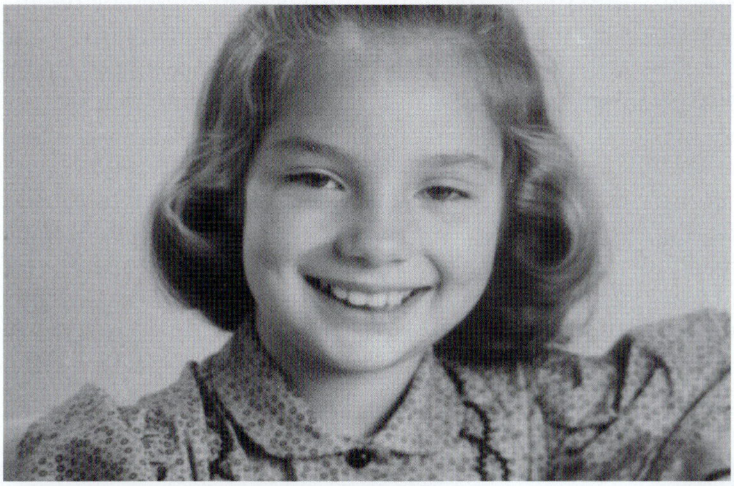
C

Figure 16–2 (**A**) Teeth are worn from aging and grinding. The upper lip has thinned. (**B**) The new smile shows a fuller lip and the teeth follow the lower lip curvature. (**C**) The patient as a child. (**D**) The patient's full face as an adult. Note the decrease in vertical dimension height. (**E**) The patient restored with veneers. The smile is made full by adding to the buccal corridor and the vertical height has been restored.

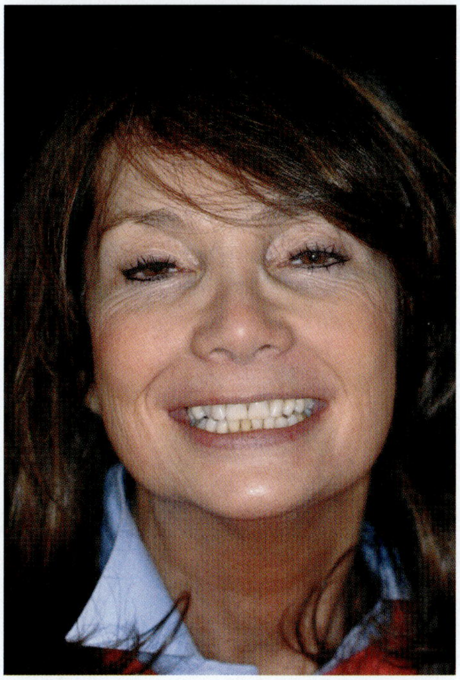
D

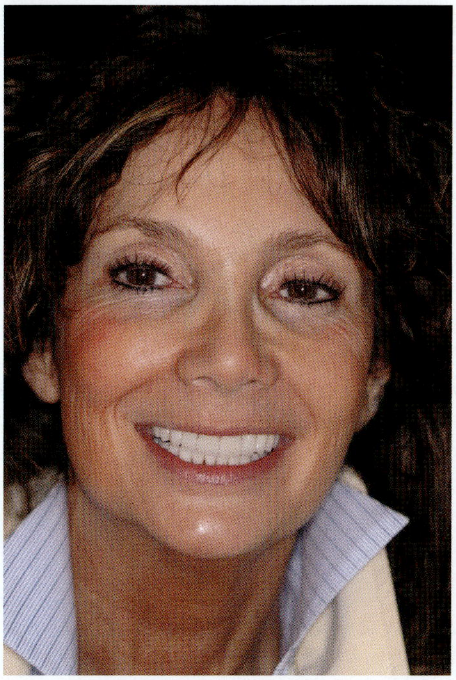
E

At certain ages, the amount of incisal edge show of the front teeth in a relaxed lip position changes. On average, a 30-year-old will show 3.5 mm of incisal edges, a 50-year-old will show 1.5 mm, and a 70-year-old will display only the edges of the front teeth. Remember, these are averages. Just as the age appearance of people differs, so does the amount of tooth wear. Therefore, it is the combination of two aging processes that causes less tooth show. The first that occurs is the loss of tooth structure. This begins from the moment teeth appear in the mouth at around 7 years of age. The amount of tooth wear that happens over the years can be accelerated in certain individuals based on grinding patterns, occlusal interferences, and the types of food that are eaten. This happens over such a long period of time that the patient may not notice that this is taking place. This can be seen in younger women with a strong bruxing habit where the upper lip elevator muscles are still strong enough to keep a perched position. The loss of tooth show is not noticed, and is therefore not accentuated, until the second process begins. Loss of upper lip muscle tonicity, which is lost due to collagen breakdown and atrophy, compounds the once-unnoticed tooth loss. Lower teeth become more noticeable. A thinning upper lip and the show of lower teeth are considered an older look. There is an indication of stress and tension when the upper teeth do not follow the gentle curvature of the lower lip. People are inclined to perceive an attractive smile as one that demonstrates full view of the upper anterior teeth that fill the buccal corridor and follow the lower lip curvature.

The aesthetic facial plastic surgeon or dermatologist should be aware of the amount of upper tooth show. The effect of the upper anterior teeth on the nasolabial groove and ridge and lip support should not be underestimated. Besides the resting position, the lipline position when the patient is smiling should also be taken into consideration. A high lipline when smiling may cause excessive gingival show, or a gummy smile, which is not desirable. On the other hand, a low lipline will not show enough teeth. The relationship between tooth lip support, lip volume, and amount of facial muscle contraction must be balanced to create the optimum aesthetic effect.

Facial Dimensions

As individuals age, there is a dimensional transformation that occurs in the lower third of the face. There is a vertical component that degenerates over time. It is a dimensional factor that varies between individuals. There is a correlation that exists between the upper and lower halves of the face. In the most ideal situations, a measurement from the tip of the brow to the ala of the nose as compared with the measurement taken from the ala to the most inferior portion of the chin should be equal. What is commonly seen in the aging patient is a bias toward the upper half of the face. There is a diminishing of the lower segment. This loss of facial height, or vertical dimension, is a result of a loss of interocclusal space. This is most dramatized in the totally edentulous patient. Many people in an aging population have been faced with the loss of their entire dentition for a multitude of reasons. Untreated carious lesions, leading to unrestorable teeth, as well as advanced forms of chronic adult periodontitis, are two of the most common ways in which teeth are lost over a lifetime.[4]

The lower third of the face can further be divided into thirds. The upper third is represented by the upper lip, and the lower two thirds by the lower lip and chin. It is the lower lip and chin area that is affected most by the loss of vertical dimension. It is here that the greatest changes can be made in rejuvenation of the aging face and dentition. Therefore, individuals who become completely edentulous will experience a total facial collapse in the lower third of the face. In a patient with no teeth present, the vertical distance is measured from a fixed point of the nose to a fixed point on the chin. In addition to this vertical component, there will also be a loss of lip support because it is the teeth that support the lips. The lips will appear to be thinner and sunken in appearance.

When a patient has teeth, vertical dimension loss is reflected by a decrease in the distance between the upper teeth and the lower teeth. Intraorally, this would be reflected as a measurement taken from the cementoenamel junction (CEJ) of the upper front incisors to the CEJ of the lower front incisors. On average this measurement is 18 mm. This measurement is taken when the teeth are fully occluded.

Support of the lower third of the face is recaptured by restoring the upper and lower teeth to their original length and interocclusal relationships. This will provide for an improved relationship between the lower third of the face components and the overall facial segments. The elimination of a deep mentolabial groove, which is an indication of age and loss of vertical height, will improve a person's looks. In addition, the loss of vertical dimension is indicative of loss of occlusal harmony. This is restored when teeth are properly positioned within the arch form and interocclusally.

◆ Conclusion

Plastic surgeons and aesthetic dermatologists have a responsibility to recognize the relationship between the teeth and the surrounding perioral area. The dentofacial relationship cannot be overlooked. Both need to be in harmony for a natural, pleasing appearance. The social

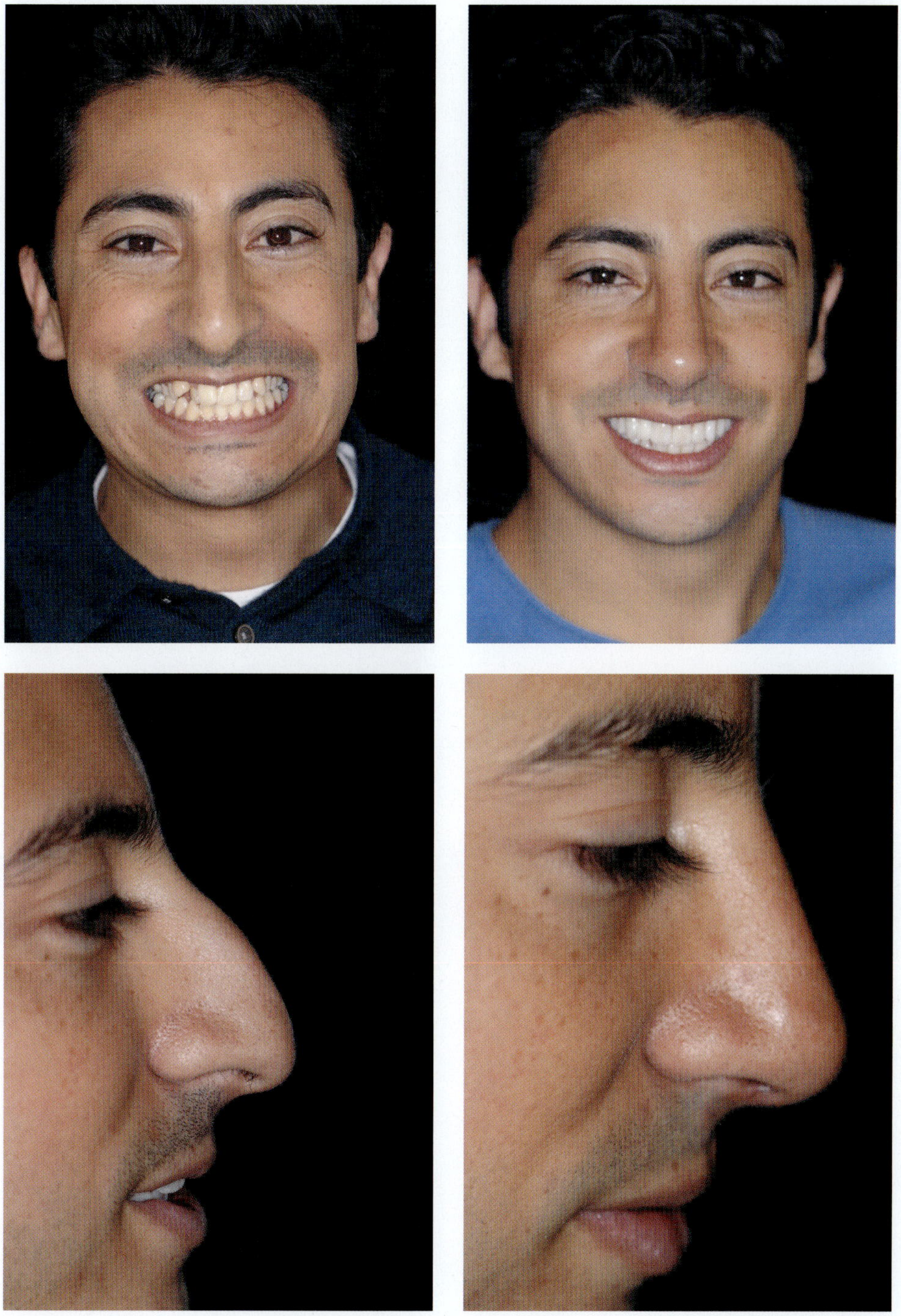

A B C D

Figure 16–3 (**A**) Preoperative. Tension in muscle contraction is exhibited when the patient is asked to smile. (**B**) Postoperative. The patient's new confidence shows a more relaxed, natural smile. (**C**) Preoperative. The nose, philtrum, lip, and teeth position is stressed. (**D**) Postoperative. A more natural relationship has been established by rhinoplasty and the placement of veneers to correct the upper lip.

importance of a beautiful, white smile cannot be underestimated. From both the functional framework and support that the teeth provide and their aesthetic contributions, today's patients seeking aesthetic enhancement can achieve much greater satisfaction than could previously be offered (Fig. **16–3A–D**).[5]

References

1. Chung WC. Gross Anatomy. 3rd ed. Baltimore: Williams & Wilkins Publishing; 1995
2. Lombardi RE. The principles of visual perception and their clinical application to denture esthetics. J Prosthet Dent 1973; 29:358–382
3. Levin EL. Dental esthetics and golden proportion. J Prosthet Dent 1978;40:244–252
4. Zarb G, Bolender C, Carlsson G. Boucher's Prosthodontic Treatment for Edentulous Patients. 11th ed. Philadelphia: Mosby; 1997
5. Rinaldi P, Marashi J. The Changing Face of Dentistry: Contemporary Esthetics and Restorative Practice. Medical World Business Press; 2004

Section IV

Complementary Treatment Modalities

17

Photodynamic Therapy for Scarless Removal of Multiple Facial Precanceroses and Superficial Carcinomas

Eckart Haneke

Skin cancer is by far the most common human malignancy. It is estimated that basal cell carcinomas (BCCs) alone are as frequent as all other organ cancers taken together. Actinic keratoses (AKs) are classical precursor lesions for squamous cell carcinomas (SCCs). There is a strong link between ultraviolet light (UVL) exposure and skin cancers; this is a direct quantitative relationship of AKs with sun exposure whereas this relationship is not so clear concerning BCCs. All patients having had one skin cancer have a risk of at least 25% of developing another primary skin malignancy, often of the same type, and patients with two or more skin cancers have a risk of over 50% to develop more. In addition, most AK patients present with multiple lesions and are prone to continuously develop more of them because the noxious effect of chronic UVL exposure continues lifelong. Thus a fair-skinned Caucasian may develop hundreds of cutaneous precanceroses and invasive carcinomas during life. Over 80% of them will be localized in the head and neck region. Surgical removal is often no challenge in the beginning, but scarring and increasing lack of movable skin may finally pose a great problem. Treatment modalities avoiding tissue loss are therefore a great advantage in the management of patients with multiple facial precancers and superficial carcinomas.

◆ Patients and Methods

Twenty-five consecutive patients with superficial malignant skin lesions—AKs, Bowen's disease, superficial BCCs—underwent photodynamic therapy (PDT) with 5-aminolevulinic acid (5-ALA) methyl ester 16% cream (Metvix). Metvix was generously applied for a minimum of 3 hours under occlusion and protected from light until treatment. The occlusive dressing was then removed, excess cream wiped off, and red light 75 J/cm^2 applied to the lesion. To avoid painful heat sensation, the patient received a cold air blowing tube that could be adjusted according to heat development and individual sensitivity. Sensitive anatomic structures, such as the eye, immediately adjacent to the treatment area were protected. Irradiation time was generally 7 to 8 minutes per field. The treated lesions were left open and the patients informed that they might have a burning sensation within the first day after treatment and would probably develop a red area corresponding to the site of Metvix absorption.

AKs were treated with one PDT, Bowen's disease and superficial BCCs with two PDT sessions. Lesions thicker than 2 mm were excluded from this treatment modality, as were nodular BCCs. Considerable hyperkeratoses were removed prior to treatment of AKs.

Patients were re-examined after 1, 2, 4, and 6 weeks, and after 6 and 12 months as well. Because all these patients have a great risk of developing more skin cancers consistent clinical follow-up once to twice a year was recommended.

◆ Results

There were 11 women and 14 men; the mean age was 56 years. Twenty patients had AKs, four patients superficial BCCs, and one patient recurrent Bowen's disease. Several AK patients had more than 10 AKs.

All 109 AKs treated reacted favorably and disappeared completely (Fig. **17–1A–C**). A second treatment

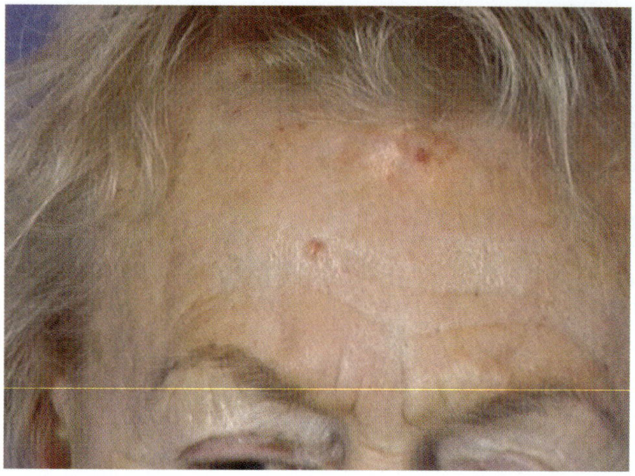

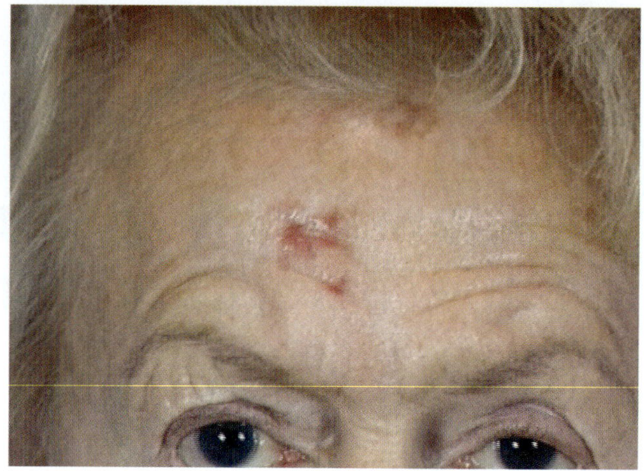

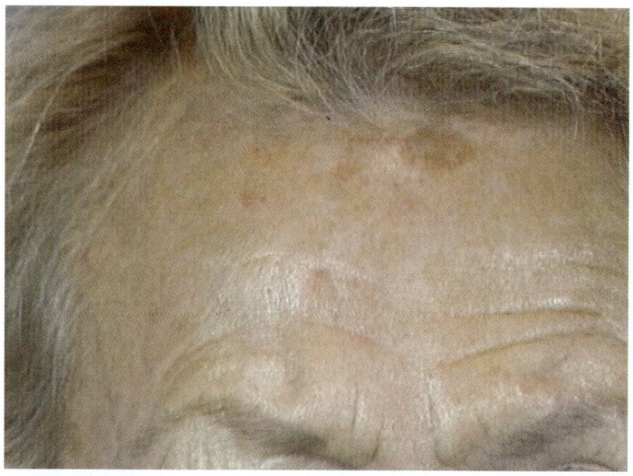

Figure 17–1 Actinic keratosis on the forehead (**A**) before photodynamic therapy (PDT). (**B**) One week after PDT, the erythema demonstrates the true extent of the lesion. (**C**) Six months after PDT.

was applied for two lesions only. The patient with Bowen's disease was initially treated once, but the lesion recurred after 8 months, so that another therapy cycle with two PDTs 4 weeks apart was instituted. Of the four BCC patients, one had a superficial recurrence on the tip of her nose after cryosurgery; she is free from recurrence 20 months after two PDTs. The other three patients together had seven superficial BCCs, which received two PDTs each.

PDT was generally tolerated very well. One patient—very fair-skinned, red-haired with freckles—reacted with very intense red spots after PDT that subsided within 2 weeks (Fig. **17–2A–C**). Most patients developed mild to moderate erythema in the area of Metvix application.

◆ Discussion

The need for skin-preserving treatment of multiple cutaneous cancers, particularly in the face, is growing because more and more patients present with multiple lesions after years of sun exposure abuse. Tangential ("shave") excision heals fast by secondary intention, yields a specimen for histopathological confirmation of the diagnosis, and allows margin control; however, many patients with multiple skin cancers do not wish to have cold steel surgery. Curettage and dermabrasion also leave open wounds. Chemocautery causes a chemical burn that takes about 2 weeks to heal. Electro- and laser surgery cause slow-healing burn wounds. Radiotherapy is not indicated for most superficial cutaneous cancers. Cryosurgery is an established and simple method for superficial lesions; however, the resultant cryonecrosis takes weeks to heal and the scar is usually hypopigmented and loses its hair follicles. Topical cytotoxic treatment with 5% 5-fluorouracil requires a 1-month treatment and must be performed until the lesions are erosive, which is often quite painful. Topical immunotherapy with imiquimod requires 6 weeks of treatment with burning and itching being almost constant adverse effects. In contrast, PDT requires only one or two treatment sessions, and untoward effects both during and after treatment are minimal to moderate. Long-term observations have shown very good healing rates and excellent cosmetic results.[1–9]

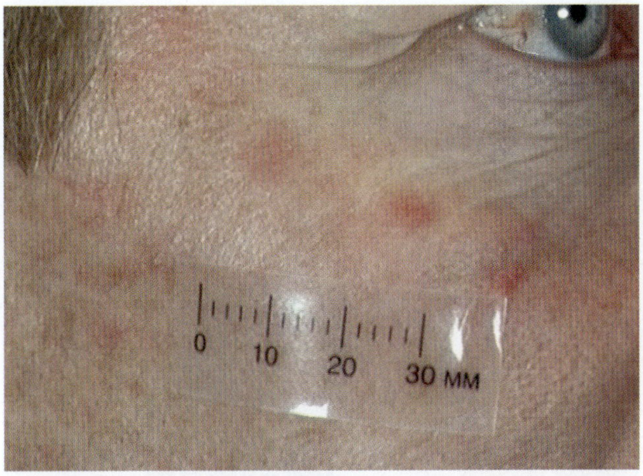

A

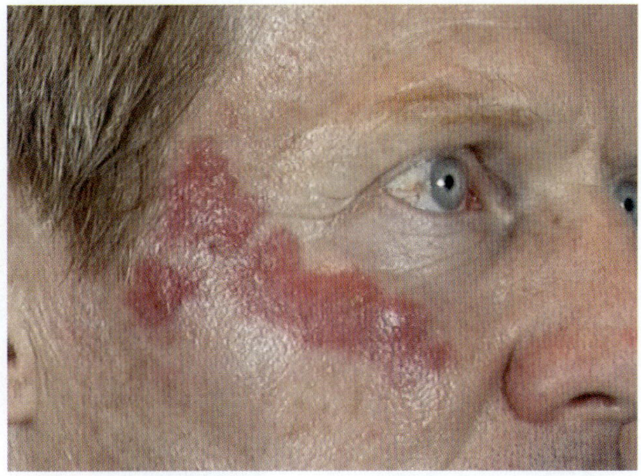
B

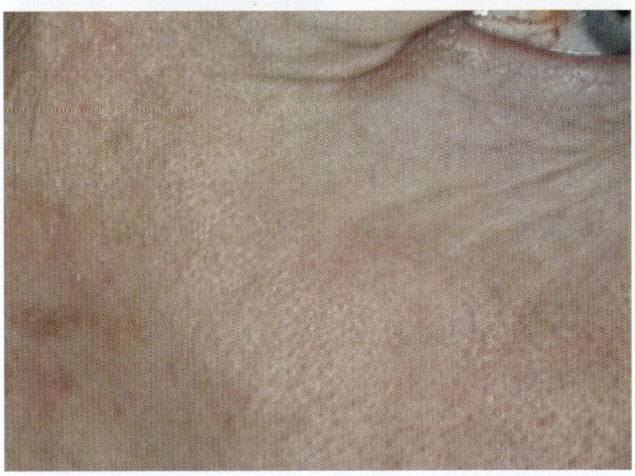
C

Figure 17–2 Multiple actinic keratoses (**A**) before treatment. (**B**) Intense erythema 1 week after photodynamic therapy (PDT). (**C**) Normal skin 12 months after PDT.

PDT is defined as the selective destruction of malignant or fast growing cells by light activation of a photosensitizing substance in the presence of oxygen (Fig. **17–3**). The preferential uptake of a completely innocuous precursor and subsequent endogenous synthesis of protoporphyrin by the target cells is the major advantage of using 5-ALA or its methyl ester (Fig. **17–4**). Irradiation with light of a wavelength capable of inducing an active state of the photosensitizer[10] stimulates the photosensitizer to generate reactive oxygen species (ROS), which then kill the target cells that preferentially took up this substance.[11] ROS induce cellular damage causing in turn cytotoxicity and immunomodulation, finally apoptosis, necrosis, and vessel occlusion (Fig. **17–3**). The role of heat during light irradiation is not yet entirely clear.[12] The method is also useful for diagnosis because the dysplastic cells exhibit a characteristic purple-red fluorescence upon irradiation with violet-blue light (Wood's light) permitting one to outline the true extent of superficial skin cancers and differentiate them from inflammatory lesions.[1,3]

PDT was first described a century ago for cancers of the skin and other organs. Skin cancer was painted with different dyes, particularly eosin, and then irradiated with sun or carbon arc light. Some viral skin diseases were treated with methylene blue and ultraviolet irradiation 50 years ago. Today, porphyrin derivatives are widely used in dermatology, ophthalmology, urology, and gastroenterology, and new indications are added in great numbers. Dermatology uses mainly the physiological porphyrin precursor 5-aminolevulinic acid (5-ALA) or its methyl ester. Living cells are capable of heme biosynthesis, which, however, is quantitatively restricted by the amount and activity of intracellular 5-ALA synthetase limiting the endogenous synthesis of 5-ALA and thus all consecutive steps of the heme synthesis. Adding exogenous 5-ALA bypasses the limiting step of endogenous 5-ALA synthesis and will therefore tremendously increase the intracellular amount of porphyrins (Fig. **17–4**). Because heme synthesis depends on the cell's activity malignant cells take up relatively more exogenous 5-ALA and produce more protoporphyrin IX rendering them more sensitive to light irradiation. Neither 5-ALA nor its methyl ester—the substances currently approved for the treatment of superficial skin cancer—are by themselves active, but are precursors of the light-sensitizing

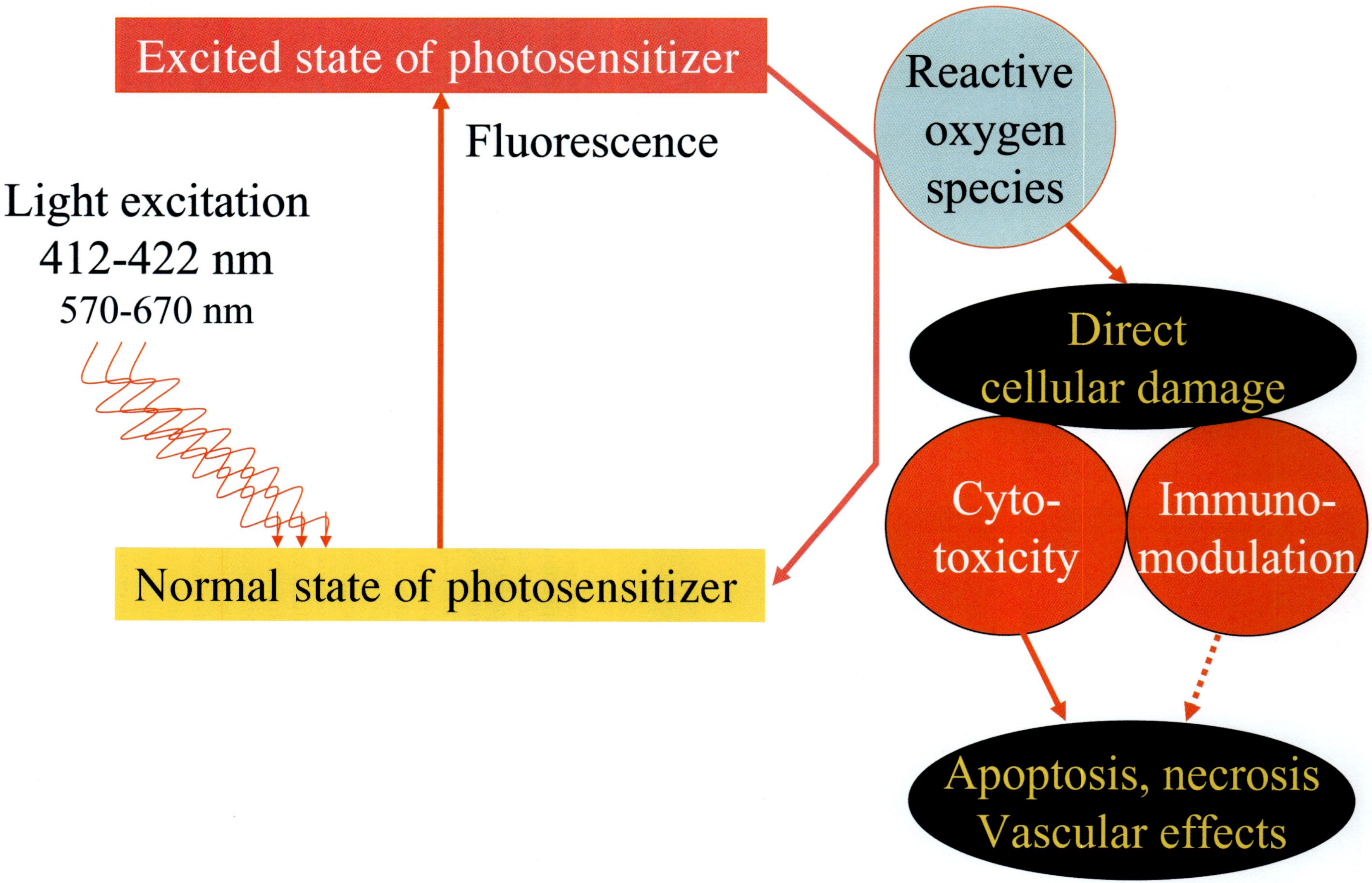

Figure 17–3 Mechanism of action of PDT: Light energy is absorbed by protoporphyrin raising it to a higher energy level. Upon return to the basic state of protoporphyrin, reactive oxygen species (ROS) are produced causing cellular and mitochondrial damage, which ultimately induces apoptosis and vascular occlusion and probably has an immunomodulatory effect.

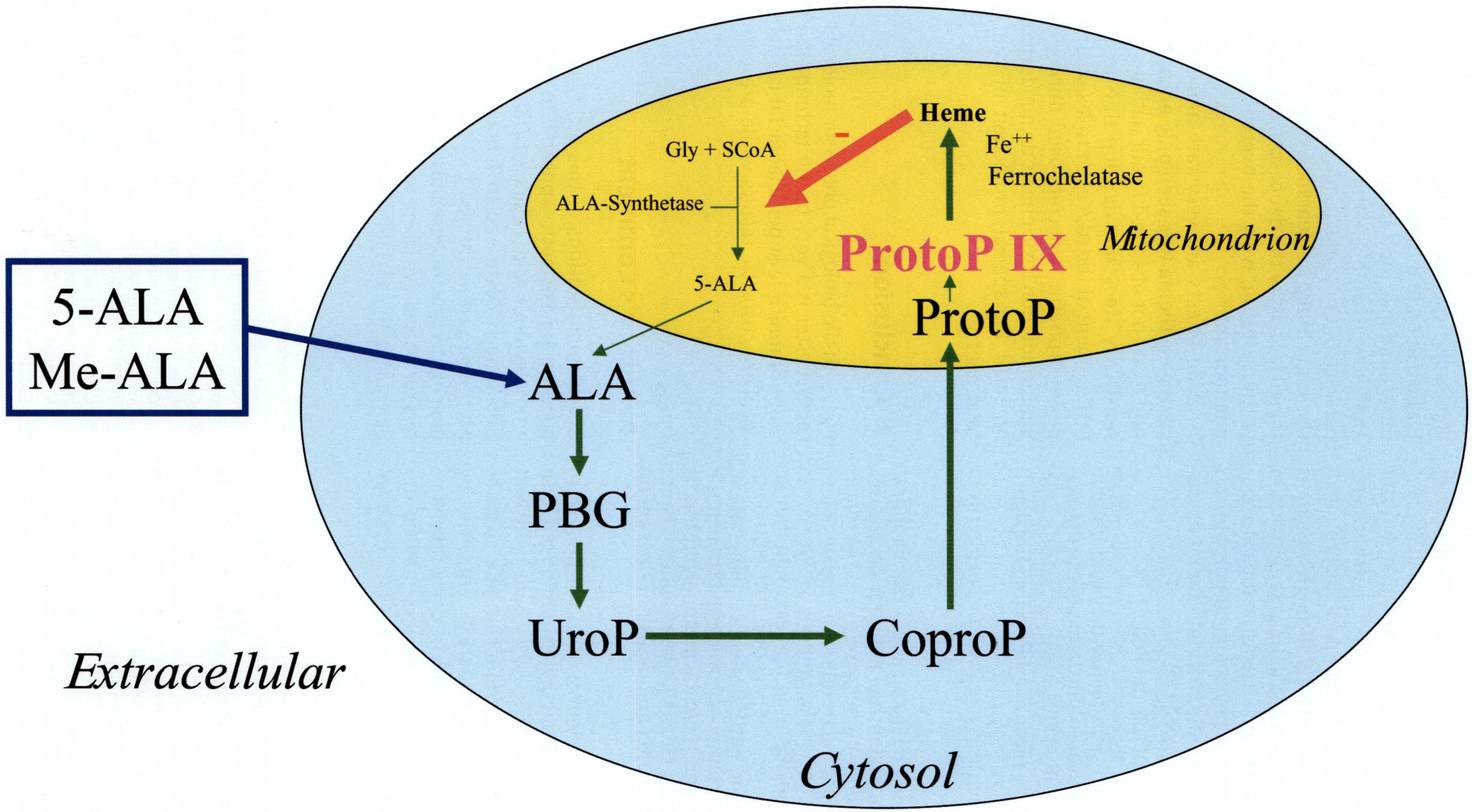

Figure 17–4 Schematic illustration of the intracellular protoporphyrin biosynthesis: 5-aminolevulinic acid is synthesized from glycine and succinyl coenzyme A by ALA synthetase, which is controlled by a negative feedback mechanism by intracellular heme concentration. When 5-ALA is added virtually unlimited protoporphyrin synthesis occurs making the cell extremely light sensitive.

compound protoporphyrin IX. Compared with normal skin, 5-ALA selectivity is ~1.5 times, ALA methyl ester selectivity is over eight times that of normal.[5,13] This allows shorter application times for ALA methyl ester cream as compared with 5-ALA cream.[14] Furthermore, nonmalignant cells are virtually left intact. Absorption of ALA and particularly its methyl ester through the skin is minimal and there is no increase in light sensitivity. In contrast to injectable photosensitizers, the topical application of the precursor of a physiological porphyrin is virtually without any systemic risk and general photosensitivity does not develop.

There are limitations of this method:

- The method is "blind" (i.e., a biopsy may therefore be necessary for histological confirmation of the diagnosis and of the treatment result).
- There are currently no means to determine the depth of penetration of the drug in routine practice. Although possible, the determination of porphyrin in living tissue[15] has not yet gained entrance into clinical practice.
- The light used to treat the lesion after cream application has only a limited depth of penetration. Ideally, violet-blue should be used because this is the wavelength of fluorescence excitation and it also can be generated without heat development. However, its penetration into the tissue is far less than 1 mm. Green light penetrates deeper, but still not deep enough. Thus red light, with the deepest penetration, up to 6 mm, is most commonly used even though the specific excitation spectrum of protoporphyrins is weak in the red range. However, laser light[16,17] is not necessary, making this technique useful for general practice.

Different studies have shown excellent long-term results with 5-ALA and ALA methyl ester plus red light for all superficial skin cancers.[1–10,16,17] Blue light that penetrates ~0.5 mm may be used for thin AKs. Hyperkeratoses should be removed before treatment, either by using 5 to 10% salicylic acid ointment or by mechanically scraping them off. Thicker tumors may be debulked by curettage 1 or 2 days prior to PDT. However, care has to be taken not to bury the lesion (i.e., treating the superficial tumor layers and leaving neoplastic tissue behind in the deeper dermis). Noninvasive pulsed ultrasound may indicate tumor resolution or recurrence and showed wide variation in the treatment response between BCCs of similar initial thickness, indicating that the probability of clearance of BCCs by PDT is determined largely by the deepest, sometimes small, regions within a lesion, with the overall area being relatively unimportant.[18]

Side effects are very rare and mild. Intense and lasting erythema was seen only once; hyperpigmentation[19] was not observed in our patients. General photosensitivity does not develop due to more selective confinement of the ALA ester to lesional skin.[20] Because protoporphyrin is decomposed during the process of light irradiation toxic effects do not develop and there is no need for special protection of the lesions after treatment.[10]

◆ Conclusion

PDT with the biological precursor molecule 5-ALA or ALA methyl ester is a very useful technique in the management of multiple superficial facial carcinomas yielding excellent cosmetic results while preserving unaffected tissue.

◆ Author's Comment

Recent modifications of this technique are further increasing its cosmetic appeal.[21] In the United States, aminolevulinic acid (Levulan, DUSA) is used. The incubation time is decreased to 1 hour, and the subsequent erythema can be limited to 1 to 3 days. In addition to blue light, either intense pulsed light (IPL) (560 or 590 filters) or pulsed dye lasers can be used for PDT. Results can be equated to 3 to 5 IPL treatments.

References

1. Wolf P, Rieger E, Kerl H. Topical photodynamic therapy with endogenous porphyrins after application of 5-aminolevulinic acid: an alternative modality for solar keratoses, superficial squamous cell carcinomas, and basal cell carcinomas? J Am Acad Dermatol 1993;28:17–21
2. Tosca A, Balas CJ, Stefanidou MP, Katsantonis J, Georgiu SK, Tzardi MN. Photodynamic treatment of skin malignancies with aminolevulinic acid. Dermatol Surg 1996;22:929–934
3. Fritsch C, Goerz G, Ruzicka T. Photodynamic therapy in dermatology. Arch Dermatol 1998;134:207–214
4. Bissonnette R, Lui H. Current status of photodynamic therapy in dermatology. Dermatol Clin 1997;15:507–519
5. Peng Q, Warloe T, Berg K, et al. 5-aminolevulinic acid based photodynamic therapy. Cancer 1997;79:2282–2308
6. Ceburkov O, Gollnick H. Photodynamic therapy in dermatology. Eur J Dermatol 2000;10:568–576
7. Kalka K, Merk H, Mukhtar H. Photodynamic therapy in dermatology. J Am Acad Dermatol 2000;42:389–413
8. Guillen C, Sanmartin O, Escudero A, Botella-Estrada R, Sevila A, Castejon P. Photodynamic therapy for in situ squamous cell carcinoma on chronic radiation dermatitis after photosensitization with 5-aminolaevulinic acid. J Eur Acad Dermatol Venereol 2000;14:298–300
9. Ceylan C, Erboz S, Özdemir F, Alper S. Topical photodynamic therapy for intraepidermal epithelioma. J Eur Acad Dermatol Venereol 2002;16:292–294
10. Braathen LR. Photodynamic therapy: when and why? J Eur Acad Dermatol Venereol 2002;16:227

11. Kennedy JC, Pottier RH, Pross DC. Photodynamic therapy with endogenous protoporphyrin IX: basic principles and present clinical experience. J Photochem Photobiol B 1990;6:143–148

12. Orenstein A, Kostenich G, Tsur H, Kogan L, Malik Z. Temperature monitoring during photodynamic therapy of skin tumours with topical 5-aminolevulinic acid application. Cancer Lett 1995;95:227–232

13. Fritsch C, Homey B, Stahl W, Lehmann P, Ruzicka T, Sies H. Preferential relative porphyrin enrichment in solar keratoses upon topical application of d-aminolevulinic acid methylester. Photochem Photobiol 1998;68:218–221

14. Xiang W, Weingandt H, Liessmann F, Klein S, Stepp H, Baumgartner R, Hillemanns P. Photodynamic effects induced by aminolevulinic acid esters on human cervical carcinoma cells in culture. Photochem Photobiol. 2001;74:617–623

15. Trepte O, Rokahr I, Andersson-Engels S, Carlsson K. Studies of porphyrin-containing specimens using an optical spectrometer connected to a confocal scanning laser microscope. J Microsc 1994;176:238–244

16. Landthaler M, Ruck A, Szeimies RM. Photodynamische Therapie von Hauttumoren. Hautarzt 1993;44:69–74

17. Svanberg K, Andersson T, Killander D, et al. Photodynamic therapy of nonmelanoma malignant tumours of the skin using topical delta-amino levulinic acid sensitization and laser irradiation. Br J Dermatol 1994;130:743–751

18. Allan E, Pye DA, Levine EL, Moore JV. Noninvasive pulsed ultrasound quantification of the resolution of basal cell carcinomas after photodynamic therapy. Lasers Med Sci 2002;17:230–237

19. Monfrecola G, Procaccini EM, D'Onofrio D, et al. Hyperpigmentation induced by topical 5-aminolaevulinic acid plus visible light. J Photochem Photobiol B 2002;68:147–155

20. Juzeniene A, Juzenas P, Iani V, Moan J. Topical application of 5-aminolevulinic acid and its methylester, hexylester and octylester derivatives: considerations for dosimetry in mouse skin model. Photochem Photobiol 2002;76:329–334

21. Goldman MP, Avram D. Effectiveness and safety of ALA-IPL in treating actinic keratoses and photodamage. Drugs Dermatol 2004;3:32–39

18

Traditional Chinese Medicine: Its Approach to Facial Beauty

Steven Schram

Beginning thousands of years ago, the practitioners of traditional Chinese medicine (TCM) developed an in-depth and very practical understanding of how the body works. As part of their understanding, they theorized a meridian system of energy channels running throughout the body. Application of this theory forms the foundation of current acupuncture techniques and it remains widely used throughout the world as a tool to help heal and balance the body. Part of this system is a subspecialty that deals with dermatology, complexion, and in particular, the face. What follows is a brief introduction to the critical concepts of TCM followed by specific techniques that help treat problems in facial complexion, including skin tone, color, lines, and texture.

◆ Overview of Facial Acupuncture

Our first focus is on the acupuncture meridians. According to TCM Channel Theory,{AQ1} these meridians are major communication conduits that run to and from the surface of the body to the organs in the deep interior. The complex interplay of organ function is assisted by the interplay and overlapping of the meridian pathways. Briefly, there are 12 major acupuncture channels, plus eight "special" channels. Half of the major channels and seven of the special ones begin, end, or traverse the face with the remaining channels exerting indirect influence.

Because the interior and exterior are so well connected, all TCM diagnostic techniques include skin examination as part of the evaluation and diagnosis procedure. And because so many channels traverse the face, it is well-accepted that the face reflects the underlying health of the person.

This means that to treat the face we must also treat the underlying health of the person. So when treating the face, not only are acupuncture needles applied directly to the face, they are also placed at other points on the body that affect health in general. This dual approach is what allows the clients' vibrant internal health to shine more robustly through to their rejuvenated face.

It is important to understand that, although facial acupuncture is often referred to as an acupuncture facelift or facial rejuvenation, it is especially effective specifically because underlying health issues are simultaneously treated through the use of body acupuncture points. Thus it is much more than a simple cosmetic procedure and is in fact a revitalization process designed to help keep the whole body looking and feeling younger.

For those who desire more comprehensive and structured discussion, I refer you to Redwingbooks.com, which maintains the most comprehensive source for a wide range of literature dealing with all aspects of Chinese Medicine.

◆ Yin/Yang and the Basics of TCM

Fundamental to any discussion of TCM are the concepts of Yin and Yang. These are energetic relationships that represent mutual paired opposites and reflect the Chinese view on the bipolar nature of the universe in general. In brief, Yin is dark, cooling, contracting, and moistening and corresponds to structure. Yang is bright, warming, expanding, and drying and corresponds to function. They are complementary, and neither can exist without the other. In fact, under TCM, the interplay between Yin and Yang forms the foundation of life.

One of the primary tenets of Yin/Yang theory is that they transform into each other. The main idea is that, in health, both exist in a relative state of mutual abundance and balance. In other words, there should not be too much of one with respect to the other. As a corollary, there should not be too little of one with respect to the other either. Applying these principles gives rise to four fundamental imbalances that a person can manifest.

1. There can be too much Yang: The person feels hot and the *face may be red.*
2. There can be too much Yin: The person feels cold and the *face may be pale.*
3. There can be too little Yang: The person feels cool and the *face may be pale.*
4. There can be too little Yin: The person feels warm the *face may have flushed cheeks.*

The first two conditions are termed excess conditions and the last two are termed deficiencies. (Although technically, the excess conditions refer to the strength of a pathogenic vector and deficiency relates to the strength of the defensive Qi, for the purpose of this chapter, we will stick to the understanding presented above.) Bear in mind that there can be many complex interactions of the four conditions among the various organ systems, and the simplistic analysis given here often evolves into multiple excesses and deficiencies among different organ systems. This is particularly so in the aged and geriatric population. The true art of TCM diagnostics lies in unraveling these complexities so the proper treatment can be designed.

◆ Disease and Diagnosis

We have already mentioned the balance of Yin and Yang. Another important concept in understanding the disease state is the concept of obstruction of the movement of Qi and Blood by external environmental pathogenic evils known as Wind, Heat, Fire, Cold, Dry, and Dampness. Qi is the Yang manifestation of the Life Force, while Blood is the Yin manifestation. In simple terms, according to TCM, disease results when an evil pathogen enters the body through any orifice or pore and proceeds to obstruct or interfere with the flow of Qi or Blood. If the response to the evil is strong, it is called an excess pattern. If the body's defensive response is too weak to fight the pathogen effectively, it becomes a deficiency pattern. The evils can enter singly or be combined into more complex patterns. When describing a pattern, one describes the organ/meridian and the evil. Common patterns include Spleen Damp, Liver Wind, Spleen Yang Deficiency, Stomach Heat, etc. There are many hundreds of patterns! The art of TCM lies in elucidating the exact pattern of disharmony.

Although this discussion of patterns of disharmony may make little sense to a Western trained medical mind, within the 3000-year-old practice of TCM, such diagnostic analysis forms the basis of many successful treatment strategies. For our purposes, we will focus on several simple aspects of facial diagnosis.

Diagnostic Relationship between Health and Facial Appearance

The Chinese were keen in observation and they were able to correlate what they saw with other symptomatic and diagnostic factors. Although there are many correlations to consider, there are a few very significant diagnostic relationships between people's health and how their face and hair looks.

Hair

- Hair loss often indicates a Blood Deficiency.
- Early graying of hair is a Deficiency of Kidney Essence.
- Dull hair with split ends may indicate a Deficiency of Lung Qi.

Face Color

- The color and moistness of the face reflect the state of Qi and Blood. It is important to distinguish between a dry and dull face versus a clear and shiny complexion. Moist, clear, and shiny, regardless of the color, are always favorable whereas dry and dull are not.
- A slight green pallor is usually a liver pattern although it could also mean interior Cold, pain, or interior Wind.
- A red face always indicates Heat. If only the cheeks are red, it is Deficiency Heat, while if the whole face is red, then it is Excess Heat.
- A yellow cast to the face indicates a Spleen deficiency or Dampness, or both. A dull yellow could be Cold Damp whereas brighter shades would represent Damp Heat.
- A white color may indicate Deficiency in Qi or Blood, Cold, or Yang Deficiency,
- Irrespective of shading, a color can be described as deep, floating, clear, dull, thin, or thick. Deep is Interior whereas floating is Exterior. Clear is a Yang condition whereas dull points to Yin. Thin represents Qi Deficiency whereas thick is an Excess condition.

Lip Color

- Very pale indicates Deficiency of Blood or Yang.
- Very red and dry indicates Stomach or Spleen Heat.
- Purple or blue indicates Blood Stasis.
- Greenish color around mouth is Stasis of Liver Blood and Rebellion of Liver Qi into the Spleen.

Table 18–1 Guidelines to Treating Areas of the Face

Facial Areas	Corresponding Organ
Forehead	Heart and Lung
Between eyebrows	Liver and Spleen
Bags under the eyes	Kidney
Bridge of nose	Heart
Upper side of nose	Gall Bladder
Lower end of nose	Large Intestine
Tip of nose	Spleen
Cheeks, upper	Liver
Cheeks, lower	Lung
Lips	Stomach/Spleen
Lateral ends of the lips	Kidney
Philtrum	Bladder
Jowls	Large Intestine
Short chin	Kidney deficiency

The different areas of the face are also diagnostically important. Table **18–1** offers some simple guidelines to areas of the face and the corresponding body area or organ one would likely treat. Note that whenever there are areas on the face that have a lot of wrinkles or deep creases, distal points on the corresponding channels should be simultaneously needled to support the local work.

◆ Acupuncture Mechanism of Action on the Skin

Skin connective tissues are primarily elastic fibers and collagen. Acupuncture needles inserted along wrinkle lines act as local irritants creating a local histamine reaction. This induces formation of collagen, which softens the wrinkle while simultaneously increasing the elasticity of the skin. They also dilate blood vessels increasing healthy circulation and stimulating cell metabolism. This enhances overall function, resulting in faster repair and sloughing of old skin cells, leaving the skin softer, smoother, and suppler with diminished lines.

◆ General Benefits

- Improves muscle tone and dermal contraction
- Improves facial color by enhancing peripheral circulation
- Reduces stress (often evident in the face)
- Promotes overall health
- Helps to bring out a person's inner beauty and radiance
- Slows down the aging process from within
- Improves hormonal balance
- Tightens the pores and brightens the eyes
- Moisturizes the skin by increasing local circulation of lymph and blood
- Opens nerve pathways in the head and the whole body, enhancing the flow of vitality throughout the whole body

◆ Practical Applications of TCM Facial Rejuvenation

Table **18–2** gives some indication for the scope of problems treated by TCM and facial acupuncture. Each of these problems is treated locally with very specific acupuncture points at the area of the problem as well as with body points that help correct the underlying health issues. General strategies and specific point recommendations follow the table.

We choose the main channels to treat based on the area of the face that has the most issues. Then, specific points on those channels are chosen, based on the underlying diagnostic pattern of disharmony discovered during the diagnostic intake session.

Strategies and Recommendations

Channel Selection

The documented use of acupuncture and herbology for facial rejuvenation by the Chinese is a longstanding tradition that goes back at least to the Song Dynasty (960 to 1270 AD), where it was used for keeping the Empress and the Emperor's concubines healthy and beautiful.

Fig. **18–1** shows the paths of the facial channels. Note how different channels govern different areas of

Table 18–2 Indications for Treatment with Traditional Chinese Medicine

Blepharoptosis	Puffy face
Bags under eyes	Sagging cheeks
Double chin	Adolescent acne
Spider veins	Red facial complexion
Graying hair	Pale facial complexion
Dry skin	Fine wrinkles
Drinker's nose	Deeper lines

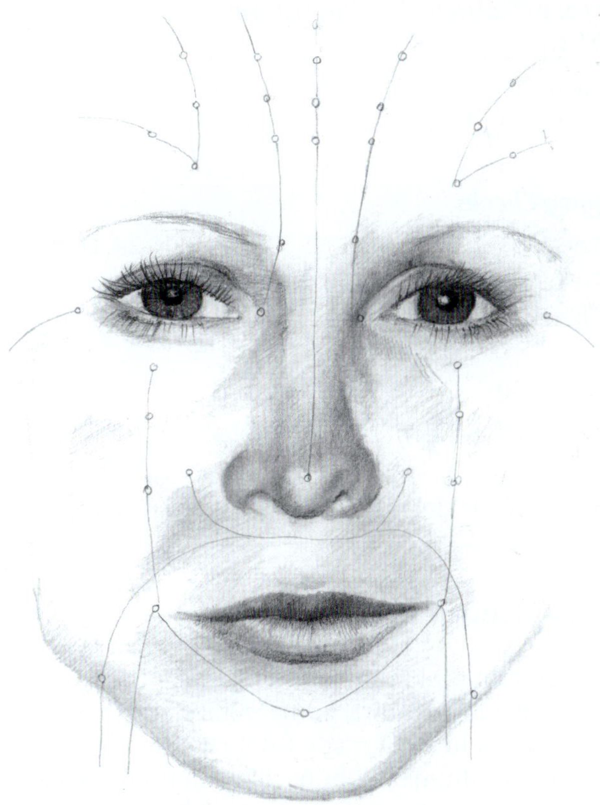

Figure 18–1 The paths of the facial channels.

the face. The value of this observation is that if you are treating a particular area of the face for rejuvenation, you will get significantly better results when you simultaneously treat the corresponding channel that runs through that area.

The main channels that reflect to the face are the Stomach/Spleen, Lung/Large Intestine, Heart, Liver/Gall Bladder, Bladder/Kidney, and Du/Ren. They will be the principle channels used to augment the facial treatments.

Point Selection

The most common point used in all facial treatments is the Command Point for the face, LI-4. In addition, points such as LU-7, REN-3, SP-6, KI-3, LV-3, and P-6 are also often used because they nourish Yin, the moistening aspect of the body.

Next chosen are the source points of the meridians that govern various facial areas. They are listed in Table **18–3.** Notice the overlap of the KI-3 and LV-3 points in this table and the list just presented.

On the ear are additional points such as Shen Men, Liver, Kidney, Spleen, and Face. There are also specific ear points for the Chin, Lips, Face, Forehead, Temple, and Sinuses. Do not discount the value of these points because they exert a powerful effect based on their embryological origin during brain and skull formation.

In general, when discussing specific conditions, general acupuncture point selection guidelines recommend that three areas always be chosen for any treatment. They include points that are local, points that are near the area, and points that are distal.

Note that the points recommended following here are by no means exhaustive or absolute because the art and science of TCM requires flexibility and creativity. It is recommended that LI-4 always be used because it is the command point of the head and face.

Also note that several points need extreme care in their usage. These are points within the orbit of the eye (BL-1, ST-1, Qui Hui) and ST-9, located near the carotid artery. And as a rule, facial points are always contraindicated for the patient population that scars or bruises easily. The following conditions are also generally contraindicated:

- Pregnant
- Sick
- Having an acute herpes outbreak
- Having an acute allergic reaction
- Intoxicated
- Fasting

Finally, patients with the following conditions must be evaluated carefully before proceeding:

- Pituitary disorders
- Heart disorders
- Diabetes mellitus
- High blood pressure
- Pacemakers (avoid electrostimulation in this case)
- Problems with easy bleeding or bruising
- Migraine headaches
- Taking corticosteroids

Table 18–3 Source Points of Meridians Governing Facial Areas

Heart	Lung	Spleen	Kidney	Gall Bladder	Large Intestine	Liver	Stomach
HT-7	LU-9	SP-3	KI-3	GB-40	LI-4	LV-3	ST-42

Specific Treatments

Blepharoptosis

Three possible disharmonies include Deficient Kidney Yang, Deficient Spleen Qi, Deficient Liver Blood with Wind.

Local: SJ-23, BL-2, Yu Yao, Yin Tang, Tai Yang, Qui Hui
Near: BL-4, ST-8, GB-14
Distal: DU-20, GB-13, GB-37, LI-4, LV-3, LI-4.

Bags under Eyes (Drain Damp, Nourish Kidney)

Local: ST-1, GB-1, BL-1, Qui Hui
Near: ST-2, ST-3, SI-18
Distal: SP-9, KI-3, LV-3, LI-4

Puffy Eyelids

Local: BL-1, ST-1, Qui Hui
Near: BL-2, Yu Yao, DU-26, SJ-23
Distal: SP-9, ST-36, ST-43, LI-4, LI-11, LU-7

Puffy Face (Drain Damp)

Local: LI-19, DU-26
Near: DU-21, DU-24
Distal: SP-9, SP-6, SP-4, ST-36, REN-8, LU-7, LI-4

Drinker's Nose

Local: DU-25 (Tip of Nose)

Pale Face (Build Blood)

Local: ST-2
Near: ST-9, SI-18, DU-23
Distal: GB-38, LI-4, ST-36, LV-8, BL-17

Red Face (Clear Heat, Regulate Yang)

Local: DU-7, ST-9
Near: ST-9, DU-20, DU-14 (Prick and Bleed)
Distal: ST-36, SP-10, LI-11, LI-4, SP-6, ST-41, GB-41, BL-19

Wrinkles on Lip

Local: DU-26, REN-24, LI-19
Near: ST-4
Distal: LI-4

Double Chin

Local: REN-23, ST-9, ST-13, ST-17
Near: GB-18
Distal: LI-4

Dry Face (Moisten Skin, Nourish Yin)

Local: ST-2
Near: ST-9
Distal: LV-8, LV-5, SP-6, ST-9, KI-6, LI-4, LI-11, LU-6

Sagging Cheeks

Local: ST-2, ST-4, ST-6, ST-7, ST-8, REN-24, LI-19
Near: DU-20, GB-13, GB-2, GB-12
Distal: SP-3

Acne (Facial)

Local: BL-1
Near: ST-9
Distal: LI-4, LI-11, SP-10, ST-9, SP-6, KI-27, BL-12, LI-1

◆ Treatment Protocol

The first step is skin preparation. Wash the face to remove makeup and dirt. Some clinics start with a hot towel soaked in a tea made from chamomile, chrysanthemum, psyllium, and mint that is left on the face for about 3 or 4 minutes. A paste made of beaten egg whites, powdered oyster shell, and pearl powder may be spread on with cosmetic applicator pads as a mask for another 10 minutes. This is taken off with a towel wet with ice water. The sum effect of this is to open the pores and clean away dead cells. It adds a nice glow to the face.

In terms of acupuncture, it is recommended to insert the ear needles first. The ear, based on its embryological origin, has a strong connection to various brain locations and acts as a cue to the body as to what areas we are focusing on. The points Shen Men and face are recommended, along with other constitutional points such as Kidney, Liver, and Spleen.

Move on to the distal points in the arms and legs and trunk and finally to the facial points. Use very fine gauge Serin needles (red or green handle). The needles are left in place for ~20 minutes after which they are withdrawn in the reverse order of insertion (Fig. **18–2A,B**). It is important that you firmly press the point when the needle is removed to minimize the likelihood of any bleeding. A chilled silver spoon and Arnica Oil can be used on any points that bleed or appear bruised upon needle extraction.

Smaller intradermal needles are used along and under any specific wrinkles. Some clinics apply a mild electrical stimulus to the needles that are in the deep crevices that lie along the muscle areas of the face. This twitches the facial muscles, which tends to enhance the collagen effect. One can also use a microcurrent stimulation, which is sensation free. Microcurrents tone

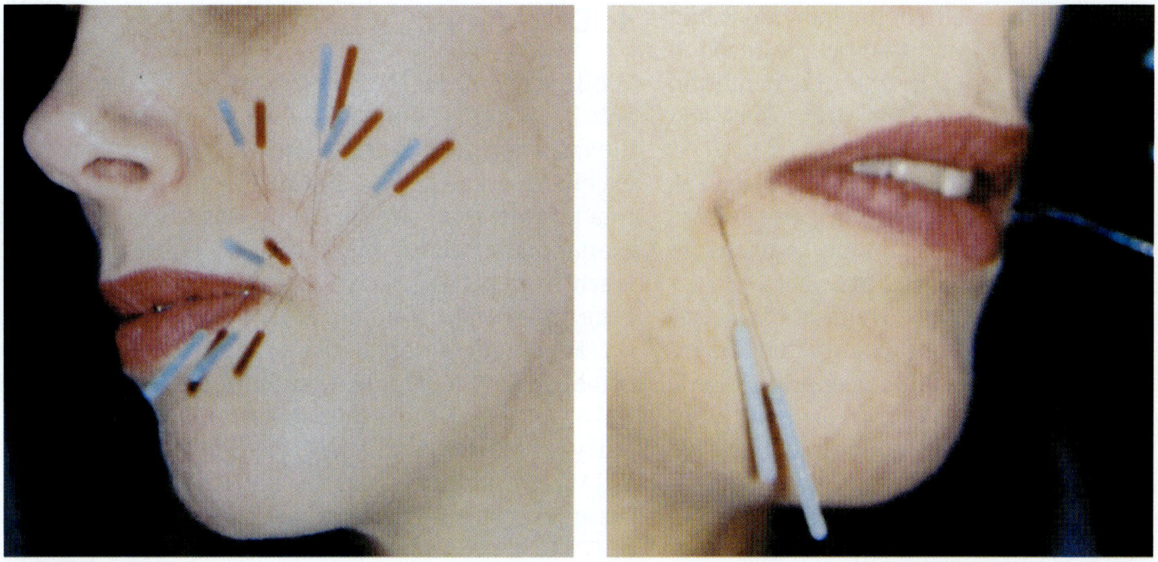

A B

Figure 18–2 Acupuncture needles in place. (A) Larger, longer, or deeper lines require more needles. (B) Smaller wrinkles or lines need fewer needles.

the muscles and improve circulation to regenerate and repair skin and heal postsurgical bruising. It also helps to improve lymphatic drainage to reduce puffiness, especially around the eyes.

◆ General Effects

The overall effectiveness of facial acupuncture is due to its direct manipulation of the body's energy system. The local effects on facial skin include increased elasticity of facial muscles, leveling of wrinkles, evening of complexion, and an overall appearance of rejuvenation that is not simply confined to the face (Fig. **18–3A,B**).

Other likely results include moisturizing of the skin with increased local circulation of blood and lymph to the face; increased collagen production, muscle tone, and dermal contraction; tightened pores; brighter eyes; improved hormonal balance to help acne; and reduced evidence of stress in the face. Fine lines may be entirely eliminated and deeper wrinkles diminished. Bags around the neck and eyes can be firmed, sagging reduced, puffiness eliminated, droopy eyelids lifted, and double chins minimized.

Typically, 10 to 15 treatments are recommended, with the actual number dependant on the age of the patient,

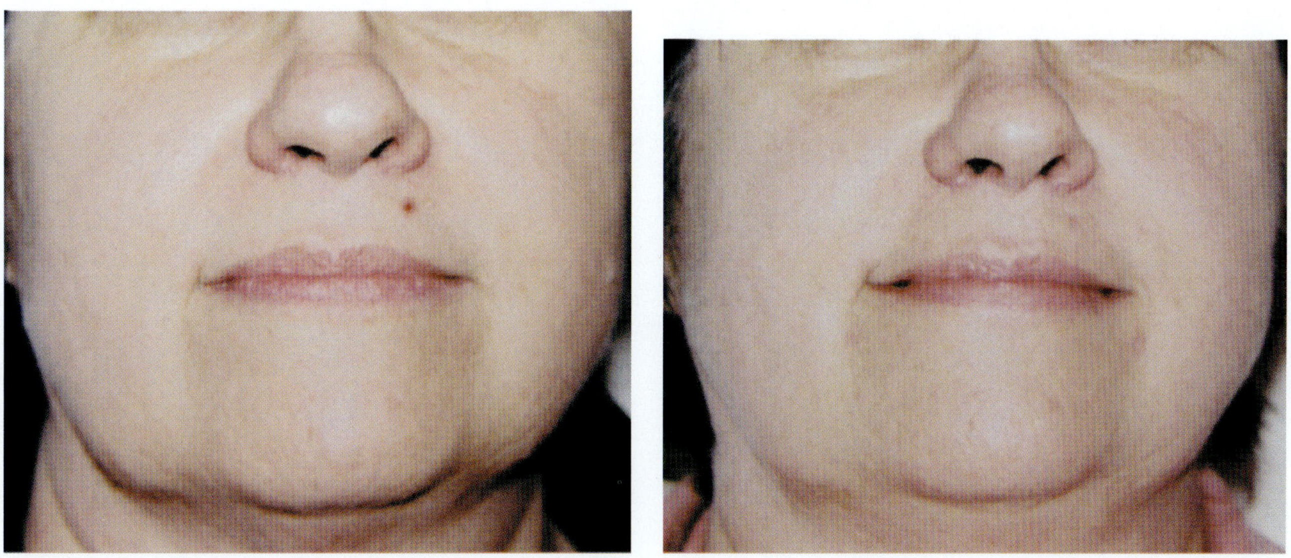

A B

Figure 18–3 (**A**) Before and (**B**) after an acupuncture session; there is improvement in facial tone and the appearance of some facial furrows.

condition of the skin, overall health of the individual, and patient compliance. Keep in mind that people respond differently depending on their lifestyle and condition prior to treatment. In general, smokers, drug users, and sun worshippers require more treatments.

Treatments are recommended to be twice a week for the first month, weekly thereafter. Once a series has been completed, monthly follow-ups are advised to maintain the effects. Results can last 2 to 5 years.

It is important to note that improvements from any one session are subtle and that most changes will be increasingly noticeable only over time. Generally, some results will be seen after three to four treatments, with more marked results seen by six. Depending on the response to treatment, the number and frequency of sessions may then be reduced to a maintenance level of one treatment every 4 to 6 weeks.

◆ Disclaimer

While most of the information presented here is available in the public domain, the actual techniques for needle insertions are the most critical element in achieving excellent results. And because acupuncture itself is much more than simple needle insertion, it is recommended that those seeking to do facial acupuncture learn from other practitioners who have both experience and specific training.

Highly recommended are the classes taught by two established teachers. They are Virginia Doran (212-769-8278), email at Workshops@luminousbeauty.com and Mary Elizabeth Wakefield (212-688-8709) email at ChiAkra@onebox.com. While both teach different treatment protocols, they each stay true to the fundamentals of TCM.

Suggested Readings

1. Deadman P, Al-Khafaji M. A Manual of Acupuncture. East Sussex, England: Journal of Chinese Medicine Publications; 2001
2. Wiseman N, Ellis A (Trans). Fundamentals of Chinese Medicine. Brookline, MA: Paradigm Publications; 1985
3. Maciocia G. The Foundations of Chinese Medicine. Edinburgh: Churchill Livingstone; 1989
4. Oleson T. Auriculartherapy Manual: Chinese and Western Systems of Ear Acupuncture, 2nd ed. Los Angeles, CA: Health Care Alternatives; 1996
5. Maciocia G. Diagnosis in Chinese Medicine. Edinburgh: Churchill Livingstone; 2004

Appendix

Rejuvenating the Skin from the Inside Out

Gary Null

Take a look in the mirror. What do you see? A lot of people, especially aging baby boomers and senior citizens, see sagging skin, wrinkles, crow's feet, lines between the eyebrows, jowls, large pores, and skin that has thickened in some areas and thinned in others. They see the veins below the skin on their face, just as on their hands. And at the same time skin deteriorates, hair becomes thinner and grayer and loses the vibrancy and luster of youth. What can one do at this point?

Most Americans do nothing at all. They are apathetic and resigned to the inevitable, that their skin and hair condition will just get worse. However, several men and women are paying more attention. They are asking two important questions: Can the damage done up to this point be reversed, and can further damage be slowed down?

Superficial remedies are available, such as topically applied night or day creams, or so-called miracle creams that promise to minimize facial lines or rehydrate the skin. Those will be adequate for some people. Others apply more makeup, and yet another group's answer is cosmetic surgery.

But a relatively small percentage of the population wants more. They first want to know why their skin became damaged. They wonder if there is much more that they can do to prevent further damage and take responsibility for their own skin and hair condition.

It is for this last group that I have written this chapter. I will make clear that it is more than the usual suspects (ultraviolet radiation, cigarette smoking, and moderate, but regular, alcohol consumption) that have contributed to skin and hair difficulties.

Before we look at the causes of wrinkled and damaged skin, let us understand more about the skin itself. Following that, we will study the causes of skin damage, and finally, solutions to these problems.

◆ The Largest Organ

The skin is the largest and most visible organ of the human body. It is an organ just like the heart, lungs, kidneys, and brain, and not just the body's covering, as many people believe. It is not merely something that must be kept in good condition so appearances won't suffer. The skin is a highly specialized organ, controlling body temperature, protecting against disease, and acting as an indicator of internal disorder. It acts as a defense, keeping out dirt, water, and other damaging substances. It is an effective barrier against germs. It is well supplied with lymph fluids, which are essential to supplying food to the cells and carrying out waste products. All in all, the skin carries a far greater burden than most of us ever realize.

The skin is made up of many different tissues. Its components include blood vessels, glands, sense organs, nerves, smooth muscle, and connective tissue. It provides resistance against mechanical shock and transmits all sorts of sensations, ranging from pain, which is a warning that something is out of order, to sexual pleasure and a sense of well-being. Indeed skin nerves are the principal organs of sexual attraction, identifying each individual by the shape of bodily contours as well as the person's skin patterns.

On the average adult, the skin covers an area of 18 to 20 square feet. Usually it is about one eighth of an inch thick, being thinner in areas such as the eyelids and thicker where more protection is needed, such as the hands and the soles of the feet. Skin is composed of a framework of elastic fibers that are well supplied with glands, blood vessels, and nerves. The skin can best be described as layered. There are three distinct layers: the epidermis, the dermis, and the subcutaneous fat. Each of these can be further subdivided into additional layers.

Each square inch of skin contains 78 nerves, 650 sweat glands, 20 blood vessels, 78 sensory apparatuses for heat detection, 13 sensory apparatuses for cold detection, 1300 nerve endings, 19,500 sensory cells at the end of nerve fibers, 160 pressure apparatuses for the sense of touch, 100 sebaceous glands, 65 hairs and 65 muscles, and 19,500,000 cells. What this means in practical terms is that an abrasion on your skin, no larger than a quarter, could cause a loss of a yard of blood vessels, four yards of nerves, and scores of other nerve endings and sweat glands, and millions of cells.

The skin of the unborn child develops very early. Suborgans such as hair, sweat glands, fingernails, and oil glands take recognizable form as early as the third month. It is at that time, for instance, that hair follicles begin to appear on a baby's head. Soon after that, more follicles can be seen on the trunk and limbs. By the time of birth, all of the hair follicles the baby will have throughout its entire life have been formed.

◆ The Skin Layers

Epidermis

The epidermis is the outermost skin layer. It provides a tough exterior surface with considerable resilience. The epidermis can be broken down into four layers:

1. The stratum corneum is the very top layer of the skin. It is composed of cells that have been manufactured in a deeper layer and have then migrated to the surface. Once these cells reach the surface, they constantly wear out or are rubbed off and so must be continually replaced.
2. The stratum lucidum is the second layer of the epidermis. This is a clear layer of cells that have lost their nuclei on their way up to become part of the stratum corneum.
3. The stratum granulosum, the third layer of the skin, is composed of cells that are undergoing chemical changes as preparation for becoming part of the outer layer.
4. The stratum germinativum is the lowest layer of the epidermis. It is sometimes called the basal cell layer. In this layer, the cells divide and form material for new skin, and just as important, for the healing of wounds.

The cell division that takes place in the stratum germinativum is a fascinating process. The basal cells are among the most vigorous in the body. After they are formed in the basal cell layer, and as they continue to grow, these cells begin to migrate upward through the epidermis toward the surface of the skin. As they move, they undergo certain significant changes. First, they begin to lose water. As they do so, the cell membranes and the internal parts of the cell make up an increasingly larger solid part of the total cell volume. Second, a substance called keratohylin is produced. This is a dark-stained chemical, which is thought to be the forerunner of carotene, the final product of the epidermis.

The initial cell migration takes ~14 days, after which the cell performs its functions in the outer layer for another 14-day period. After that time, the cell is discarded. As you can see, this process is one of constant renewal.

Another function of the epidermis is the production of melanin, a substance involved in skin pigmentation. This chemical darkens the skin when it is exposed to the sun and is thus responsible for the tan that many people desire for social reasons. Interestingly, tanning is nothing more than a byproduct of a much more important function that protects the skin and the body from the destructive effects of ultraviolet radiation. The primary purpose of melanin is to absorb this radiation before it can cause harm.

Melanin is produced by the melanocytes, evenly distributed cells found in the basal cell layer. Melanin secretion is triggered by the presence of ultraviolet radiation. The quantity of melanin produced is not fixed by the melanocytes. It varies considerably from one person to the next. That is why we all have different degrees of tanning.

Dermis

The dermis is located immediately under the epidermis. It is the second major layer of skin, and, like the upper layer, serves basically as protection. It varies in thickness in different areas of the body, being thicker wherever the skin is used more or where there is heavier pressure. It is not ordinarily visible to the unassisted eye. It supports the epidermis, binding it to the underlying bone and muscle tissue. In the dermis are located the nerves, the blood vessels, and the various secreting lymph cells, together with the sweat and sebaceous glands.

Collagen

The dermis is made primarily of a substance called collagen. This is a tough, elastic fiber, made up of protein. It grows in bundles and is one of the most abundant proteins in the animal world. The dermis is richly supplied with blood. In fact, the blood supply system is far more complex and widespread than that of the top layer of the skin.

Sweat Glands

The sweat glands, together with the sebaceous glands, are some of the most important structures to be found in the dermis. Their activities are what make the skin qualify as an organ of excretion because these glands are designed to carry waste material out of the body, particularly when kidney function and waste disposal through urination are impaired.

A major task of the sweat glands is to regulate the body's temperature. This is a very sophisticated function involving the evaporation of the excreted liquid on the skin's surface. Basically, we sweat to cool the skin. As the liquid evaporates, we cool down. Sweat glands are found almost everywhere in the body. However, they are concentrated in the palms of the hands and soles of the feet.

It has been calculated that the average person has roughly 2.5 million sweat glands. They vary greatly in size and shape. Some are merely straight tubes passing through the skin. Others are odd corkscrew shapes, especially those glands in the hands and feet. The largest sweat glands are under the armpits and in the groin area whereas the fewest are found in the skin covering the back and the shoulders. Interestingly, earwax is a product of modified sweat glands, as are growths on the eyelids such as a sty. Each gland is equipped with a blood supply and nerve endings as well as a duct through which the sweat is secreted.

Sebaceous Glands

In addition to the sweat gland ducts, the skin is penetrated by another type of opening, a cylindrical indentation for the hair follicle. Each hair follicle is usually accompanied by a sebaceous gland, which explains why sebaceous glands may be found wherever hair grows. These glands produce a substance called sebum, which is essentially a fat produced to lubricate the skin and the hair. Each hair is attached to a small muscle called the arrector pili. The other end of this muscle is attached to the skin. Whenever the muscle contracts the gland is compressed and sebum is forced out. The secretion varies in quantity and is affected by a lot of outside forces, such as heat and cold.

Sebaceous glands are larger in certain areas of the body such as the nose and the muscles stretching between the hair and the skin, producing the effect commonly known as goose flesh or goose bumps. Sebum is a very complex substance consisting of acid and salts, as well as oil, water, and worn out fragments of skin cells. Unlike sweat, sebum is usually produced at a steady rate. As it moves up the sebaceous duct against the hair shaft, both the skin and the hair benefit from its lubricating qualities.

The activity of the sebaceous glands varies greatly during your lifetime. The glands, which are quite large in the newborn, become dormant during childhood. Their activity increases dramatically during puberty and contributes to the teenage problem of acne.

Subcutaneous Fat

The lowest, but certainly not least, major layer of the skin is the subcutaneous fat. It is located between the dermis and the internal body. The boundary between the two lower layers is not well defined and varies widely in thickness. Basically the subcutaneous fat layer is composed of closely packed cells containing fat. This layer serves several purposes, one of which is providing skin plasticity. It also acts as an insulator, preventing heat loss from within the body. It provides mobile bedding upon which the skin rests. This permits the skin to move small distances in any direction if it is pushed or pulled.

In summary, we must understand the skin's structure to understand its real purposes. Then we can understand what we are doing daily that might cause it to age prematurely.

◆ Skin Functions

The skin covers the entire body, with the possible exception of the eyes and the mouth, thus making it the body's largest single organ. It serves as our first line of defense against all forms of bacterial and other invading organisms. It is a barrier against objects that might penetrate the softer inner tissues and viscera of the body. The skin also helps keep our internal organs in place. It is, thus, a protective organ as well as a type of waste disposal system. It serves as a supplement to the lungs' expulsion of unwanted gases. Most of these functions are obvious, but the skin has many less obvious functions essential to our health.

Body Temperature

As already mentioned, it is one of the most important factors in regulating body temperature. This is a never-ending task. In order for the body to remain in good health, a constant temperature between 97° and 99°F must be maintained. Because outside temperatures keep changing, a constant balance is necessary. The main components in the skin that control these factors are the blood and the sweat glands.

Blood Vessels

The blood vessels are controlled by a heat-regulating center in the brain. This center acts upon the network of blood vessels in the dermis. This network has an attached series of capillary loops extending upward, nearly to the surface of the skin. Although the main function of this system is the transport of nutrients and oxygen to the cells and the removal of waste and carbon dioxide for eventual excretion, these capillaries also carry heat away from the inner parts of the body.

When the body is enveloped in higher temperatures, the brain heat-regulating center causes the capillaries to relax and enlarge, allowing more blood to pass through, thus carrying more heat to the surface for disposal. On the other hand, when the body is exposed to low temperatures, these capillaries constrict, and less blood can flow through, thus conserving the body's heat and maintaining a higher internal temperature. As small as they are, capillaries seem to possess extremely muscular walls. These walls are under the control of the brain and the nervous system, and they bring about the desired cooling and warming of the body.

Sweat Glands

As the body temperature rises, the sweat glands become increasingly active. There are literally millions of these tiny glands beneath the surface of the skin. Each one is connected to the surface by a small duct. Even under ideal temperature conditions, these glands constantly excrete water and other types of waste materials from the body. But if you are in a sauna, working out, or running a race, for example, and the surrounding temperature rises, these glands excrete more and more water. This leads to more evaporation, and, thus, more cooling of both the skin's surface as well as the blood flowing in the capillaries underneath.

These may seem to be simple processes, and under ordinary circumstances they are. However, any unnatural occurrence causes the body temperature to vary dramatically, thus indicating something is amiss in the body's interior. Of course, perspiration is essential to this warning system. This vital function of the skin is too often taken for granted.

There are three types of perspiration: ordinary, sensible, and profuse perspiration. The first type is normal, daily perspiration, which is almost imperceptible. Sensible perspiration is enough for you to notice. You may feel damp. With profuse sweating, you can lose a lot of water. When I ran the New York City Marathon in 2002, I lost about 7 pounds during the race. It was all water weight. I rehydrated later.

Perspiration also plays an important role in cleansing and detoxifying the body. When we indulge in unhealthy daily habits, such as using the wrong oils and cosmetics, which clog up the pores, we impede the skin's circulation. This prevents normal perspiration, which is dangerous because it prevents perspiration from ridding the body of toxins. Certain acids, such as uric acid, are eliminated from the body in this manner, as are other substances such as sugar in diabetics and some types of bile from other diseases.

Blood Pressure Regulation and Gas Exchange

Two rather surprising functions of the skin are its help in blood pressure regulation and its breathing. Blood vessels in the skin are equipped with sphincter-like muscles that serve to shut off the flow of blood through the capillaries. The blood then bypasses the capillaries and flows directly into the small arteries and into the veins. This mechanism acts like a safety valve when blood pressure rises to dangerous or damaging levels.

Skin breathing is limited, but there is, nevertheless, a certain amount of gas interchange through the skin. This, of course, is a supplement to the principal breathing through the lungs. It is, however, healthy to take this into consideration in a total program for skin care. In Europe, for decades, the practice of nudity has allowed the body to breathe. In America, however, we tend to overdress, and do not, in general, encourage nudity, even at home. However, nudity promotes the skin's health.

◆ Summary

Here is a brief summary of what we have learned up to this point: The skin is a very unique organ. It is the largest organ, with lots of blood vessels, lymphocytes, specialized nerve endings, hair follicles, and various types of sweat glands. Besides temperature regulation, containment of the internal organs, protection against foreign objects and organisms, the skin is a barrier against radiation. It is also the body's largest sense organ. The intricate structure of the skin can be most readily understood in terms of three basic divisions: the epidermis, the dermis, and the subcutaneous fat.

The epidermis, the outer surface, is the part of the skin that can be seen and touched. It is invisibly coated with a protective acid mantle and contains the pigmentation that determines the coloring of the complexion. The epidermis is constantly being renewed. Invisibly, but consistently, the top layer is flaking off. The dermis, the middle layer, contains sebaceous glands that produce sebum, the skin oil that lubricates and controls the texture of the complexion. The subcutaneous tissue is the deepest skin layer. It contains the sweat glands, hair roots, blood vessels, and nerves. From the sebaceous tissue, the body's internal messages are transmitted to the visible skin.

◆ Causes of Damaged and Prematurely Aging Skin

What are the reasons that this wonderful miracle of life becomes damaged? Today, even young people may have bad skin. Various techniques to alleviate the problem are available, such as blue lasers, derma peels, retinoic acids, skin grafting, or skin tightening. There are probably 30 different procedures. Sometimes even teenagers are using them. Why? We will look here at the causes of aging skin.

Glycation

The principal reason our skin ages is glycation. The results of this process are known as advanced glycation end products (with the fortuitous acronym AGE). Glycation occurs when excess proteins and sugars interact.

In today's fast-food world, we consume too much protein and too much sugar. Nearly 100 million American adults and children are overweight, with a high percentage of outright obesity. The amount of protein they are putting into their system far exceeds what the body can handle. We also consume sugar and refined carbohydrates like pastas, breads, and pastries in quantities far greater than what is healthful.

A normal blood sugar level is ~79, but the average American's is closer to a level of 125. Many Americans, and all diabetics, have an even higher level! Anything above the absolutely necessary blood sugar level will cause serious metabolic problems: When you have elevated sugar levels, your body ceases, or severely limits, the production of human growth hormone. Your insulin level increases, throwing your body into a fight or flight response. This is the body's way of instantly giving you a greater sense of strength, speed, sight, sound, and sensation. However, it is definitely not a benefit under these circumstances. The truth is, you do not need to fight or flee, but the body assumes you do and goes through a biological process to prepare you for it. In doing this, it prevents the normal secretion of healthy hormones, which are precisely the ones you need. Instead, putting the body on such an alert increases stress hormones like cortisol, epinephrine, and adrenaline. These adversely affect a healthy metabolism, including the skin's metabolism.

Here is an example of what an increase in stress hormones can do. Let us look at an average woman who is on a high protein diet because she is overweight. She is stressed because of her overweight condition and other factors over which she has no control. Both high fat and high protein produce estrogen. Together with her stress, these conditions cause estrogen dominance, which can lead to a higher incidence of breast cancer. And just when she most needs progesterone, the protective hormone that balances estrogen, her high cortisol level (from being stressed) will adversely affect the secretion of that balancing hormone.

More important for our discussion is what is happening to her skin. As already mentioned, excess fat and protein reacts with elevated blood sugar to form protein-like structures called advanced glycation end products. These AGEs are completely useless to the body. The main result of AGEs is a stiffening of the skin and many other internal and external tissues. Stiffening, of course, is one of the main signs of aging.

Picture a chicken before it goes into an oven. It is soft and pliable. Its skin is resilient. After it comes out of the oven it is stiff. It is very firm. There is no pliability. That is exactly what happens to our skin and other tissues with glycation. It is as if you were baking your head in an oven, making it stiff and wrinkled, except that glycation is a slow, gradual process. Because we are unaware of its existence, or choose to do nothing about it, we allow it to spread, day by day. The causes of glycation, such as a bad diet, are similar to those for other dangerous processes like free radical proliferation. For example, the more sun you are exposed to, the more glycation, as well as free radical damage, will occur.

Free Radicals

Collagen, as mentioned earlier, is protein-rich connective tissue found in the dermis. It is the matrix that holds the body together. But it can be dangerously altered by free radicals. These unstable molecules, with unpaired electrons in their outer orbits, are produced in many different ways: food allergies, environmental background pollutants, air and water pollutants, ultraviolet radiation from the sun, industrial chemicals, exercise and emotional stress, drinking any amount of alcohol, and smoking. These last two activities constrict capillaries, diminishing blood flow to the skin, thus creating conditions of inefficient disposal of waste products. All this creates enormous numbers of free radicals. Free radicals damage body tissue by causing oxidative stress; that is, by starting infections that become inflammations. The skin is among the tissue damaged in this manner.

A major way of creating free radicals is to eat denatured, highly processed, and allergy-producing foods, such as dairy foods, wheat, corn, sugar or artificial sweeteners, caffeine, colas, chicken, and beef—the nine foods that represent probably 90% of what people consume in a day.

When you indulge in hamburgers, sodas, French fries, hot dogs, sugarcoated cereals, coffee, and the like, you set the stage for both glycation end products and inflammatory responses all over your body. One of the most susceptible areas is your skin.

Glycation provokes allergenic immune modulators. Unfortunately, these cause local inflammation. Some proinflammatory markers are homocysteine, fibrinogen, C-reactive protein, and cytokines. These last trigger prostaglandin E2 (a bad prostaglandin), which heightens inflammatory processes. They are all destructive to the skin.

The human body has over 200 trillion cells, with each cell undergoing ~100,000 DNA gene mutations every day. In addition, free radicals attack the cells hundreds of billions of times a second. DNA is not always repaired when the body lacks sufficient repair enzymes and nutrients. If the cell's altered DNA is not repaired, the cell could become mutagenic or carcinogenic.

Biochemistry is limited in what it can do to protect the cell. There are over 100,000 synthetic chemicals that can attack the cells. If you have a bad diet, smoke, do not exercise, drink alcohol and coffee (which is just another drug), work in a polluted environment, and are in the sun, you are greatly increasing the odds that your body will lose the fight against free radicals. It is like going into a fight against 2500 muggers with your arms tied behind your back and one leg tied behind your other leg!

Free radicals increase with every single negative thing you do, no matter how inconsequential it may seem. Thus eating a single candy bar produces some free radicals, as does smoking one cigarette or breathing polluted air for only a few minutes.

Attacks by free radicals and other inflammatory agents often result in the cell being deprived of nutrients, especially oxygen. At the same time, the lymph and circulatory systems cannot properly remove the byproduct of cell respiration, carbon dioxide, and other cell debris. This leads to pollution of the cell, just like in a clogged toilet that cannot flush. Cleansing or detoxifying the cell is therefore of paramount importance and has a direct impact on the health of the skin.

◆ Reversing the Damage

Diets are usually chosen for their impact on weight control, not on what they can do for the skin. People therefore starve themselves or restrict certain types of foods to control their weight, never realizing that they are also starving the body of essential nutrients.

The body needs antioxidants, phytochemicals, trace elements, quality protein, complex carbohydrates, essential fatty acids, and more. What you do daily has a great effect on the skin. For example, if you habitually have a cigarette and coffee upon waking, then rush off to work, breathing pollutants all day, drinking alcohol and eating steak, by the time you have finished your day you haven't done one single thing to help your body's cells, its immune system, its hormonal system, and its skin. Instead, day by day, you are adding to the growing disease processes in your body. And then one day you will go to a plastic surgeon in need of some treatment. This was definitely preventable. But is it reversible? It is, if you follow a strict, accurate protocol. To do it correctly you have to do a lot of things:

Elimination

First, and foremost, you must go through an elimination process. You must stop what is causing the problem. For a lot of people this is a very difficult task because they are so used to their bad habits. They are used to their coffee or sugar.

Ask yourself some questions: Do you drink coffee? Do you smoke? Do you consume refined sugar, in any of the hidden ways it is in our foods? Do you drink any alcohol? Are you addicted to any drugs, including marijuana? This would include even occasional usage. Remember, this is a comprehensive program. Unlike superficial remedies, this one will bring glowing good health, in addition to beautiful, healthy skin and hair. Thinking of the complexity and interrelatedness of body systems, including the skin, already outlined here, and the unremitting onslaught of free radicals that our cells are up against, it should be apparent why only a total program will work. Assuming you can motivate yourself to begin this protocol for hair and skin health, it is crucial that major habits like smoking and alcohol use be curbed in order for this program to have any chance of working. There is a lot to do, not all of it easy, even after these major habits are conquered.

The elimination diet must be set in motion: Gradually, one by one, or all together, eliminate the following: all meat and poultry, all dairy foods, all yeast and wheat bread, all other wheat products, all sugar and artificial sweeteners, all caffeine and carbonated beverages. As soon as possible, buy mainly organically grown food. The reason: A pesticide's only job is to attack the cell and kill it.

Get tested by a holistic practitioner. Do you have parasites? Do you have viral and bacterial infections? Do you have local focal infections? Have your homocysteine, C-reactive protein, and cytokine levels determined. Have your thyroid balance checked.

Water

Most people are dehydrated. Lack of thirst is no indication whatsoever that your body is getting enough water. In fact, a lot of people suffer from either hydradypsia or polydypsia, and do not know when their water level is correct. People are actually dying in nursing homes because they are not drinking enough liquids.

Take a simple impedance test to determine your body's percentage of water. It should be ~74 percent. Hydration is the bringing of water into the body in sufficient quantity to fully perform all its functions. With proper hydration from pure distilled or spring water and organic juices, your face and skin will immediately show an improvement. Dehydration is one of the very first things that destroys your skin. The older we get, the fewer liquids we consume. That is why senior citizens frequently have extremely damaged skin. It is often primarily a matter of not consuming enough water.

Hydration helps nutrients enter the cells and helps bring out the waste products. There are no tasks more crucial than these. Hydration also assists with proper electrical transmission of nerve impulses to the cells. It frees up our lymphatic system, allowing it to flow. After all, the lymph system, unlike the circulatory system, has no pump.

Drink about 1 gallon of water a day, but space the water throughout the day.

We have now begun an elimination program. This stops the substances that cause many of our problems. We are hydrating the body every day. We will, eventually, rebuild any damaged tissue, but first we must detoxify the tissue.

Detoxification

Detoxification is the second step in rejuvenating the skin. Take 50 g of high-quality fibers daily, from grains, nuts, seeds, legumes, berries (blueberries, raspberries, strawberries, cherries) apples, prunes, apricots, and figs. These are all excellent foods for sweeping debris out of the intestines. Emptying the intestines of fermenting and putrefying waste products frees up the immune system, enabling it to concentrate on other parts of the body.

The liver is crucially important for eliminating waste. Taking caprylic acid (a fatty acid that has antifungal properties), grape seed extract, and the juices of lemon and lime with some olive oil in the morning helps stimulate proper bile flow and releases toxins out of the liver.

Nothing is better at getting easily absorbed nutrients into the body than drinking green vegetable juices. Juicing is central to any detoxification program. You should use juices to cleanse the body throughout the day.

Take an 8 to 14 ounce glass of the juices of celery, cabbage, cucumber, ginger, and garlic in the morning. The amount of ginger and garlic in the juice can vary according to your tolerance or need for these strong, burning, but wonderful detoxifiers, but, in general, it should be a much smaller amount than the other ingredients.

Chlorophyll is the single most important blood purification substance. It is also an antimutation agent and fights free radicals. Chlorophyllin is a byproduct of chlorophyll. Studies show that chlorophyllin suppresses mutagenic activity by more than 90%. In some human breast cells, chlorophyllin inhibited DNA adduct formation by 65%. DNA adducts occur in response to gene mutation. Preventing these adducts from forming dramatically lowers cancer risks. The best sources of chlorophyll are green vegetable juices. You also get chlorophyll from red, yellow, green, and other colored fruits and vegetables.

Red fruits—raspberries, strawberries, watermelon, cranberries, blood oranges, pink grapefruit, pomegranates, currants—taken as juices or concentrates have special phytochemicals that are phenomenal at enhancing the enzyme repair mechanism within the cell and thus can reverse skin damage.

Garlic is the great detoxifier for the body. It greatly helps the skin. Generally it is taken at 1000 to 2000 mg of garlic extract. Bee propolis is also very good at cleansing and helping the body reregulate. Chinese green tea protects cells and stops cell mutation, including those in the skin.

Protein and Other Nutrients

You are now cleansing the body with chlorophyll and fiber throughout the day. You also need protein, but not too much. The best quality sources are grains like brown rice, millet, quinoa, and amaranth. Complete protein, consisting of all eight essential amino acids, may be gotten from grains together with the bean, or legume, family. There are over 70 varieties of beans. For example, you can choose from black beans, navy beans, adzuki beans, soy beans (often in the form of tofu or tempeh), lima beans (for a buttery texture), black eyed peas, split peas, turtle beans, lentils, and canoli beans.

Walnuts, almonds, pine nuts, and pistachios have very good oils and proteins as well. Sunflower, pumpkin, chia, and sesame seeds are very good sources of protein and oils when eaten raw. Soak them in water for a few hours to make them more easily digestible.

Start the day with a rice protein shake. One or two scoops in water, juice, or soy milk, will provide 20 to 40 g of protein that does not tax the digestive system.

Almost everyone with poor skin has poor digestion. It is therefore important to take digestive enzymes with your meals, especially the nutrient L-glutamine, at 2000 to 3000 mg per day. This amino acid repairs damage to the cells in the intestines. It stops leaky gut syndrome and enhances the body's absorption of nutrients. It is also a great energy provider to the cells.

Take 100 mg of B complex with extra non-flush niacin and B6 and folic acid. Take trimethyl glycine 500 mg twice a day, 1000 μg of B12, 100 mg of B6, and 1000 μg of folic acid daily.

Oxygen or methylating agents help rejuvenate the skin because they bring oxygen to the cells. Take vitamin E from gamma tocopherol, at 400 to 800 units, plus tocotrienols. The tocotrienols are the specific fractions of the tocopherol that are terrific for oxygenation.

Antioxidants

However, just as the body must bring oxygen to the cells, so, too, must it guard against too much oxygen, which leads to free radicals and inflammation. Antioxidants help neutralize free radicals produced in the skin. Vitamins C and E are the most well known antioxidants. However there are many others.

Coenzyme Q10 is a superstar of antioxidants. It is essential for anyone who wants a healthy body. A dosage of 200 to 300 mg daily is not too much to take if we want to gain an edge over our toxic environment.

Take 2000 mg n-acetyl cysteine, 1000 alpha lipoic acid, and grape seed extract. These are three superstar antioxidants, but their most important benefit is that they allow the creation of glutathione. Glutathione is the cell's number one internal antioxidant. Almost everyone who has prematurely aged or damaged skin is deficient in glutathione. Glutathione protects all the cells of your body.

Inflammations and Fish Oils

Chronic inflammation can manifest in different places and cause different diseases and conditions. For example, an inflammation in your arteries could lead to arterial sclerosis. In your cells, an inflammation could result in DNA damage that could lead to cancer. In your joints, it produces arthritis. Inflammations on the skin result in all forms of skin eruptions, acne, psoriasis, and other conditions.

According to scientific literature, fish oils turn off all forms of inflammatory processes, including those on the skin. Omega-3 fatty acids (DHA) come from fish and from flaxseed oil as well. You should have ~1000 to 15000 mg of omega-3 fatty acids daily.

Your skin will suffer if you do not have the correct balance between omega-6 and omega-3 fatty acids. Flaxseed oil, more so than fish oil, contains the correct balance of omega-6. Balance is significant when it comes to fatty acids. The proper balance of omega-6 (n-6) to omega 3 (n-3) fatty acids enables the body to reduce inflammation, lower blood pressure, prevent irregular heartbeat, and promotes healthy blood flow. There should be twice as much omega-6 oil as omega-3 oil. Omega-6 oils are available in flaxseed oil, oil of primrose, and borage seed oil, at 1000 to 1500 mg.

L-Carnosine

The single most important nutrient for the skin is L-carnosine (not to be confused with L-carnitine). Carnosine helps wherever there is a blood supply to a given organ, whether it is the skin or the brain.

A dangerous situation develops when fat oxidizes. This is called lipid peroxidation and can take place anywhere in the body, such as the skin, brain, arteries. L-carnosine reduces the level of lipid peroxidation, thus lengthening the lives of organs and protecting other tissue. It is known that carnosine also protects against one step in the glycation process. In addition, it increases the flowability of cell membranes. This means that nutrients can get into, and waste products out of, the cell with ease, when l-carnosine is present.

Carnosine helps limit attacks on cell DNA. These attacks speed up the cell's aging process. Substances called excitotoxins, such as artificial sweeteners, additives, or airborne chemicals, increase the rate of cell death. Carnosine slows down the entire process. Excitotoxins trigger a cascade of events, such as membrane polarization, which end in the death of the cell. Carnosine can stop the process and extend the lifespan of cells throughout the body.

In summary, L-carnosine is the primary antiaging nutrient for the skin and the whole body. It will stop free radicals, glycation, oxidative stress, and lipid peroxidation. It is the best single agent for quenching the hydroxyl free radical, a very destructive protein-oxidizing substance. L-carnosine does this better than vitamins E and C. Take 1000 to 2000 mg of L-carnosine daily.

Collagen Synthesis and Vitamin C

You can clearly tell when your skin is aging. Glycated skin is wrinkled skin. It is sagging skin. It forms crow's feet. The sagging and wrinkling of aging skin is due to very poor collagen sysnthesis. Collagen, as mentioned, is the connective tissue of the skin, and is made primarily from the synthesis of vitamin C. Therefore, the more vitamin C you have, the more collagen you can synthesize and the stronger and more resilient the skin becomes. In effect, you are pulling the skin back together. It is, thus, very important to take a large amount of vitamin C. Start with ~500 mg and build up to bowel tolerance (the amount of vitamin C at which you get diarrhea). Then, of course, reduce the amount slightly. Thus your vitamin C intake may be anywhere from 3000 to 20,000 mg, divided into five doses a day. Always take 2000 mg bioflavonoids together with vitamin C.

You can also take lycopene, lutein, β-carotene, and quercetin. Quercetin is another superstar. When taken together with vitamin C, this bioflavonoid will greatly increase collagen synthesis.

Topical Applications

You do not have to bake in the sun to have sun-damaged skin. An average exposure to sunlight is sufficient. Included among topically applied skin creams are vitamin A and retinoid analogs that stimulate skin cell renewal by increasing the rate of mitotic cell division. Vitamin A induces a signaling agent to stimulate the binding of epidermal growth factors to skin cells. Almost everyone who has sun-damaged skin, which includes most people who have been in the sun, has reduced collagen synthesis. But vitamin A and retinoic acid will help by increasing skin turnover. This means that the damaged skin will be removed, so the next layer under it will have a better opportunity to be undamaged. This increases fibroblast growth and collagen synthesis while reducing levels of collagen degradation. The skin enzyme metalloproteinase is reduced.

Hyaluronic acid helps the skin retain its moisture. It is important to protect your skin with a moisture-based topical application that contains antioxidants, especially one that delivers nutrients to the lower layers of the skin (lysomal delivery.) This protects the skin from the damaging effects of aging.

Alpha glycolic acid significantly reduces wrinkling and other types of skin damage by sun exposure, alcohol consumption, or smoking. Take *Ginkgo biloba* at 100 to 300 mg. It signals the fibroblast activity in the skin to increase the synthesis of collagen, and it also turns off inflammatory agents. Dimethyl amino ethanol (DMAE) has been shown to protect the skin's firmness. It functions as a cell membrane stabilizer.

◆ Summary

In summarizing this program, our three main activities have been elimination, detoxification, and rebuilding. Our three goals have been to eliminate new damage to the skin, to reverse the effects of past damage, and to maintain healthy conditions in the body for the future.

Suggested Readings

1. Amagase H. Intake of garlic and its components [abstract 4]. Nutritional and Health Benefits of Garlic as a Supplement Conference, Newport Beach, CA, 1998
2. Baynes JW. From life to death—the struggle between chemistry and biology during aging: the Maillard reaction as an amplifier of genomic damage. Biogerontology 2000;1:235–246
3. Block G, Patterson B, Subar A. Fruit, vegetables and cancer prevention: a review of the epidemiological evidence. Nutr Cancer 1992;18:1–29
4. Borek C. Maximize Your Healthspan with Antioxidants. New Canaan, CT: Keats Publishing; 1995
5. Bringold F, Serrano M. Tumor suppressors and oncogenes in cellular senescence. Exp Gerontol 2000;35:317–329
6. Darr D, Combs S, Dunston S, Manning T, Pinnell S. Topical vitamin C protects porcine skin from ultraviolet radiation-induced damage. Br J Dermatol 1992;127:247–253
7. Campisi J. The role of cellular senescence in skin aging. J Investig Dermatol Symp Proc 1998;3:1–5
8. Ciechanover A. The ubiquitin-proteasome pathway: on protein death and cell life. EMBO J 1998;17:7151–7160
9. Ford HL, Pardee AB. Cancer and the cell cycle. J Cell Biochem 1999;(Suppl 32–33):166–172
10. Grune T, Reinheckel T, Davies KJ. Degradation of oxidized proteins in mammalian cells. FASEB J 1997;11:526–534
11. Halliwell B, Gutteridge JMC. Free Radicals in Biology and Medicine. 3rd ed. New York: Oxford University Press; 1999
12. Hennekens HH, Buring JE, Manson JE, et al. Lack of effect of long-term supplementation with beta carotene on the incidence of malignant neoplasms and cardiovascular disease. N Engl J Med 1996;334:1145–1149
13. Hipkiss AR, Michaelis J, Syrris P, et al. Strategies for the extension of human life span. Perspect Hum Biol 1995;1:59–70
14. Horning MS, Blakemore LJ, Trombley PQ. Endogenous mechanisms of neuroprotection: role of zinc, copper, and carnosine. Brain Res 2000;852:56–61
15. Horton JW, White DJ, Maass DL, Hybki DP, Haudek S, Giroir B. Antioxidant vitamin therapy alters burn trauma-mediated cardiac NF-kappaB activation and cardiomyocyte cytokine secretion. J Trauma 2001;50:397–408
16. Huang X, Cuajungco MP, Atwood CS, et al. Cu(II) potentiation of Alzheimer abeta neurotoxicity: correlation with cell-free hydrogen peroxide production and metal reduction. J Biol Chem 1999;274:37111–37116
17. Imai J, Ide N, Nagae S, Moriguchi T, Matsuura H, Itakura Y. Antioxidants and free radical scavenge effects of aged garlic extract and its constituents. Planta Med 1994;60:417–420
18. Stewart MS, Cameron GS, Pence BC. Antioxidant nutrients protect against UVB-induced oxidative damage to DNA

of mouse keratinocytes in culture. J Invest Dermatol 1996;106:1086–1089

19. Lau BHS. Detoxifying, radioprotective and phagocyte-enhancing effects of garlic. Int Nutr Rev 1989;9:27–31

20. Lykkesfeld J, et al. Age-associated decline in ascorbic acid concentration, recycling, and biosynthesis in rat hepatocytes-reversal with R alpha lipoic acid supplementation. FASEB J 1998;12:1183–1189

21. Merker K, Sitte N, Grune T. Hydrogen peroxide-mediated protein oxidation in young and old human MRC-5 fibroblasts. Arch Biochem Biophys 2000;375:50–54

22. Munch G, Mayer S, Michaelis J, et al. Influence of advanced glycation end-products and AGE-inhibitors on nucleation-dependent polymerization of beta-amyloid peptide. Biochim Biophys Acta 1997;1360:17–29

23. Navarro JF, Mora C, Rivero A, et al. Urinary protein excretion and serum tumor necrosis factor in diabetic patients with advanced renal failure: effects of pentoxifylline administration. Am J Kidney Dis 1999;33:458–463

24. Petropoulos I, Conconi M, Wang X, et al. Increase of oxidatively modified protein is associated with a decrease of proteasome activity and content in aging epidermal cells. J Gerontol A Biol Sci Med Sci 2000;55:B220–B227

25. Podda M, Grundmann-Kollmann M. Low molecular weight antioxidants and their role in skin ageing. Clin Exp Dermatol 2001;26:578–582

26. Price DL, Rhett PM, Thorpe SR, et al. Chelating activity of advanced glycation end-product (AGE) inhibitors. J Biol Chem. 2001;276:48967–48972

27. Sander CS, Chang H, Salzmann S, et al. Photoaging is associated with protein oxidation in human skin in vivo. J Invest Dermatol 2002;118:618–625

28. Upritchard JE, Sutherland WH, Mann JI. Effect of supplementation with tomato juice, vitamin E, and vitamin C on LDL oxidation and products of inflammatory activity in type 2 diabetes. Diabetes Care 2000;23:733–738

29. Van der Meide PH, Schellekens H. Cytokines and the immune response. Biotherapy 1996;8:243–249

30. Ward PA. Cytokines, inflammation, and autoimmune diseases. Hosp Pract 1995;30:35–41. Department of Pathology, Texas Tech University Health Sciences Center, Lubbock, TX, 79430

31. Wei Z, Lau BHS. Garlic inhibits free radical generation and augments antioxidant enzyme activity in vascular endothelial cells. Nutr Res 1998;18:61–70

32. West MD. The cellular and molecular biology of skin aging. Arch Dermatol 1994;130:87–95

33. Winrow VR, Winyard PG, Morris CJ. Free radicals in inflammation: second messengers and mediators of tissue destruction. Br Med Bull 1993;49:506–522

Index

Pages followed by an "f" or "t" indicate that the entry is in a figure or a table, respectively.

D

E

F

N

O

T

U

V

W

Y

Z